Dairy Technology

VOLUME – 1

Dairy Technology

VOLUME – 1

Milk and Milk Processing

Shivashraya Singh
Former Joint Director-cum-Dean and Emeritus Scientist
National Dairy Research Institute
Karnal – 132 001, Haryana

NEW INDIA PUBLISHING AGENCY
New Delhi – 110 034

NEW INDIA PUBLISHING AGENCY
101, Vikas Surya Plaza, CU Block, LSC Market
Pitam Pura, New Delhi 110 034, India
Phone: + 91 (11)27 34 17 17 Fax: + 91(11) 27 34 16 16
Email: info@nipabooks.com
Web: www.nipabooks.com

Feedback at feedbacks@nipabooks.com

ISBN: 978-93-83305-08-7 (Volume -01)

ISBN: 978-93-83305-09-4 (Volume -02)

ISBN: 978-93-81450-99-4 (Set)

Composed and Designed by NIPA

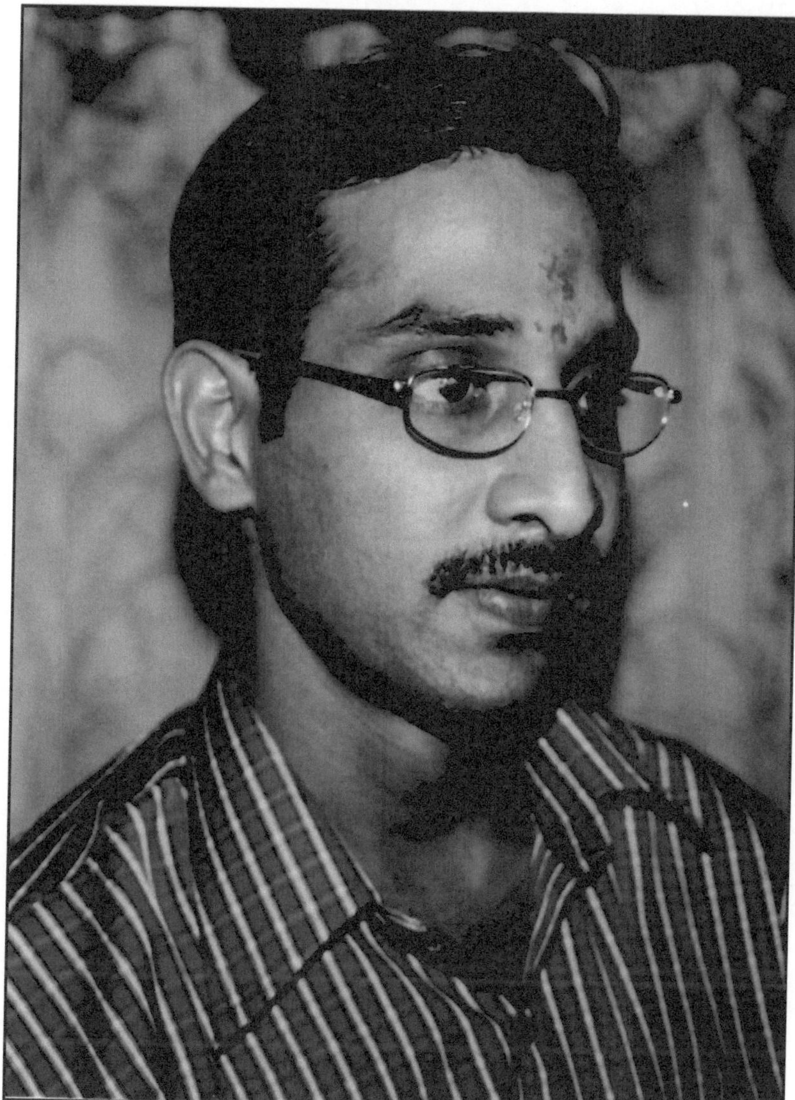

Dedicated in the sweet memories of my beloved son, Shri Anil Singh (May 1976 – April 2007)

Foreword

Milk is considered an ideal food for neonates, adolescents, adults and geriatrics and hence every attempt has been made by mankind to preserve this wholesome food by various processing operations. In the recent decade, the focus of attention has been on improving the quality, particularly sensory, nutritional and functional qualities of foods and at the same time, minimizing the processing and post harvest losses through technological and biotechnological interventions. Recent advancements in dairy technology have also offered the opportunity not only to control the existing food processes in better way, but also to adopt entirely novel approaches to quality control and newer product development. Meanwhile, an ever-increasing variety of specialized dairy products from whole and skim milks to creams, cheeses, yoghurts, whey products and specialty powders are opening up tremendous opportunities for growth. In search of efficiency, the dairy industry, a major sector of the food industry at a national level, is constantly seeking to improve the working practices, and the advances in process technology are an integral part of this trend.

Growing awareness towards the beneficial role of milk and milk products in maintaining human health has led to the development of a wide range of novel functional foods, health foods, neutraceuticals, mood elevating and refreshing foods. In the advanced countries the dairy industry is rapidly diversifying its product to produce a range of dairy foods that are targeted to reduce the role of medicines in maintaining the human health. In addition, there are also vast opportunities of development of new milk products for improving their functional and nutritional attributes by the use of food biotechnology. Biotechnology may have immense impact in all areas of food processing, starting from raw material production to improving the shelf life, and enhancing the acceptability and nutritive value of foods. Further the knowledge of physicochemical and microbiological characteristics of milk is most important to understand the properties of food, improving its quality and storage stability and controlling its behavior during handling.

I found this an excellent textbook on physicochemical and microbiological characteristics of milk, processing and preservation of milk, manufacturing of various dairy products and quality assurance. This book will be very useful to students as well as faculty in the universities and institutes. In addition to enhancing the quality of instruction it will also be of great value to food scientists.

Professor (Dr.) Singh is eminently qualified to write the book on Dairy Technology because of his in-depth knowledge, understanding and dedication to the subject of dairy and food science research and education. This book provides comprehensive coverage of all topics related to dairy technology, suitable for students in the discipline of dairy and food science and technology.

I congratulate Professor (Dr.) Singh for this accomplishment and wish him all success in his endeavour.

Prof. (Dr.) A.K. Srivastava
Director & Vice Chancellor
National Dairy Research Institute
(Deemed University), Karnal

Foreword

I had the privilege of reviewing the complete text of the book titled' Dairy Technology' authored singularly by Prof. (Dr) Shivashraya Singh, former Joint Director-cum-Dean and Emeritus scientist (ICAR) of National Dairy Research Institute, Karnal (India). I very much appreciate and compliment the author for this Herculean task for the benefit of dairy fraternity of India, may it be the student, the teacher, the researcher, the dairy processor or even a freelance knowledge seeker. We have been contemporary while in education and thereafter our thinking invariably matched on almost all academic matters. In our early service career we had felt that there is a dire need of a book which is easily comprehensible to Indian students. In fact we all faced the dilemma of not having one for ourselves and reading voluminous treatises containing plethora of unabsorbable subject matter on individual products/processes unduly texed. Hence, I also tried twice first in English and subsequently in Hindi language for Dairy Chemistry. But both attempts could not fulfill the requirements of all concerned. The present book is a marvelous feat as it is going to fulfill the long cherished desire of the author to benefit the dairy students at large by giving one comprehensive yet detailed and up to date text book in their hands. I remember that two foreign authors wrote and published their books on dairying while being in India some five decades back, but both lost their usefulness as time passed by. Hopefully, the present book has since been nicely structured and crafted incorporating the details of the latest technological facts established by research will go a long way to serve the purpose of the elite for a decade at least when incorporation of some revision may become imminent. I do hope the text book finds its due place and overwhelmingly applauded for its quality so that the author feels himself rewarded for this noble work. My best wishes to the author for his acomplishment.

I wish the text book will prove its usefulness in times ahead.

Prof. V.B. SINGH
Former Vice Chancellor
Maharana Pratap University of Agriculture & Technology
Udaipur (Raj.)

Preface

Dairy Technology is the industrial, non-farm phase of the tremendously large, dynamic and complex dairy industry. This phase represents a combination of science, engineering, business, and art as applied to all dairy and dairy-type foods and their industries. Dairy and dairy-type foods represent a major segment of the vast and varied food industry.

Processing of milk into various dairy foods, i.e. Dairy Technology, is underpinned by disciplines such as chemistry and biochemistry, microbiology and process engineering. Strong emphasis on public health aspects and product quality demands that proper attention be given to the points in the production and processing chain where both pathogenic and spoilage microorganisms can be controlled effectively.

Keeping above points in view, a very comprehensive book has been written encompassing entire gamuts of chemical, physical and microbiological characteristics of milk, processing and preservation of milk, manufacture of dairy products, functional foods, utilization of dairy byproducts, cleaning and sanitization and quality assurance.

The entire material has been presented in two volumes. The 1st volume consists of physicochemical and microbiological characteristics of milk and processing and preservation of milk. The 2nd volume deals with the manufacture of dairy products and quality assurance. The whole material has been consolidated in 20 chapters.

The main objective of the book is to provide the latest information in a consolidated form at one point to meet the requirements of not only undergraduate and postgraduates students but also teachers and dairy professionals. I am sure it will not only serve as a textbook on Dairy Technology for students and teachers but also as a reference book for the entire dairy industry. This book will prove to be very useful not only to the academic community but also to the researchers, planners, plant managers and extension workers.

Acknowledgement: Well, to say this is my book will be totally untrue. At best this is my dream. There are people in this world, some of them so wonderful, that made this dream become a product that you are holding in your hand. I would like to thank all of them from the bottom of my heart.

I am indebted to the authors, editors and publishers of various scientific books, periodicals and pamphlets from which the information presented here have been gathered to supplement the basic content of this textbook. These are too numerous to be named individually, however, to mention some of them as follows:

- Encyclopedia of Dairy Sciences, edited by Hubert Roginski, *et al.* (2003).
- Technology of Indian Milk Products by R.P. Aneja, *et al.* (2002).
- Dairy Technology by P. Walstraw, *et al.* (1999).
- Dairy Handbook by Alfa-Laval.
- Principles of Dairy Chemistry by R, Jenness and S. Patton (1969).
- Lecture compendiums prepared under the aegis of Centre of Advance Studies, Division of Dairy Technology, NDRI, Karnal.
- Lecture notes of Dairy Technology Diploma course, IGNOU.
- Dairy India, 2007, 6th edition.
- Other subject matter specialized books on individual dairy products such as condensed and dried products, frozen products, etc.

I offer my sincere thanks to the faculty members of the Dairy Technology Division, NDRI, Karnal whom I consulted freely on scientific matters included in this book as and when required. I would like to place on record my special thanks to Dr. A.A. Patel, Head, Dr. S.K. Kanawjia, Principal Scientist, Dr. R.R.B. Singh, Principal Scientist and Dr. A.K. Singh, Sr. Scientist for their unstinted support and cooperation in accomplishing this mission. I also thank all the staffs of Dairy Technology Division who helped me directly or indirectly in accomplishing this mission.

I am also thankful to Prof. (Dr.) A.K. Srivastava, Director, NDRI for permitting me to use the facilities of the institute and for continued interest and encouragement in this endeavour. Sincere thanks are also due to Prof. (Dr.) V.B. Singh, former Vice Chancellor, Maharana Pratap University of Agriculture and Technology, Udaipur (Rajasthan) for reviewing the manuscript and giving valuable suggestions. I would like to place on record the contribution of Dairy Technology Society of India under the aegis of which I could get enough time and support to complete this mission.

I will fail in my duty if I do not recognize the contribution of my family members, relatives and friends. I am grateful to my beloved grandson, Dr. Vishwendra Singh who taught me computer application after my retirement, as a result of which the whole manuscript was typed by me. The contribution of my wife, Indira, daughter, Saroj and son, Sunil are duly recognized. Thanks are also due to the publishers of this book, since without their kind cooperation and support this mission would have not been accomplished.

Shivashraya Singh

Contents

Contents — Vol 2

Dairy Products and Quality Assurance

Part I: Manufacturing of Dairy Products

Part II: Quality Assurance

PART I
Physicochemical and Microbiological Characteristics of Milk

1

Definition and Composition of Milk

1.1. General Discussion of Milk

"The cow is the foster mother of the human race. From the days of the ancient Hindoo to this time have the thoughts of men turned to this kindly and beneficent creature as one of the chief sustaining forces of human life".

William Dempster Hoard (1836-1918)
Former Governor, State of Wisconsin, USA (1889-1891)
Founder of Hoard's Dairyman (1885)

The oldest written records of the human race are in Sanskrit and are preserved in India. At the time these records began, about 6,000 years ago, milk had already become an important article of food. In fact, so important was the cow to these early people of South and Central Asia that wealth was measured in numbers of cattle, and the cow was in time made a sacred animal and is still so considered in India.

According to the best authorities, the domestication of cattle must have occurred somewhere between 6,000 and 10,000 years ago. The cow was worshipped in Babylonia, and in Egypt about 20,000 B.C. Over fifty references to cows and milk are found in Old Testament and the Promised Land was described as "a land flowing with milk and honey".

Milk is the only food of the young mammal during the first period of its life. The substances in milk provide more energy and the building materials necessary for growth. Milk also contains antibodies which protect the young mammal against infection. A calf needs about 1000 litres of milk for growth, and that is the quantity which the primitive cow produces for each calf. There has been an enormous changes since man took the cow into his service. Selective breeding has resulted in dairy cows which yield more than 5,000 litres of milk per calf, i.e. five times as much as the primitive cow. Some cows can yield 10,000 litres or more.

Milk has been a part of diet of Indian society since times immemorial. Our scriptures are full of references on importance and value of milk for human life. And the only milk, apart from mother's milk, known to Indians was cow milk which has been equated with the *'Amrita'*. There are innumerable such references in all ancient Indian scriptures from Vedas to Mahabharatha and Charak or Sushenta which state that cow milk and milk products have been in use in ancient India not only as a source of nutrition but also as a curative and prophylactic food/medicine. It is because of these qualities of cow's milk that cow has been revered as "Cow Mother", a provider of Amrita, provider of health, wealth, prosperity, fame and respect.

Milk is an important human food. It is palatable, easy to digest and highly nutritious. Milk is one of the few foodstuffs consumed in its natural state. It is only article in diet with exception of honey, whose sole function in nature is to serve as food. Practically everything else we eat fulfills some other function in the animal and vegetable world. Thus most vegetables are root or leaves of plants, fruits or parts of plants containing seeds, and meat comes from the body of the animals.

Nowadays common expression used in reference to nutrition is that, milk is the most nearly perfect food. It is one foodstuff upon which all nutritionists agree concerning its value for the proper growth and development of children and young animals. Not only it is the sole source of subsistence for everyone during the critical period of early infancy, but in one form or other it continues in our normal diet throughout life. In sickness specially, it is the one food most often called upon to sustain and nourish the body. No other single substance can serve as a complete substitute for milk in diet. From the very beginning milk has served as a foundation for the study of nutrition.

1.1.1. Definition of milk

Milk is a complex biological fluid, secreted by mammals explicitly for the nourishment of their young ones. It is a dynamically balanced mixture of fats, proteins, carbohydrates, salts and water co-existing as emulsion, colloidal suspension and true solution. Alteration of these relationships either by removal of or by changing the ratio of one or more of the components is used to the advantage for the preparation of a variety of milk products. Milk constituents can be broadly classified into two phases, viz. continuous and dispersed. The continuous phase may be considered to be an aqueous solution of soluble proteins, lactose, inorganic salts as well as various organic substances in small amounts and the dispersed phase is composed of fat, caseinate phosphate complex and colloidal calcium phosphate.

On account of high nutritional value it has been studied in detail from different aspects, chemical, physical, physiological and bacteriological. Various definitions for milk have been suggested from time to time, some of which are presented as follows:

A. Biological Definition

Milk is the natural secretion of the special gland of the female intended for the nourishment of the newly born offspring.

B. Commercial Definition

1. Milk is the integral product of entire and uninterrupted milking of milch cows in good health and well nourished and not over worked. It ought to be collected in the proper manner and contain no colostrums. ***(Geneva Congress)***

2. Milk is the whole, fresh, lacteal secretion obtained by the complete milking of one or more healthy cows, excluding that obtained within 15 days before and 5 days after calving, or such longer period as may be necessary to render the milk practically colostrum free. The milk should not contain less than 3.25% fat and 8.5% solids-not-fat (S.N.F.). ***(U.S. legal definition)***

The above definitions are not according to the Indian conditions. The fat and SNF in milk of Indian cows are higher than that of foreign cows. In addition, a major share of milk in India is from buffaloes, which contains higher milk solids than Indian cows. Therefore, Bureau of Indian Standards (BIS) has given following definitions:

Milk is normal, clean and fresh lacteal secretion obtained by complete milking of one or more healthy cow, buffalo, goat or sheep excluding that obtained within three days of calving or such longer period when it has become colostrum free whether it is processed or not.

Except Orissa and Punjab the milk fat in cow milk should not be less than 3.5% and SNF not less than 8.5% in whole of India. In Orissa, fat should not be less than 3% and in Punjab not less than 4%. In case of buffalo milk fat should not be less than 5.0% and SNF not less than 9.0% except in Punjab, Haryana, Delhi, UP, Bihar, West Bengal, Assam, Maharashtra, and Gujarat, where fat should not be less than 6% .In case of goat and sheep milk, the fat should not be less than 3% and SNF not less than 8.5% except in Madhya Pradesh, Maharashtra, Kerala, Punjab and UP where fat should not be less than 3.5%. In addition, other than normal milk some modified milks have also become important commodity of trade for Indian dairy industry which are defined as follows:

Standardized Milk: Standardized milk means cow milk or buffalo milk or sheep or goat milk or a combination of these milks that has been standardized to requisite fat and SNF percentage by adjustment of milk solids. It shall be pasteurized and shall show negative phosphatase test. It contains not less than 4.5% fat and 8.5% SNF.

Toned Milk: Toned milk means the product prepared by admixture of cow or buffalo milk or both with fresh skim milk; or by admixture of cow or buffalo milk or both, that has been standardized to requisite fat and SNF percentage, by adjustment of milk solids. It shall be pasteurized and shall show negative phosphatase test. When fat or dry non-fat-milk solids are used, it shall be ensured that the product remains homogenous and no deposition of solids takes place on standing. It contains not less than 3.0% fat and 8.5% SNF. It is prepared by skimming part of the whole milk or by blending skimmilk with whole milk according to calculation. Reconstituted skimmilk powder can also be used.

Double Toned Milk: Double toned milk means the product prepared by admixture of cow or buffalo milk or both with fresh skim milk; or by admixture of cow or buffalo milk or both, that has been standardized to requisite fat and SNF percentage, by adjustment of milk solids. It shall be pasteurized and shall show negative phosphatase test. When fat or dry non-fat-milk solids are used, it shall be ensured that the product remains homogenous and no deposition of solids takes place on standing. It does not contain less than 1.5% fat and 9% SNF.

Full Cream Milk: Full cream milk means milk or a combination of buffalo or cow milk or a product prepared by combination of both that has been standardized to requisite fat and SNF percentage, by adjustment/addition of milk solids. Full cream milk shall be pasteurized. It shall show negative phosphate test. It shall be packed in clean, sound and sanitary containers properly sealed so as to prevent contamination.

Skimmed Milk: Means the product prepared from milk from which almost all the milk fat has been removed. It shall contain not more than 0.5% fat and not less than 8.7% SNF.

Mixed Milk: Means the product of combination of milk of cow, buffalo, sheep, goat or any other milch animal and may be combination of any of this milk, which has been made and conforms to the standards. It shall contain not less than 4.5% fat and not less than 8.5% SNF.

Flavoured Milk: By whatever name called, may contain nuts (whole, fragmented or ground), chocolate, coffee or any other edible flavour, edible food colours, and cane sugar. Flavoured milk shall be pasteurized, sterilized or boiled. The type of milk shall be maintained on the label.

Recombined milk: Means the homogenized product prepared from milk fat, non-fat milk solids and water. Recombined milk shall be pasteurized and shall show negative phosphatase test.

C. Chemical Definition

Chemically milk is regarded as heterogeneous product in which fat, protein, sugar, minerals and other constituents are held in solution, colloidal suspension or emulsion in a major constituents of continuous water phase.

1.1.2. Composition of milk

All the constituents found in milk can be classified in two major groups as follows;

a) Major

b) Minor

Major constituents: Water, fat, protein, lactose, minerals

Minor constituents: Vitamins, enzymes, pigments, non-protein nitrogenous compounds, gases and different cells.

All the constituents together other than water are called Total Solids (T.S.). All the total solids other than fat are called Solids-not-fat (S.N.F.). If fat is removed from the milk the remaining portion is called milk plasma or skim milk. If fat and casein both are removed from milk then the remaining liquid is called milk serum such as whey which is obtained during the manufacture of cheese, paneer and chhana.

Milk has well defined physical equilibrium among its various constituents that exist mainly in three forms: true solution, colloidal suspension and emulsion.

True Solution: Those constituents whose particle size is less than 1 mm, viz. lactose, all cations and anions, undissolved salts, vitamins and other hydrophilic minor organic components.

Colloidal Suspension: A state of subdivision of matter (particle size), intermediate between molecular dispersion and visibility under light microscope. The particle size under this group is reported to be between 10^{-4} to 10^{-5} mm. The colloidal phase consists of casein micelles, calcium phosphates and globular proteins.

Emulsion: An emulsion is a system of two immiscible liquids, one of which is dispersed throughout the other in small drops. The particle size of the dispersed phase is larger than that of colloidal particles (10^{-2} to 10^{-3} mm). Milk is an emulsion of oil-in-water where water is continuous phase and fat is dispersed phase.

The composition of milk changes from time to time even in the same animal, hence it is by no means easy to give an absolutely fair estimate of the average composition of milk even for one country. It is impossible to examine the milk of every cow in any country at each milking on any given day. Hence there is always an element of doubt and error in the results, the average composition of milk is based on the results of a number of examinations, taking into account all the possible variations.

Due to the wide variations in the climatic conditions of the different regions of the world, different types of animals have been domesticated for milk production. The world milk production in 2008 is estimated at 684 million tonnes, 2.1 per cent or 13.9 million tonnes more than in 2007. The annual growth rates in 2006 and 2007 were 2.5 and 1.3%, respectively. Between 1997 and 2007 the world milk production was expanded by 122 million tonnes or 22%, which equals an average annual growth of 1.9 per cent. Out of this, cow milk will account for 576 million tonnes. The growth in cow milk production representing 84% of the total milk production, has slowed down again after a peak in 2005. The production in India is estimated at 104 million tonnes. The major species supplying milk to consumers in the world are 1339 million cows, followed by 172 million buffaloes and 1,172 million sheep and 783 million goats (FAO, 2004). Approximately 84%, 13%, 2% and 1% of global milk production is from, cows, buffaloes, goats and sheep, respectively; although the other dairying species- camel, yak and mithun are important in certain regions, they are of very little significance globally (Fox, 2003). The worldwide production of buffalo milk is estimated at 83 million tonnes in 2007 and continues to grow. It increased on an average by more than 3 per cent annually during the last ten years. Almost 90 per cent of the total volume is produced in India and Pakistan with strong annual growth every year.

However, by far the largest production of milk is from cow. In India buffalo is very popular as milch animal and accounts for nearly 58% of the total milk production of the country. Goat has also been reared as milk animal and it is particularly adopted for mountainous regions. It is thus natural that by far the most widely produced, the most generally known and studied milk is that of the cow and the term "milk" usually refers to cow milk unless otherwise stated.

The composition of milk varies according to the species of milch animals. The nature has created milk especially to meet the nutritional requirements of newly born offspring. The level of growth and development of newly born offspring is different in different species. Therefore, the food requirement of the newly born offspring is quite different in different species at the time of birth. Accordingly, the composition of milk of different species varies considerably. The composition of milk of some species is given in Table 1.1.1.

Table 1.1.1. Average composition of milk of mammalian animals

Species	Water	Total Solids	Fat	Protein	Lactose	Ash	References
Cattle (zebu)	86.5	13.5	4.7	3.2	4.9	0.7	Epstein (1974)
Cattle (exotic)	87.5	12.5	3.8	3.3	4.7	0.7	Jenness (1974)
Buffalo	82.8	17.2	7.4	3.8	4.8	0.7	Blanc (1981)
Goat	85.2	14.8	5.6	3.8	4.8	0.7	Jenness (1974)
Sheep	80.7	19.3	7.4	5.5	4.8	1.4	Jenness (1974)
Camel	86.63	13.37	3.78	4.0	4.9	0.95	Ohri & Joshi (1961)
Yak	82.07	17.93	6.43	5.94	4.68	0.87	Gupta *et al.* (1997)
Human	88.5	11.5	3.3	1.3	6.8	0.2	—

The above account gives only broad classification of milk constituents. These classes have been further subdivided into individual components. Numerous studies in the past century have revealed the presence of a wide array of constituents in normal milk.

1.1.3. Colostrum

The first milk that a milch animal produces after calving is called colostrum. It differs greatly from normal milk in composition and general properties (Table 1.1.2). It has yellowish to brownish–yellow colour, a peculiar smell and a rather salty taste. It is very thick in nature with high viscosity. It has a high concentration of immunoglobulins, β-lactoglobulin, albumin, chloride, and low lactose content. This results in colostrum coagulating when heated. Its fat content may be higher or lower than that of milk. Of the minerals, Ca, Na, Mg, P and Cl are higher but K is lower in colostrum than in milk. Colostrum from different cows and buffaloes varies much more in composition than does milk. The content of catalase and peroxidase is high.

The biological function of colostrum is to provide the newborn at its most vulnerable phase of life with immune protection against pathogens and to boost its physiological performance, growth and development. Colostrum contains plenty of immunologically and physiologically active components. These include immunoglobulins, leucocytes, lactoferrin, lysozyme, cytokines and other immunomodulatory factors (casein derivatives), growth factors, hormones, *etc.* These bioactive substances have in the past attracted an increasing interest in commercial exploitation of colostrums for pharmaceutical and dietary uses. Thus colostrum contains antibodies which protect the calf from infection until its own immunity system has been established. The proportion of whey proteins is substantially higher in colostrum than in milk. The foremost protein fraction of colostrum is the immunoglobulins (IgG, IgM, IgA). The β-lactoglobulin concentrations in bovine colostrum ranges from 8-30 g per litre, the average being 14 g per litre in the 1st milking and falling thereafter sharply to 8 g per litre at the 2nd and 4th milkings. Then the decrease is slower up to the 16th milking, the average being 5g l^{-1}. The level of α-lactalbumin decreases from 2 g l^{-1} in the 1st milking to 1.4 g l^{-1} in the 16th milking (Marnila and Korhonen, 2003).

Immune Protection by Colostrum: Passively acquired immunity from colostrum is important for the health of a neonate. Newborn calves and piglets that do not receive colostrum show high mortality and poor weight gain during the first weeks of life. Calves deprived of colostrum or given colostrum of poor quality suffer severe long scour episodes. Colostrum from the first two milkings is most important since the concentrations of immunoglobulins and lactoferrin decrease steeply after the first milkings.

Colostrum also contains an active complement system which participates in the immune defense of the udder. It is not known whether the colostral complement system provides any immunological protection to the newborn.

Most farm animals do not have *in utero* transport of immunoglobulins to the foetus and their newborns are born virtually without protective anti-bodies. In humans, the IgG transport via the placenta is very efficient and therefore the human infant is born with serum concentrations of IgG equaling that of the mother. Mammals can be divided into species with extensive placental transfer (e.g. human, rabbit), species with no placental transport but extensive lacteal transport (e.g. cow, goat, sheep, horse, pig), and species that use both pathways (e.g. dog, mouse and rat).

Colostral Ig and complement proteins are quite resistant to gastric acids but sensitive to the trypsin. On the other hand, bovine colostrum contains a trypsin inhibitor which neutralizes the trypsin activity and allows absorption of Ig.

Colostral Ig represents the mother's specific immune response to antigens encountered in the past. This immunological memory is mediated to the next generation via colostrum. In addition, colostrum contains also components which carry non-specific antimicrobial and immune-enhancing properties. Such factors are lactoferrin (LF), lysozyme (LZM), lactoperoxidase (LP) and leucocytes.

Human colostrum is particularly rich in LF, the concentration ranging from 5 -10 g l^{-1}. The concentration decreases in transition to normal milk to about 0.1 g l^{-1}. In cows' colostrum the LF concentration varies from 1-2 g l^{-1}, decreasing soon after parturition to the level of about 0.1 g l^{-1} in normal milk. LF is synthesized in the mammary gland, but also in other exocrine glands. LF and especially its cleavage products have a broad bacteriostatic and bactericidal spectrum and they also modulate inflammatory reactions.

LP is an effective antimicrobial enzyme which can be exploited for preservation of raw milk and also for the improvement of the growth of newborn calves. Cows' colostrum contains about 30 mg l^{-1} LP, the same level as in the normal milk. in human colostrum, practically all of the peroxidase activity is derived from the myeloperoxidase of leucocyte origin, and only a trace amount of it is from LP. In human infants, the salivary peroxidase may compensate the paucity of LP in colostrum.

LZM is a potent antibacterial component of human colostrum and milk and influences the intestinal bacterial flora of the neonate. Human colostrum contains LZM at about 0.36 g l^{-1}; the concentration of LZM decreases to 0.30 g l^{-1} in transition and normal milk. in bovine colostrum, the LZM level is from 0.3- 0.8 mg l^{-1}, declining to 0.1 mg l^{-1} in normal milk.

Living leucocytes are an integral part of the normal bovine and human colostrum and milk. Their concentration is highest in colostrum and declines gradually in transition to normal milk. The leucocytes defend the breast or udder against pathogens. The leucocytes may also enhance the newborn's defense against gastrointestinal infections. There is evidence from experimental animal studies that milk lymphocytes are able to enter the tissues of the neonate. Thus, maternal immunological memory may be transmitted to the offsprings. However, thus far only little is known about the influence of colostral leucocytes on immunological reactions in the neonate.

The protein composition of human colostrum and milk differs considerably from that of bovine. Human colostrum does not contain β-lactoglobulin and the major Ig class is IgA. The major casein content of human colostrum is β-casein instead of α-casein, which is the predominant casein fraction in bovine colostrum.

With successive milkings, the composition rapidly approaches that of milk and variability decreases (Table 1.1.2). The transition from colostrum to a composition within the range of variation of normal milk is complete in about 4-5 days, the protein content being slowest to complete the transition.

Table 1.1.2. Composition of colostrum

Colostrum	Total Solid %	Fat %	Total Protein %	Lactose %	Ash %	Specific Gravity
1st milking	24.55	3.89	16.76	2.50	1.33	1.0604
2nd milking	18.00	3.84	9.33	3.52	0.97	1.0437
3rd milking	16.79	3.11	7.06	3.85	0.96	1.036
4th milking	15.21	3.82	6.17	4.23	0.88	1.0372

Industrial Utilization of Colostrum: Colostrum is normally produced in amounts that exceed the need of the newborn. At present, dairy or food industries do not exploit bovine colostrum commercially on large scale due to technical and hygienic problems related to collection and processing. In many countries, colostrum must be excluded from the bulk milk collection during the first 5 days postpartum. The low clotting temperature of colostrum interferes with pasteurization and the high protein content leads to problems in industrial processes. Further, the high content of anti-microbial components in colostrum may slow down or inhibit fermentation processes. This fact also affects the antibiotic residue tests based on microbial growth, causing false positive results.

Bovine colostrum is utilized on minor industrial scale and in households in many countries, e.g. in Scandinavia, in form of cheese baked in an oven. Also, the casein fraction of renneted colostrum is baked and used as fresh cheese. In India, colostrum is blended with *jaggery* and the mixture is heated and poured in a plate. After cooling it gets converted into a solid mass. The desired size pieces are cut and consumed as a sweet dish.

Immunoglobulin preparations designed for farm animals are commercially available and some colostrum-based products are being marketed for humans as dietary supplements. Immune milk preparations have proven effective in prophylaxis against infections caused by a variety of gastrointestinal pathogens. Cheese whey- and colostral whey-based antibody preparations are commercially available in many countries as feed supplements or colostrum substitute for farm animals. They are prepared mainly for neonate calves and pigs and have shown variable efficacy in the prevention of diarrhoeal diseases caused by, for example, rotavirus and enterotoxigenic *E. coli* strains. Increasing interest is focused on the development of so-called 'immune milk' preparations made from the colostrum of hyper-immunized cows. Such preparations may target both humans and domestic animals for prevention and treatment of specific gastrointestinal diseases. A few preparations, e.g. against rotavirus and *E. coli,* are already on the market.

Bovine colostrum has many well established health benefits. Colostrum has been used for various illnesses in India for thousands of years and its medical importance is described in the ancient medicine, Ayurveda. In U.S., colostrum was in use for its antibacterial activity before the discovery of antibiotics. The pharmaceutical and biotechnological industries have recently shown interest in bovine colostrum as a source of growth factors and other specific bioactive components. Colostrum is emerging as the most potent natural immune booster for human beings. It is a rich source of immune components and growth factors. It contains more protein, immunoglobulins (Ig), fat, vitamins and minerals than milk. Evidence suggests the beneficial effects of supplementation of bovine colostrums in improving health, athletic performance, diarrhea in persons with immune deficiency syndromes, NSAID (Non-steroidal anti-inflammatory drug) - induced gastrointestinal disturbances, and aspects of the acute phase response that occurs secondary to surgery. Colostrum-based growth media have been developed for culturing cells. Also, a multitude of health products and foods made from various colostrum fractions, e.g. drinks and chewing gums for athletes, have been launched on the market. Currently, there is increasing pharmaceutical research under way to examine the potential related to the use of colostrum –derived preparations for a wide range of gastroenterological conditions.

1.2. Cow Milk

'Charak Shastra' is one of the most ancient books in the history of medical science. 'Rishi Charak' was an eminent Indian Physician and his book 'Charak Shastra' is followed even today by practitioners of Indian system of medicine- the Ayurveda. Charak has described the cow milk to be tasteful, sweet, has a fine flavour, is dense, contains fat, but light, easily digestible, and not easily spoiled. It gives us tranquility and cheerfulness.

Milk ranges in colour from a bluish-white to an almost golden-yellow, depending upon the breed of cattle, the amount of fat and solids present, and, most of all, upon the nature of the feed consumed by the cow. In large quantities, milk appears entirely opaque, while in thin layers it is somewhat transparent. The milk from which fat has been removed or that is naturally very low in fat and other solids shows a bluish tint.

It is supposed to have a typical, clean, full, slightly sweet taste and should also have a typical clean smell. Any pronounced taste is abnormal. Freshly drawn milk has a characteristic, but not very pronounced, odour which is quite volatile and which practically disappears when milk is exposed to the air. Other odours are abnormal.

Constituents

Milk is a complex mixture of various constituents. The Table 1.2.1 gives a tabulation of individual constituents that have been identified in normal cow milk as it is drawn from the udder. Some of these constituents actually have been isolated, others have been identified by specific tests. A few materials have been included in the table, whose presence in milk is not entirely certain. Milk fat, lactose, caseins, β-lactoglobulin, α-lactalbumin, and probably some of the other proteins are specifically characteristic of milk being synthesized in the mammary gland. The other constituents, however, are not specific for milk but are found in other biological sources. The distribution of constituents of cow milk is also illustrated in Fig. 1.2.1

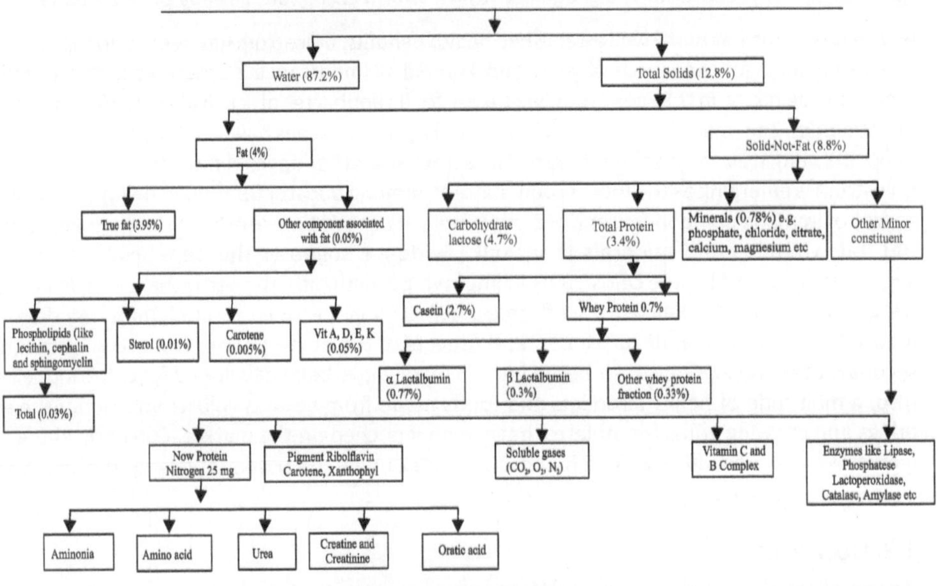

Fig. 1.2.1. Distribution of constituents of cow milk

Milk is one of the most precious natural materials and has been a basic component of human food for a long time. It is one of the oldest foods and at the same time the most important one. It is a complex mixture of innumerable precious nutrients. It has been reported that bovine milk fat contains up to 400 fatty acids (more than any other fat), resulting in several thousand triglycerides and complex lipids. In addition to the eight main proteins (α_{s1-}, α_{s2-}, β-and κ-caseins, β-lactoglobulin, α-lactalbumin, blood serum albumin and immunoglobulins), there are at least 80 minor proteins including ~ 60 enzymes. The ash fraction contains at least 30 elements, which are important from technological, stability and nutritional standpoints. Milk contains all known vitamins, some at very high concentrations.

Table 1.2.1. Approximate concentration of the constituents in normal cow milk

Constituents	Approximate concentration (Weight/ litre of milk)
1. **Water**	860-880g.
2. **Lipids in emulsion phase**	
a. Milk fat (a mixture of mixed triglycerides)	30-50g.
b. Phospholipids (lecithins, cephalins, sphingomyelins, etc.)	0.30g.
c. Cerebrosides	?
d. Sterols	0.10g
e. Carotenoids	0.10-0.60mg.
f. Vitamin A	0.10-0.50mg.
g. Vitamin D	0.4mg.
h. Vitamin E	1.0mg.
i. Vitamin K	trace
3. **Proteins in colloidal dispersion**	
a. Casein (a,b,g fractions)	25g.
b. b- lactoglobulin(s)	3g.
c. a-lactalbumin	0.7g
d. Albumin probably identical to blood serum albumin	0.3g
e. Euglobulin	0.3g
f. Pseudoglobulin	0.3g
g. Other albumins and globulins	1.3g
h. Mucins(?)	?
i. Fat globule protein (?)	0.2g
j. Enzymes (?)	
1. Catalase	
2. Peroxidase	
3. Xanthinoxidase	
4. Phosphatases (acid and alkaline)	
5. Aldolase	
6. Amylases (a and b)	
7. Lipases and other esterases	
8. Proteases	
9. Carbonic anhydrase	
10. Salolase(?)	
4. **Dissolved materials**	
a. Carbohydrates	
1. Lactose (a and b)	45-50g
2. Glucose	50 mg
3. Other sugars traces	
b. Inorganic and organic ions and salts	
1. Calcium*	1.25g
2. Magnesium *	0.10g
3. Sodium	0.50g
4. Phosphates* (As $PO_4^{a''}$)	2.10g
5. Citrates* (as citric acid)	2.00g

(Contd.)

Constituents	Approximate concentration (Weight/ litre of milk)
6. Chloride	1.00g
7. Bicarbonate	0.20g
8. Sulphate	0.10g
9. Lactate(?)	0.02g
c. Water soluble Vitamins	
1. Thiamine	0.4mg
2. Riboflavin	1.5mg
3. Niacin	0.2-1.2mg
4. Pyridoxine	0.7mg
5. Pantothenic acid	3.0mg
6. Biotin	50mg
7. Folic acid	1.0mg
8. Choline (total)	150mg
9. Vitamin B-12	7.0mg
10. Inositol	180mg
11. Ascorbic acid	20mg
d. Nitrogenous materials not proteins or vitamins (as N)	250mg
1. Ammonia (as N)	2-12mg
2. Amino acids (as N)	3.5mg
3. Urea (as N)	100mg
4. Creatine and creatinine (as N)	15mg
5. Methyl guanidine (?)	?
6. Uric acid	7 mg
7. Adenine	
8. Guanine	
9. Hypoxanthine (?)	
10. Xanthine (?)	
11. Uracil- 4- carboxylic acid (Orotic acid)	50-00mg
12. Hippuric acid	30-60 mg
13. Indican	0.3-2.0mg
14. Thiocyanate (?)	
e. Gases (milk exposed to air)	
1. Carbon Dioxide	100mg
2. Oxygen	7.5mg
3. Nitrogen	15.0mg
f. Miscellaneous	
1. Esters of phosphoric acid not yet identified (as phosphorous)	0.10g
5. **Trace elements (form of occurrence not elucidated)**	
Usually present	
Rb, Li, Ba, Sr, Mn, Al, Zn, B, Cu, Fe, Co, I	
Occasionally present or questionable	
Pb, Mo, Cr, Ag, Sn. Ti, V, F, Si	

(?) Presence, identity, or concentration uncertain.

* Partly in colloidal dispersion

(Jenness & Patton, 1969)

A detailed study of the constituents of milk is essential to understand the nature of milk, its physicochemical characteristics and nutritive value. They have an important role in processing of milk and manufacture of milk products. The study of each constituent helps in understanding the chemistry, microbiology and technology of milk.

1.2.1. Fat

Fat is one of the most important constituents of milk. Milk fat has always had an important bearing on the economics of milk and milk products. It has been only in recent past that the true worth of the non-fat milk solids has been recognized. Previously most price plans for milk were based largely, if not solely, on the milk fat content. Although this picture has changed considerably in recent years, milk fat still plays a very significant role in determining the price of milk and milk products. Since milk fat is still relatively expensive compared to the other milk constituents, it is obvious that the cost of dairy products that contain milk solids will depend to a considerable extent on the amount of milk fat which they contain.

Milk fats are very important from nutritional standpoint. It serves as a rich source of energy, yielding approximately 9 kilocalories per gram. It also serves as a carrier of the fat soluble vitamins A, D, E and K. Milk fat contains significant amount of essential fatty acids.

The most significant role which the milk lipids play in dairy products concerns flavour. The rich pleasing flavour of milk lipids is not adequately duplicated by any other type of fat. For this reason, milk fat in the form of butter, ice cream, coffee and whipping cream has stood up remarkably well under the competitive onslaught of cheaper fats. It is also notable from a practical standpoint that the milk lipids are significant in many of the flavour problems of dairy products. The subject of body and texture in dairy products is closely related to flavour so far as consumer acceptability is concerned. Undoubtedly the fine body and texture in most dairy products is one factor which makes them so appealing to most consumers. This characteristic in many instances is determined primarily by the milk lipids. They impart soft, smooth, and rich tasting qualities and overcome flat, hard, grainy, or watery characteristics which are normally encountered in their absence.

Thus it is clear that the milk lipids are of diverse practical importance. Moreover, it is evident that the contribution of this material in dairy products is interrelated. The fine flavour and physical properties which milk lipids impart to dairy products, and to food products in general, are important factors in the economics of milk. In addition, since milk lipids undoubtedly enhance the consumer acceptability of foods, they also serve the best interest of human nutrition through the incentive of eating what tastes good.

Composition of Milk Fat: The bulk of the fat in milk exists in the form of small fat globules, which average approximately 2-5μ in size. This is an oil-in-water type emulsion. The surface of these fat globules is coated with an adsorbed layer of material commonly known as the fat globule membrane. This membrane contains phospholipids and proteins in the form of a complex. In addition to stabilizing the emulsion of the fat in milk and preserving the individual identities of the fat globule, the phospholipid-protein complex is important in number of processes and problems of milk and milk products. Small quantities of lipids also occur in milk serum, presumably in combination with protein. Thus, milk lipids are found in three distinctly different phases of milk; namely the fat globules, the membrane surrounding these globules, and the milk serum.

The total fat content of milk, which reflects the energy requirements of the newborn, ranges from 3.5% (cow, woman) to 50% (aquatic mammals) according to the species, and varies with breed, age of animal, stage of lactation, and type of feed. The lipids associated with the milk fat globule are mostly (98%) triglycerides; the other lipids amounts to less than 2% of the total, and of this, about 0.5% is diacylglycerols and monoacylglycerols, the balance being made up of phospholipids, sterols, free fatty acids, and traces of other substances such as the fat-soluble vitamins. Table 1.2.2 presents the various lipid materials in milk, their level of occurrence, and their disposition in milk with respect to the three categories mentioned.

Table 1.2.2. Composition of milk lipids*

Constituent	Amount (wt.%)	Location in Milk
Triacylglycerols	98.3	Fat globules
Diacylglycerols	0.3	Fat globules
Monoacylglycerols	0.03	Fat globules
Free fatty acids	0.1	Fat globules, serum
Phospholipids`	0.8	Globule membrane, serum
Sterols	0.3	Fat globules, globule membrane, serum
Carotenoids	Trace	Fat globules
Fat soluble vitamins	Trace	Fat globules, FGM, serum
Flavour compounds	Trace	Serum

*Walstra and Jenness (1984)

Classification of Lipids: The lipids can be classified on the basis of their reaction with base in following two categories:

A) Saponifiable Matter,

B) Unsaponifiable Matter

Saponifiable Matter: The saponifiable lipids are hydrolyzed with base. Since in most fat the greater portion is made up of glyceride esters, the saponifiable material is large relative to the unsaponifiable matter. In addition to the triglycerides the saponifiable matter includes the phospholipids and other esters, such as those of cholesterol. Although not saponifiable in the classic sense, free fatty acids bind base and thus are disposed with the saponifiable matter.

Triacylglycerols: Triacylglycerols are relatively simple molecules consisting of a glycerol backbone to which are esterified three fatty acid molecules (Fig 1.2.2). They are non-polar molecules and hence insoluble in water. Although not highly reactive, triacylglycerols can undergo hydrolytic and oxidative reactions at ambient temperature. They are by far the most important class of compounds in milk fat, from a quantitative viewpoint, accounting for about 98% of the total fat Table 1.2.2). As a result, the triacylglycerols have a major influence on the properties of milk fat, e.g. density and melting profile.

$$
\begin{array}{llll}
CH_2OH & & CH_2OOC_{17}H_{35} & \\
| & & | & \\
CHOH + 3C_{17}H_{35}COOH & \rightarrow & CHOOC_{17}H_{35} & + 3H_2O \\
| & & | & \\
CH_2OH & & CH_2OOC_{17}H_{35} & \\
\text{Glycerol}\ \ \text{Stearic acid} & & \text{Stearin} & \text{Water}
\end{array}
$$

Fig. 1.2.2: Triacylglycerol formation

There are many different types of triacylglycerols in milk fat which vary considerably in molecular weight and degree of unsaturation. This complex mixture is a direct result of the large number and variety of constituent fatty acids which vary in chain length from 4 to 18 carbons.

The distribution of fatty acids at the three positions of the triacylglycerol molecule (position sn-1, sn-2 and sn-3, Fig 1.2.1) is not random. This is because mechanism involved in the biosynthesis of triacylglycerols in mammary exert some selectivity over the placement of fatty acids. Indeed, one of the distinctive features of milk fat is the almost exclusive esterification of short-chain fatty acids, butyric and caproic, at position sn-3. As a result of this highly specific distribution, the major triacylglycerols consist of two broad structural types: those containing various combinations of three long- chain fatty acids and those containing two long-chain fatty acids and a short chain-fatty acids.

Phospholipids: Phospholipids are a small but important lipid class in milk. They are present in fat globule membrane (about 60% of the total) and in other membranous material of the skim milk phase (about 40% of the total). The total phospholipid content of buffalo milk fat averages 21.04 mg/100 ml of milk, whereas for cow milk the corresponding value is 33.71 mg/ml. The Table 1.2.3 shows the concentration of various fractions of phospholipids present in buffalo and cow milk.

Table 1.2.3: Concentration of phospholipid fractions in buffalo and cow milk.

Phospholipid	Concentration(mg/100 ml)	
	Buffalo milk	Cow milk (Zebu)
Lecithin	7.29	10.01
Cephalin	9.12	15.57
Sphingomyelin	4.63	8.13

Source; Aneja, *et al.* (2002)

The glycerophospholipids constitute about 75% of the total, while the sphingolipids account for most of the remainder. Glycerophospholipids consist of a glycerol backbone to which are attached two fatty acids at position sn-1 and sn-2 and a phosphate group at position sn-3. Different side chains are attached to the phosphate group. The major glycerophospholipids are phosphatidylcholine (Fig.1.2.3) and phosphatidylethanolamine. Two other glycerophospholipids, namely phosphtidylserine and phosphtidylinositol, are present in small amounts.

The two charged groups in the glycerophospholipids give the molecules a polar part. The remaining part is nonpolar and hence they are amphiphilic and can accumulate at an oil-water interface. This explains their presence in membrane material.

The glycerophospholipids, phosphatidylethanolamine and phosphtidylcholine, have greater proportions of unsaturated fatty acids (47% $C_{18:1}$ and 13% $C_{18:2}$ in the case of phosphatidyl ethanolamine) than triacylglycerols (25% $C_{18:1}$ and 2% $C_{18:2}$) and hence they are more susceptible to oxidation. This has led to postulation that fat oxidation in milk may begin with the glycerophospholipids in the fat globule membrane.

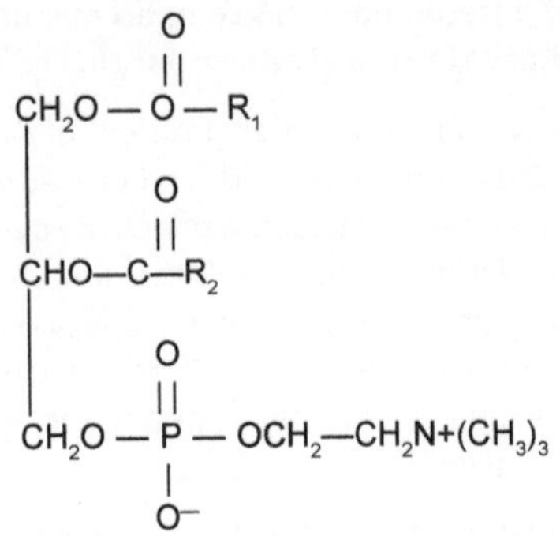

Fig. 1.2.3: Lecithin (α-glycerolphosphorylcholine)

Sphingolipids contain a ceramide, which consists of sphingosine base and a fatty acid. When a phosphorylcholine group is esterified at position 1 of the ceramide sphingomyelin, which is the major sphingolipid in milk, is formed. Sphingomyelin also exhibits amphiphilic properties.

Trace amounts of the glycosphingolipids, cerebrosides and gangliosides are also present in milk. Cerebrosides consist of a ceramide linked to a sugar group while the more complex gangliosides contain a ceramide, a number of sugar groups and sialic acid. These molecules are important biological compounds.

Diacylglycerols, Monoacylglycerols and Free Fatty Acids: Directly after milking, milk contains only small amounts of di- and monoacylglycerols and free fatty acids (Table 1.3). On storage, however, triacylglycerols in milk fat may be subjected to enzymatic hydrolysis by either milk lipase or bacterial lipases which can significantly increase the quantities of these compounds. For example, free fatty acids can increase from 0.1% to greater than 1%. Such an increase normally leads to a rancid flavour in milk which is caused by the lipases releasing short-chain fatty acids.

The small amounts of diacylglycerols present in fresh milk are largely sn-1, 2 diacylglycerols. Since the sn-3 position is the last to be acelated during the biosynthesis of triacylglycerols, these diacylglycerols are probably intermediates in this process. They are unlikely to be the products of lipolysis because the lipases preferentially attack the sn-1 and sn-3 positions of the triacylglycerol molecule, thereby forming a mixture of sn-1, 2 and sn-2, 3 diacylglycerols.

The profile of free fatty acids in freshly drawn milk differs somewhat from the profile of the fatty acids esterified to triacyglycerols (e.g. there appears to be very little free butyric acid), indicating that they also are unlikely to be the products of lipolysis.

Although diacylglycerols have a free hydroxyl group, their physical properties are broadly similar to those of triacylglycerols in that they are only slightly polar and show little surface activity. In contrast, monoacylglycerols can be considered relatively polar molecules. Those containing long-chain fatty acids are amphiphilic, and thus surface active, while those with short-chain fatty acids are partially soluble in water. Free fatty acids in the undissociated state have broadly similar properties to monoacylglycerols; long chain fatty acids are surface active, while short-chain fatty acids are partially soluble in water. However, at the pH of fresh milk (6.7), free fatty acids are predominantly in the dissociated form, which markedly increases their solubility in water.

Unsaponifiable Matter: The unsaponifiable matter is represented by the ether extract obtained after the hydrolysis of fat with alcoholic base by boiling. The ether extract, after some washing to remove impurities, is evaporated and dried to constant weight. This dry residue represents the unsaponifiable matter which for milk fat generally falls within the range of 0.30-0.45% by weight. The unsaponifiable matter consists of cholesterol and related sterols, the fat soluble vitamins A, D, E and K, traces of squalene, unidentified waxes and an homologous series of n-alkyl methyl ketones containing odd numbers of carbons, C_3 to C_{15}.

Sterols: Although sterols are a minor component of milk fat (0.30-0.45%), they are the major part of unsaponifiable matter. Cholesterol ($C_{27}H_{45}OH$) (Fig 1.2.4) is the principal sterol component, accounting for about 95% of the total sterols (0.25-0.40%). Small amounts of other sterols, such as lanosterol and b-sitosterols, are also present. It should be noted that a small proportion of cholesterol exists in the esterified form and these cholesterol esters are saponifiable.

The basic structure of sterols is a four-membered ring system, termed cyclo-pentenophenanthrene ring. Various side chains are attached to this ring system to give different sterols. These compounds are very nonpolar but, interestingly associate with phospholipids.

Cholesterol is an important biological compound that appears to play a role in controlling lipid and protein transitions and conformations in membranes. It is also a precursor for a number of hormones. Cholesterol has been implicated in a number of diseases which afflict humans, such as atherosclerosis, cholesterol gallstones and certain inherited disorders.

An interesting aspect of cholesterol is that, in direct contrast to cow milk fat and other animal fats, there are only trace amounts of cholesterol in vegetable oils. This has important commercial implications, since food products containing only vegetable oils can be labeled as cholesterol-free.

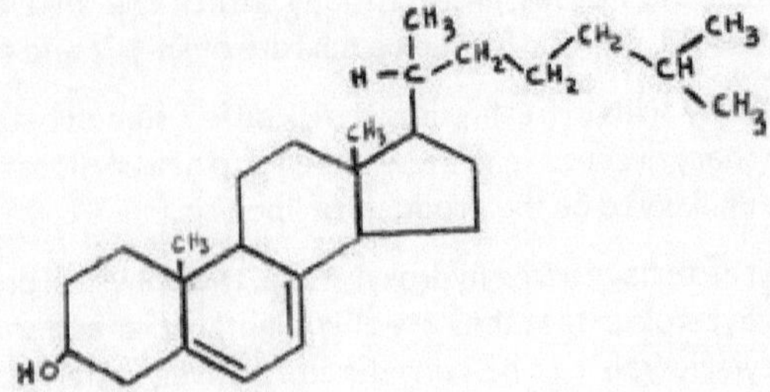

Fig. 1.2.4: Cholesterol

Carotenoids: The principal colour component in milk fat is - carotene, accounting for about 95% of the total carotenoids present. It is highly unsaturated hydrocarbon, containing a series of conjugated double bonds which absorb at about 450 nm. The concentration of β-carotene in milk fat varies considerably, with levels ranging from 2.5-8.5 mg / g fat.

The β- carotene content is dependent upon diet and breed of cow. Jersey cows produce milk fat with a higher colour than Friesian cows, while cows fed a diet of hay and concentrate tend to produce milk fat with a lower colour than pasture-fed cows. This latter finding is not surprising as carotenoid pigments are abundant in green plant materials.

Fat-Soluble Vitamins: A significant nutritional aspect of fats and oils is that the vitamins A, D, E and K are dissolved in liquid fat or oil phase. Milk fat is considered to be a major source of vitamin A but is a poor source of vitamin D, E and K.

Vitamin A is considered to exist in two forms: preformed vitamin A (retinol and retinyl esters) and provitamin A (β-carotene). The vitamin A activity of these different compounds varies considerably, ranging from 100% for all- *trans* retinol, 75% for 1,3- *cis* retinol and just 17% for β-carotene. Levels of all-*trans* retinol in milk fat range from 8-14 mg / g fat with typical values of about 10g / g fat. The value for 1,3- *cis* retinol is much lower, about 1mg / g fat. The total vitamin A activity can be obtained by summation of the concentrations and activities of all *trans*- retinol, 1, 3-*cis* retinol and β-carotene. This gives an average value for milk fat of approximately 11.5 retinol equivalent / g fat or 40 IU/ g fat.

Vitamin D activity is derived from a number of compounds, namely 25-hydroxycholecalciferol (25-hydroxy vitamin D_3), which accounts for about 65% of the total activity, cholecalciferol (vtamin D_3) and ergocalciferol (vitamin D_2). The level of vitamin D in milk is very low, about 0.01-0.02 mg / g fat, which equates to 0.4-0.8 IU / g fat. There is evidence to suggest that vitamin D levels in cows are affected by the amount of sunlight to which cows are exposed, with greater levels present in summer than during winter months.

A series of compounds termed tocopherols and tocotrienols, contribute to vitamin E activity. In milk fat, α-tocopherol accounts for virtually all the vitamin E and is present at a concentration of about 35 mg / g fat (range is 25-50 mg / g fat). This is equivalent to approximately 0.05 IU / g fat. The amount of tocopherol can vary during the dairying season: lush spring pastures result in greater levels than mature summer pastures. It is generally accepted that tocopherols act as antioxidants by reacting with free radicals, thereby protecting unsaturated fatty acids and β-carotenes from oxidation.

Vitamin K which is required for the synthesis of blood-clotting compounds, is present in milk at low concentrations. The amount of phylloquinone (vitamin K_1) is about 0.1- 0.2 mg /g fat.

Flavour Compounds: The desirable flavour of milk fat is one of its main attributes. The flavour is very complex, with a large number of compounds contributing to the overall aroma and taste. Approximately 120 volatile compounds have been identified in milk fat and, although many are present at concentrations below their individual threshold values, some may interact in synergistic manner and contribute to the overall flavour profile. Variations in the concentration of individual volatile compounds can also affect the perceived flavour, e.g. some aldehydes are thought to contribute buttery flavours at very low concentrations but are the source of oxidized flavours at higher levels.

The main classes of volatile compounds which are considered to contribute to the overall flavour of butter are: fatty acids, aldehydes, lactones and methyl ketones.

Short-and medium-chain fatty acids ($C_{4-}C_{12}$), which are present in fresh milk fat at concentrations at or below their threshold values, are thought to act synergistically to provide key flavour components in milk fat. Most of these fatty acids tend to impart unpleasant flavours at higher concentrations and hence lipolysis of triacylglycerols, which releases fatty acids, will inevitably lead to undesirable, rancid flavours.

Aliphatic aldehydes in milk fat originate from oxidation of unsaturated fatty acids in triacylglycerols. Thus, the concentrations of these aldehydes in high- quality, fresh milk fat are extremely low. However, these aldehydes have very low flavour threshold values, in the range 0.05-1.0 mg / g fat for saturated aliphatic aldehydes and as low as 0.001mg / g fat for unsaturated aldehydes. Thus, slight oxidation of milk fat can increase concentrations of aldehydes to levels where they can contribute sensorily. Generally, aldehydes are the source of 'oxidized' flavours but there is evidence that certain aldehydes, at very low concentrations (i.e. at or below their flavour threshold levels) may contribute buttery and deep-fried flavours.

In milk fat, small amounts of 4- and 5-hydroxy acids are esterified in triacylglycerols. These acids act as precursors for a series of four-carbon ring (g) and five-carbon ring (d) lactones which are important flavour components. A proportion of these hydroxy acids rearrange spontaneously at ambient temperature to give a concentration of lactones in the range 10-30 mg/g fat in fresh milk fat. It has been reported that three lactones, namely C_8 lactone, d C_{10} lactone and g C_{12} lactone, which have flavour threshold values between 1 and 3 mg / g fat, are present at sufficient concentrations to impart sweet, fruity flavours to fresh milk fat. When milk fat is heated, all hydroxy acids are converted to lactones to give a total concentration of 80-150 mg/g. Virtually all the lactones exceed their flavour threshold values and contribute to the rich flavour associated with baked goods containing butter. Lactones also contribute to the rich flavour of highly heated milk and ghee.

Milk fat also contains trace amounts of b-keto acids esterified to triacylglycerols. At high temperature, they are hydrolyzed and decarboxylated to form methyl ketones which, at low concentrations, are thought to contribute to cooked butter flavours.

In addition to the four classes of compounds discussed above, there are several other volatiles that contribute to the aroma and taste of milk fat. They include diacetyl (a diketone), phenol and cresol (aromatic alcohols) and skatole.

Fatty Acids: The major components of fats are the fatty acids. In the case of milk fat, the fatty acids account for over 85% and the glycerol for approximately 12.5% of the weight. Glycerol is a non-varying component of all fats, whereas the fatty acids represent the significant variable. Consequently the chemistry of a particular fat depends primarily on its component acids.

Bovine milk fat contains a great number of fatty acids. However, many of these are found in extremely small quantities and there are only 15 or 16 fatty acids present at concentrations at or above 1%. The main saturated fatty acids, which account for 62-70% of the total fatty acids, are straight-chain molecules which vary in length from 4 to 18 carbon atoms. The principal unsaturated fatty acid is oleic acid (about 20% of the total). The acid composition of milk fat is affected by factors such as the diet of the cow and the stage of lactation.

The fatty acid composition of bovine milk fat is to a large extent the fatty acid composition of its constituent triacylglycerols because the triacylglycerols make up approximately 98% of milk fat. Small quantities of fatty acids are also esterified to mono- and diacylglycerols and to phospholipids and there is about 0.1% unesterified or free fatty acids in milk fat. The fatty acids of triacylglycerols account for a large proportion of the molecular weight of the triacylglycerol molecule (85-95%). Furthermore, unsaturated fatty acids contain double bonds which are reactive sites. Thus, it is not surprising that the fatty acids have a marked effect on the physical and chemical properties of triacylglycerols, and subsequently on the properties of milk fat. Examples of the influence of fatty acids are: the melting characteristics of milk fat and the rate at which fat oxidation occurs.

Bovine milk fat is regarded as one of the most complex naturally occurring fats and oils because of the large number and wide variety of fatty acids it contains. It has been reported that about 400 fatty acids are found in milk fat though only 15 or 16 are major ones constituting about 95% (Table 1.2.4).

There is an empirical classification of these major acids on the basis of the length of the hydrocarbon chain; namely short-chain C_4 to C_6, medium-chain C_8 to C_{14} and long-chain C_{16} to C_{18}

Table 1.2.4. Major fatty acids of bovine milk fat

Fatty Acid	Percent (wt/wt)	
	Cow milk	Buffalo milk
Butyric $C_{4:0}$	3.20	4.36
Caproic $C_{6:0}$	2.11	1.51
Caprylic $C_{8:0}$	1.16	0.78
Capric $C_{10:0}$	2.57	1.28
Lauric $C_{12:0}$	3.6	1.78
Myristic $C_{14:0}$	11.93	10.81
Myristoleic $C_{14:1}$	2.12	1.27
Palmitic $C_{16:0}$	29.95	33.08
Palmitoleic $C_{16:1}$	2.16	1.99
Stearic $C_{18:0}$	10.07	11.97
Oleic $C_{18:1}$	27.42	27.15
Vaccenic $C_{18;1}$	4.2	-
Linoleic $C_{18:2}$	1.49	1.51
Linoleic (conjugated) $C_{18:2c}$	1.1	-
Linoleic (alpha) $C_{18:3}$	0.9	-
Minor acids	4.4	-

Source: Aneja, *et al.* (2002)

Types of Fatty Acids

Saturated Fatty Acids: The major saturated fatty acids are molecules with unbranched hydrocarbon chains containing an even number of carbon atoms; the length of the molecules vary from 4 to 18 carbons. These saturated fatty acids account for approximately 65-70% (w/w) of the total fatty acids. The most important saturated fatty acid from quantitative viewpoint is palmitic acid which accounts for about 25-30% of the total, while two other fatty acids, myristic and stearic, constitute 10-12% each.

The amount of short-chain fatty acids, butyric and caproic, are reasonably high when their proportion are expressed on as molar percentages (approximately 9.5 and 4.5%, respectively). Interestingly, these short-chain fatty acids are esterified almost exclusively at position sn-3 on the glycerol molecule, which means that approximately 42% (3x14%) of bovine milk fat triacylglycerols contain a short-chain fatty acid in combination with two other fatty acids. Short-chain fatty acids are responsible for the characteristic dairy flavour and aroma, and they can contribute either to the desirable aromas of some cheeses or to rancid flavour.

Two reasons have been postulated to explain the relatively high proportion of short- and medium-chain fatty acids in bovine milk fat. Firstly these fatty acids are absorbed rapidly as free fatty acids from the intestine into the portal blood stream and are quickly metabolized in the liver. Hence, they can make rapid and direct contribution to the energy metabolism of the new born calf. Secondly, short-chain fatty acids and, to a lesser extent, medium-chain fatty acids, lower the melting point of triacylglycerols and thus their presence helps to keep milk fat liquid at physiological temperatures.

Unsaturated Fatty Acids: The principal monounsaturated fatty acid is oleic acid (*cis*-9-octadecenoic acid) which constitutes 17-25% (w/w) of the total fatty acids but the percentage can vary with the feed of the animal (higher in summer with pasture). There are also relatively small but significant contributions from other monounsaturated acids, namely, myristoleic (about 1.0%), and palmitoleic (about 1.5%) and vaccenic acid (*trans*- 11-octadecenoic acid). The latter is formed as a result of biohydrogenation in the rumen and its proportion in milk fat is markedly affected by the cow's diet; a mixture of hay and concentrate gives a low level (about 1.5%) whereas pasture results in a high value (about 5%).

Because of the biohydrogenation reactions in the rumen, there are only low concentrations of the polyunsaturated fatty acids, linoleic and linolenic, in milk fat. The level of polyunsaturated fatty acids is lower in ruminant milk than monogastric milk. In particular, cow milk fat contains low level of polyunsaturates,C18:2 linoleic (2.4%) and C18:3 linoleic (0.8%). The level of linoleic acid is of interest because it is an essential fatty acid. Despite its low level, the newborn calf appears to be able to build up reserve of this acid. However, there have been concerns that an infant formula made solely from whole milk may not contain sufficient linoleic acid to meet the requirements of the human infant. Thus, commercial infant formulae are supplemented with vegetable oils to raise the level of linoleic acid.

In milk a small amount of *trans* fatty acids (unsaturated fatty acids with at least a double bond in *trans* configuration) occurs; their presence is due to the hydrogenation action of the microorganisms of the rumen (Jahreis, *et al.*,1999). Generally, *trans* fatty acids have been found to increase low-density lipoprotein (LDL) cholesterol and decrease high–density lipoprotein (HDL) cholesterol, and a relationship between risk of coronary heart disease and high intake of *trans* fatty acids has been hypothesized.

In contrast, *Butyrivirus fibrisolvens*, a microorganism of the rumen, is able to convert linoleic acid into 24 isomers, most of which, such as 9-*cis*, 11-*trans* octadecadienoicacid (rumenic acid) - the main isomer in ruminant milk fat, are responsible for beneficial effects (conjugated linoleic acid (CLA)) (Sebedio, *et al.*, 1999). Actually, in the last decade, several favourable biological activities of CLA have been hypothesized. CLA is thought to possess anticarcinogenic properties and capacity to modify lipid metabolism and postglandin production in specific tissues. Milk fat is a good source of CLA (0.6%); according to Creamer and MacGibbon New Zealand milk contains the highest level, probably due to feeding cattle mainly on pasture. In addition the acid may be able to regulate energy metabolism so that the body fat may be reduced.

An important difference between *cis and trans* unsaturated fatty acids is that the *cis* configuration of the double bond puts a significant 'kink' in the hydrocarbon chain whereas the *trans* configuration causes only a slight distortion. This has a major impact on the packing density of triacylglycerols in crystal lattices. Triacylglycerols containing *cis* unsaturated fatty acids have a lower packing density than triacylglycerols containing either *trans unsaturated* or saturated fatty acids and as a result have lower melting points. Thus, the relative levels of *cis and trans* unsaturated fatty acids can exert a considerable influence on the melting characteristics of milk fat.

1.2.2. Proteins

Proteins constitute an extremely important class of naturally occurring compounds that are essential to all living processes. They perform a variety of functions ranging from structure to reproduction in living organisms. Milk, the natural food of young mammals, contains a number of proteins that serve their nutritive requirements. Milk proteins also represent one of the greatest contributions of milk to human nutrition. With the development of more sophisticated analytical techniques over the years, more than 200 types of proteins have been characterized in bovine milk. The proteins in cow milk are the most widely studied in terms of their isolation, characterization, structural properties, functions and biosynthetic pathways. Hence, unless otherwise stated, the term 'milk protein' generally refers to the bovine species.

Composition: Proteins are polymers of certain L-α-amino acids* that are formed by living organisms. Some of them contain non-amino acid constituents as well, but the basic and overwhelmingly important units are amino acids. Of all the vast number of different α-amino acids that are conceivable or that can be produced in the laboratory, only 20 occur regularly in proteins. One of these, hydroxyproline, seems to be absent from milk proteins. It should be reemphasized that the amino acids found in proteins possess the common features that they are all α'(i.e., that the amino group is on the carbon atom next to the carboxyl) and that they are all, with the exception of glycine which has no asymmetric carbon atom, of the L-configuration. The latter statement does not mean that they are all levorotatory; as a matter of fact, some of them are dextrorotatory. It merely means that the arrangements of groups on the asymmetric carbon is analogous to L-glyceraldehyde which serves as the stereochemical standard for the sugars and amino acids. The general formula for a-amino acids of L-series is therefore:

COOH
|
H_2NC —— H ——
|
R

*Proline of course is a cyclic *imino* acid, but otherwise similar in structure to α-amino acids.

They differ in the R-group that they possess. The R-groups of the 19 amino acids found in milk proteins are given in Table 1.2.5. The chemistry of proteins is to a large degree concerned with the reactivity of these functional groups. They may be grouped into the general types of aliphatic hydrocarbon, alcohol, acid, amide, bases, thiol (or sulfhydryl), disulfide, thioether, aromatic and heterocyclic as is indicated in Table 1.2.5.

Table 1.2.5. Amino Acids of milk proteins.

Amino Acid	Formula	Reactive Group
Glycine	$\mathrm{NH_2\text{-}CH_2\text{-}COOH}$	
Alanine	$\mathrm{CH_3\text{-}CH\ (NH_2)\text{-}COOH}$	Aliphatic hydrocarbon
Valine	$\mathrm{(CH_3)2\text{-}CH\text{-}CH\ (NH_2)\text{-}COOH}$	Aliphatic hydrocarbon
Leucine	$\mathrm{(CH_3)2\text{-}CH\text{-}CH_2\text{-}CH\ (NH_2)\text{-}COOH}$	Aliphatic hydrocarbon
Isoleucine	$\mathrm{CH_3\text{-}CH_2\text{-}CH\ (CH_3)\text{-}CH\ (NH_2)\text{-}COOH}$	Aliphatic hydrocarbon
Serine	$\mathrm{CH_3\text{-}CH_2\text{-}CH\ (CH_3)\text{-}CH\ (NH_2)\text{-}COOH}$	
Threonine	$\mathrm{CH_3\text{-}CH\ (OH)\text{-}CH\ (NH_2)\text{-}COOH}$	
Asparatic Acid	$\mathrm{HOOC\text{-}CH_2\text{-}CH\ (NH_2)\text{-}COOH}$	
Asparagine	$\mathrm{H_2N\text{-}CO\text{-}CH_2\text{-}CH\ (NH_2)\text{-}COOH}$	
Glutamic Acid	$\mathrm{HOOC\text{-}(CH_2)2\text{-}CH\ (NH_2)\text{-}COOH}$	
Glutamine	$\mathrm{H_2N\text{-}CO\text{-}(CH_2)2\text{-}CH\ (NH_2)\text{-}COOH}$	
Arginine	$\mathrm{HN{=}C(NH_2)\text{-}NH\text{-}(CH_2)3\text{-}CH(NH_2)\text{-}COOH}$	
Histidine	$\mathrm{NH\text{-}CH{=}N\text{-}CH{=}C\text{-}CH_2\text{-}CH\ (NH_2)\text{-}COOH}$	
Lysine	$\mathrm{H_2N\text{-}(CH_2)4\text{-}CH\ (NH_2)\text{-}COOH}$	
Cysteine	$\mathrm{HS\text{-}CH_2\text{-}CH\ (NH_2)\text{-}COOH}$	
Methionine	$\mathrm{CH_3\text{-}S\text{-}(CH_2)2\text{-}CH\ (NH_2)\text{-}COOH}$	
Phenylalanine -	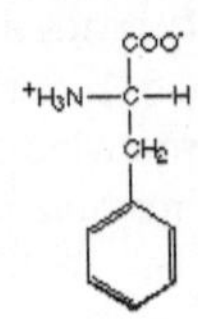	
Tyrosine	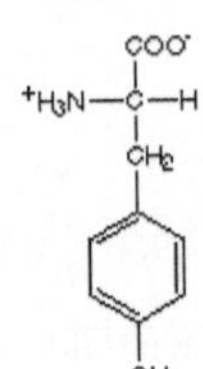	
Tryptophan	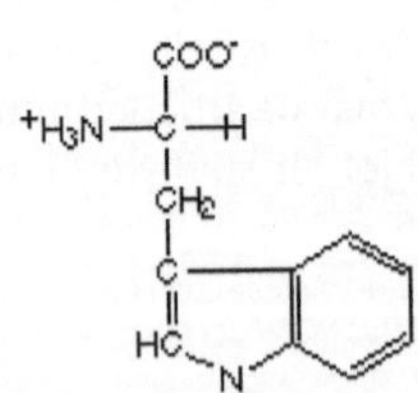	
Proline*	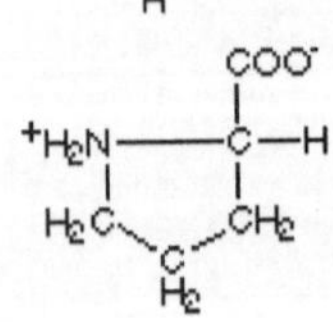	

*Imino acid

The fundamental linkage involved in proteins is the peptide linkage formed by the reaction of an amino and carboxyl group.

$$\underset{\text{R' CH-COOH}}{\overset{NH_2}{|}} + \underset{\text{R' CH-COOH}}{\overset{NH_2}{|}} \longrightarrow \begin{matrix} NH_2 \ \text{O H COOH} \\ \text{|| |} \\ \text{R CH-C-N-CH-R'} \end{matrix}$$

With difunctional units such as the amino acids, long-chain polymers can be built up in this way. Thus the protein consists of long chain polymers or polypeptides formed by a succession of peptide linkages and having the R groups attached along the chains. Such a polypeptide chain may be represented as follows:

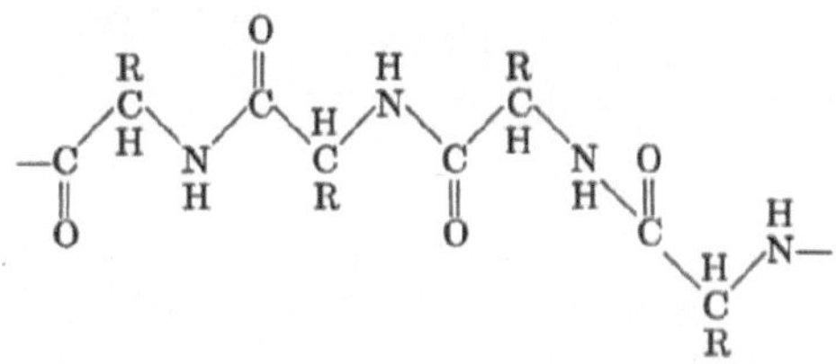

Classification: When raw skim milk is adjusted to pH 4.6, a precipitate containing approximately 80% of the protein of the cow milk is formed. This precipitation procedure has been used as the basis for the classification of milk proteins into two main groups, with casein in the precipitate and whey proteins (non-casein protein) in the supernatant. Milk protein is a very heterogeneous group of molecules and, for ease of description, could be classified into following two groups:

A. Major

B. Minor

The major group consists of the caselns and whey proteins; and minor group consists of enzymes, fat globule membrane proteins and other miscellaneous minor proteins.

A. Major Proteins

Caseins: Typical of milk proteins, caseins display a distinctive structure as well as physical, biological and nutritional properties. Casein, the principal protein in milk, exists in colloidal form along with a divalent ion to form a stable micelle. Casein in its original form occurs in milk as a large colloidal particle, containing calcium and phosphate as the prominent inorganic ions. The particle size of casein varies from 30 to 300 μm. The casein micelle consists of about 94% protein and 6% minerals.

Bovine milk contains four types of casein denoted as a_{s1-}, a_{s2-}, b- and k-casein, all of which are product of specific genes (Table 1.2.6). However, alkaline PAGE of whole casein preparations resolves in excess of 20 protein bands. Several of the electrophoretic bands represent post-translational products of one of the four caseins.

Table 1.2.6: Different proteins in bovine milk

Protein	Concentration in Milk		
	Indian Cow	Western Cow	Buffalo
α_{S1} -casein	1.04- 1.3	1.2- 1.5	1.44-1.8
α_{S2} - casein	0.26- 0.34	0.3-0.4	0.22- 0.28
β-casein	0.94	0.9-1.11	1.26- 1.58
γ-casein	0.15	0.1- 0.2	0.16
κ-casein	0.30-0.37	0.3- 0.4	0.43-0.54
β-lactoglobulins	0.31-0.38	0.2-0.4	0.39
α-lactalbumins	0.71-0.1	0.1-0.15	0.14
Protease peptone	0.24	0.6-1.8	0.33
Serum albumins	-	0.1-0.4	0.029
Lactoferrin	0.005	-	0.032

Source: Aneja *et al.* (2002)

The caseins which are synthesized in the mammary gland, are proteins containing ester-bound phosphate and due to their high content of proline, they tend to have very little secondary structure. The primary structure of a_{s1-} casein contains 199 amino acid residues. It has no cysteine residue and eight phosphates attached to serines.

The α_{s2-} casein contains 207 amino acid residues. It has 10 prolines, more phosphoserines and more lysines than the other caseins, and has two cysteins at positions 36 and 40. Several forms α_{s2-} casein are discernible by PAGE due to different degree of phosphorylation which range from 10 to 13 phosphate groups. These forms have been identified as α_{s2-}, α_{s3-}, α_{s4-}, α_{s5-}, and α_{s6-} casein.

There are 209 amino acids in β-casein. It is the most hydrophobic casein, has no cysteine, and a high proportion of proline (35 residues), which has a profound effect on its structure. At milk pH, the N-terminal 21-residue segment is highly negatively charged while the rest of the molecule, which is very hydrophobic, has no net charge. The amphipathic nature of the b-casein molecule is the reason why it forms micellar aggregates in solution. The β-casein has been shown to consist of six proteins with an identical amino acid sequence, but with 0-5 phosphate groups attached to the serine residues. The γ-caseins, which have been known for a long time, are the hydrolytic products of β-casein, produced by the action of plasmin. Gamma-caseins corresponding to residues 29-209, 106-209 and 108-209 of β-casein are present in the precipitate during isoelectric precipitation of whole casein at pH 4.6. Other fragments of β-casein (residues 1-28, 1-105 and 1-107) are found in the whey and they constitute part of a fraction formerly known as 'proteose peptone'.

Kappa-casein, which constitutes 10-12% of whole casein, plays a crucial role in stabilizing the casein micelles in milk, and after enzymatic cleavage, destabilizing the colloidal casein system. The enzymatic cleavage that brings about this transformation is important for the nutrition of suckling calf and for production of many cheese varieties. This is achieved by the molecule having two distinctly different domains that can be separated by cleavage of a bond that is hydrolyzed by an acid protease at neutral pH. The N-terminal domain (residues 1-95) carries a net positive charge, is very hydrophobic and interacts strongly with the other casein molecules. The C-terminal domain (residues 113-169) carries a net negative charge and contains a preponderance of polar residues. These domains are joined by a peptide (residues 96-112) that carries a net positive charge, is generally predicted to be β-strand, is generally well conserved in most species and contains a motif that is readily recognized by chymosin and rapidly and specifically cleaved to give a large hydrophobic peptide (para-kappa casein; κ-casein (1-105) and a smaller hydrophilic peptide (caseinomacropeptide), also called glycomacropeptide

Kappa-casein is the only protein of the casein family that is glycosylated. The different degrees of glycosylation, as revealed by up to seven bands during PAGE, are related to the number of negative charges on the N-acetylneuraminic acid residues. The primary structure of the carbohydrate-free portion of Kappa-casein contains 169 amino acids. Kappa-casein is the target for chymosin and it is the most extensively studied milk protein. It stabilizes casein micelles against calcium precipitation and loses this protective role when the Phe 105 - Met 106 bond is cleaved by enzymes to form two peptides: *para* -k-casein (residues 1-105), which is the hydrophobic portion and precipitates with the casein micelles, and caseinomacropeptide (residues 106-169), which remains in solution due to its high polarity and high content of negative charges. The amphipathic character of k-casein encourages it to form micelles in solution. Unlike other caseins, k-casein does not bind calcium extensively and is not sensitive to precipitation by Ca.

Heterogeneity of the caseins also arises from their interactions with one another and with other proteins and small ions. With the calcium phosphate present in milk, the caseins exist as micelles.

Caseins are heat stable. Heat has little or no effect on casein molecules since they exist naturally in an open and extended state at higher temperatures. However, heating of milk at elevated temperatures for a long time may result in hydrolytic cleavage of peptide and phosphate bond, which affects the stability of the complex, contributing to the coagulation of milk.

The ε-amino group of lysine present in casein interacts with the aldehyde group of lactose at elevated temperature, leading to the formation of brown pigments (Maillard reaction). This explains browning of heat desiccated products during storage.

As compared to cow milk, buffalo milk is richer in total proteins, particularly the casein and whey proteins. However, the proportion of various protein fractions is similar in milk of both species. Distinct differences exist in the physicochemical make-up of casein in cow and buffalo milk. The proportion of micellar casein is nearly 100% in buffalo milk, while that of soluble casein is very low whereas in cow milk, the micellar casein is of the order of 90-95 per cent. The voluminosity of the buffalo milk casein is 2.68-3.72 ml/g. The hydration (solvation) of the buffalo micelle is lower (2.60-2.90 g water/g casein) as compared to 3.48 g water/g casein for cow micelle. The particle size of the buffalo casein micelles is larger in diameter (110-160 nm) than that of the cow casein micelles (70-110 nm). The buffalo milk casein micelle is more opaque (about three times, when suspended in a different medium) than the cow micelle. The buffalo casein has superior whitening as compared to that of cow casein due perhaps to a higher proportion of calcium present in it. However, the sialic acid and hexose content in buffalo milk is lower than that of cow milk.

Whey Proteins: The whey protein fraction, which accounts for approximately 20% of the total protein, comprises the non-casein proteins that remain soluble when caseins have been isoelectrically precipitated at pH 4.6. Whey proteins are even more heterogeneous group of compounds than the caseins and share few characteristics, other than being soluble under conditions that render the caseins insoluble. Unlike the caseins, which lack secondary structures, the whey proteins have more organized secondary and tertiary structures and most are globular proteins. Four major proteins denoted as β-lactoglobulin, α-lactalbumin, serum albumin and immunoglobulins as shown in Table 1.2.7, account for > 95% of the non-casein proteins. Both β-lactoglobulin and α-lactalbumin are synthesized in the mammary gland whereas serum albumin is transported to the mammary gland via the blood serum.

More than half of the whey protein is β-lactoglobulin. Its primary structure contains 162 amino acids. It has five cysteine residues capable of forming disulphide bonds between residues 66 and 160,119 and 121, or 106 and 119. At pH 3 to 7 it self- associates to form dimmers. The buffalo milk β-lactoglobulin displays molecular weight of about 38,500 daltons, as compared to that of 37,600 daltons observed in the cow milk β-lactoglobulin. In milk of Indian cattle breeds, mainly two genetic variants (A&B) of β-lactoglobulin are found, whereas in western dairy breeds C and D variants have also been reported. Milk of Murrah buffalo shows the predominant presence of two genetic variants of β-lactoglobulin. Their electrophoretic mobility is similar to that of A and C variants of cow milk β-lactoglobulin. Buffalo milk also shows the presence of yet another variant of β-lactoglobulin, which has faster electrophoretic mobility than the A variant of cow milk β-lactoglobulin.

Alpha-lactalbumin is the smallest of the major whey proteins. It plays a very important role in the biosynthesis of lactose by being the modifier in the lactose synthetase complex. It contains 123 amino acids in its primary structure. All the eight cysteine residues in α-lactalbumin are connected by disulphide bridges between position 6 and 120, 28 and 111, 61 and 77, and 73 and 91. Several studies indicate that α-lactalbumin binds calcium, phospholipids and membranes. Minor forms of α-lactalbumin have been shown to contain a carbohydrate moiety consisting of mannose, galactose, fucose, N-acetylglucosamine, N-acetylgalactosamine and N-acetylneuraminic acid. The α-lactalbumins present in buffalo and cow milks display almost similar attributes. The molecular weight of buffalo and cow α-lactalbumins has been observed to be 16000, 14176 daltons, respectively. There are two genetic variants of α-lactalbumins - variants A and B- both in cow and buffalo milk. They have almost similar electrophoretic mobility.

Milk serum albumin is physically and immunologically identical to blood plasma albumin. It contains a sequence of 582 amino acids. All of the 35 cysteine residues (except cys 34) form intra-chain disulphide bonds. The molecule is considered to have three major domains, each consisting of two large double loops and a small double loop, and assumes an ellipsoidal shape. The N-terminal region is more compact than the C-terminal region. There are different domains, varying in hydrophobicity, net charge and ligand-binding sites. Isoelectric focusing patterns of serum albumin show evidence of considerable microheterogeneity of the protein.

The largest (molecular wt. >1000 kDa) and most heterogeneous of the major whey proteins belongs to a group collectively known as the immunoglobulins, which have been classified as IgG, IgA, IgM, IgE and IgD. They all exist as either monomer or polymers of a basic unit made up of two light and two heavy chains, each containing about 200 and 450-600 amino acid residues, respectively. The various classes of immunoglobulins found in milk are similar to immunoglobulins from other sources in terms of structure and functions. The N-terminal half (residues 1-115) of the light chain is known as the variable region because of its highly variable amino acid sequence. The C-terminal half is known as the constant region because the sequence of amino acid is not as variable. The heavy chains also contain a variable segment (residue 1-115) and a constant region (residue 310-500). The variable regions of the light and heavy chains are responsible for antigen binding, whereas functions of complement fixation, membrane transport, catabolism and mediation of immediate- type hypersensitivity have been attributed to the constant region of the heavy chains.

The immunoglobulins are antibodies synthesized in response to stimulation by specific antigens. These offer non-specific humoral response to Gram- negative enteric and respiratory bacteria. Of the five immunoglobulin classes, IgG is the most predominant fraction in buffalo and cow milk, comprising about 90% of the total colostral immunoglobulins. The average immunoglobulin content of buffalo milk is appreciably higher as compared to cow milk, 76.2 mg/100g whey proteins in first milking post-partum. It decreases to 43.4mg /100g on the sixth day milking post-partum. The total concentration of immunoglobulins in Zebu cattle averages about 41.1mg/ml immediately after calving and it declines to 045 mg/ml on the eighth day post-partum.

The average level of proteose-peptone in buffalo milk at about 330.5 mg/100 ml is significantly higher when compared to 240 mg/100 ml in cow milk.

The average range of whey proteins in buffalo milk is found to be between 0.70-0.74% as compared to 0.50-0.53% in cow milk. The average level of proteose-peptone in buffalo milk (330.5 mg/100 ml) is significantly higher than that in cow milk (240 mg /100 ml).

Milk proteins display significant functional characteristics (Table1.2.7), due to which they have become important ingredients in various foods.

Table 1.2.7. Functional characteristics of milk proteins.

Functionality	Casein or caseinates	Whey proteins
Water binding	Very high, minimum at pH 4.6	Water-binding capacity increases with denaturation of protein
Solubility	Insoluble at pH 4.6	Soluble at all pH levels. If denatured, insoluble at pH 5.
Viscosity	High at or above pH 4.6	Low for native protein. Higher if denatured
Gelation	No thermal gelation except in the presence of Ca^{+2} micelles gel with rennin	Heat gelation at 70 C or higher, Influenced by pH and salts
Emulsification	Excellent at neutral and basic pH	Good at pH 4-5, if heat denatured
Foaming	Good overrun, κ-casein best followed by α- and β_{s1}- casein. Poor foam stability.	Good overrun. β-Lactoglobulin better than β-lactalbumin.
Flavour binding	Good	Retention varies with degree of denaturation.

Source: Aneja, *et al.* (2002).

B. Minor Proteins

Enzymes: Amongst the minor proteins present in milk, milk enzymes play a vital role in assessing the quality and shelf life of milk. Milk being a repository of several enzymes it is a popular starting material for the isolation and purification of certain enzymes. Enzymes are a group of proteins produced by living organisms. They have the ability to trigger chemical reactions and to affect the course and speed of such reactions. Enzymes do this without being consumed. They are therefore sometimes called biocatalysts. An enzyme probably takes part in a reaction, but is released again when it has completed its job.

The action of enzymes is specific; each type of enzyme only catalyses one type of reaction. Two factors which strongly influence enzymatic action are temperature and pH. As a rule enzymes are most active in an optimum temperature range between 25 and 50°C. The activity drops if the temperature is increased beyond optimum, ceasing altogether somewhere between 50 and 120°C. At these temperatures the enzymes are more or less completely inactivated. The temperature of inactivation varies from one type of enzyme to another- a fact which has been widely utilized for the purpose of determining the degree of pasteurization of milk. Enzymes also have their optimum pH ranges, some function best in acid solutions, others in an alkaline environment.

The enzymes in milk come either from the cow's udder or from bacteria. The former are normal constituents of milk and are called *indigenous* enzymes. The latter, *bacterial enzymes*, vary in type and abundance according to the nature and size of the bacterial population.

The first reported enzyme in milk was lactoperoxidase and, to date, over 60 enzymes have been reported as being indigenous to milk and, as a group, they account for less than 1% of the total milk protein. Enzymes are heterogeneously distributed in milk, e.g. catalase and lactoperoxidase, ribonuclease and glucosaminidase are found mainly in the whey fraction while proteinases and lipases are associated with the casein micelles, and xanthine oxidase is found in the milk fat globule membrane. Many enzymes, e.g. catalase, are present predominantly in one component of milk, but are not confined exclusively to that component. This may be due to redistribution of the enzymes in the milk system. Alpha-lactalbumin, a major whey protein, may be classified as an enzyme because of its involvement in lactose synthesis.

Several of the enzymes in milk are utilized for quality testing and control. Among the more important ones are peroxidase, catalase, phophatase, lipase and lactase.

Peroxidase transfers oxygen from hydrogen peroxide (H_2O_2) to other readily oxidizable substances. Lactoperoxidase is the principal enzyme present in fresh milk. Activation of lactoperoxidase results in enhancement of shelf life of raw milk. This enzyme is inactivated if the milk is at 80°C for a few seconds, a fact which can be used to prove the presence or absence of peroxidase in milk and thereby check whether or not a pasteurization temperature above 80°C has been reached. This test is called Storch's peroxide test.

Catalase splits hydrogen peroxide into water and free oxygen. By determining the amount of oxygen that the enzyme can release in milk, it is possible to estimate the catalase content of the milk and learn whether or not the milk has come from an animal with a healthy udder. Milk from diseased udders has a high catalase content, while a fresh milk from a healthy udder contains only an insignificant amount. There are, however, many bacteria which produce this kind of enzyme. Catalase is destroyed by ordinary HTST pasteurization (75°C for 60 seconds).

Phosphatase has the property of being able to split certain phosphoric acid esters into phosphoric acid and the corresponding alcohols. Alkaline phosphatase is one of the most important milk enzymes. The presence of phosphatase in milk can be detected by adding a phosphoric acid ester and a reagent that changes colour when it reacts with the liberated alcohol. A change in colour reveals that the milk contains phosphatase. Phosphatase is destroyed by pasteurization, so the phosphatase test can be used to determine whether the pasteurization temperature has actually been attained. The routine test used in dairies is called phosphatase test.

The phosphatase test should preferably be performed immediately after the heat treatment. Failing that, the milk must be chilled below 5°C and kept at that temperature until analyzed. The analysis should be carried out the same day, otherwise a phenomenon known as reactivation may occur, i.e. an inactivated enzyme becomes active again and gives a positive test reading. Cream is particularly susceptible where this is concerned.

Lipase splits fat into glycerol and free fatty acids. Excess free fatty acids in milk and milk products result in a rancid taste. The action of this enzyme seems, in most cases, to be very weak, though the milk from certain cows may show strong lipase activity. The quantity of lipase in milk is believed to increase towards the end of lactation cycle. Lipase is, to a great extent, inactivated by HTST pasteurization, but higher temperatures are required for total inactivation. Many microorganisms produce lipase. This can cause serious problems as the enzyme is very resistant to heat.

Lactase hydrolyses lactose into glucose and galactose. The principal enzyme is β-galactosidase which hydrolyzes lactose leading finally to the formation of lactic acid. The extent of lactic acid present in milk denotes about the quality of milk.

Milk Fat Globule Membrane Protein: The fat globules of milk are stabilized by a complex membrane consisting of proteins and phospholipids; these proteins are designated as milk fat globule membrane proteins. A large number of proteins are present in milk at relatively low concentrations and are not isolated with either the casein or whey protein fractions but belong to a separate group known as the milk fat globule membrane proteins. These proteins were traditionally classified on the basis of their relative mobility on SDS-PAGE. The protein bands were numbered consecutively from the point of sample application in order of increasing mobility. Confusion arose with regard to the naming of the specific proteins because of inconsistencies in the use of the numbering system and different electrophoretic procedures used by different researchers. It has been recommended that the practice of identifying the milk fat globule membrane proteins by number be abandoned and be replaced by specific names because they are characterized by molecular cloning and sequencing techniques. For example, the term 'butyrophilin' is used to denote a protein which has been known under the following names: band IV/ glycoprotein E, component IV, component V/glycoprotein 6, component 12/IV, band 4/1 and CB5/PAS5.

Minor Miscellaneous Proteins: Proteins that do not fall into the classification of caseins, whey proteins, enzymes or milk fat globule membrane proteins are categorized as miscellaneous minor proteins and include transferrin, lactoferrin, ceruloplasmin, lactollin, glycoprotein-a, kininogen, M-1 glycoprotein, epidermal growth factor, glycolactin, angiogenin, *etc.* A wide range of biological functions has been assigned to those minor proteins present at concentrations in the mg/kg range.

Two iron-binding proteins, transferrin and lactoferrin (formerly known as 'red protein'), have been identified in milk. Lactoferrin is a nonhaem glycoprotein consisting of a single polypeptide chain of 690 amino acid residues with a molecular mass of about 80 kDa. Lactoferrin, a glycoprotein displays a strong inhibitory effect towards Gram-negative enteropathogenic bacteria by virtue of its ability to bind free ionic iron, which is essentially required for the growth of enteropathogenic microorganisms. Apart from the antibacterial effect, a nutritional role in iron metabolism has also been ascribed to lactoferrin. The average lactoferrin content of buffalo milk is relatively higher at 0.32-0.5 mg / ml than the average of 0.15-0.32 mg / ml for cow milk.

Ceruloplsmin is a copper-binding protein which has been detected in milk, colostrums and blood serum. Also present in milk serum are several proteins that bind other nutrients and components, such as folate, vitamin B_{12} corticosteroids and immunoglobulins; b_2-microglobulin, also known as lactollin, is part of the histocompatibility complex. The 98 amino acids of b_2-microglobulin, with a molecular mass of 11636 Da, have been sequenced. With the development of more sensitive analytical techniques, other proteins are being identified and added to the list of minor proteins. Recently, it was reported that a novel protein, denoted as 'glycolactin' and with a molecular mass of about 64 kDa, has been isolated from milk.

1.2.3. Lactose

Lactose, milk sugar, is the major carbohydrate of milk. Although trace amounts of glucose, galactose and other sugars are present, lactose is the only sugar in milk in significant quantities. Moreover, in most mixed milks lactose is the solid constituent present in the greatest quantities. It generally ranges between 4.7 and 4.9 per cent. It is true that in milk of high fat -testing breeds, indigenous cows and buffaloes, milk fat content may exceed the amount of lactose present. The most important factor affecting the level of lactose in milk is the condition of udder infection. Mastitis promotes an increased level of chlorides in the milk and depresses secretion of lactose. However, from an osmotic pressure stand-point, these changes are compensating and the osmotic pressures of normal and mastitic milk are generally the same. As suggested by these relationships, the lactose content of milk is inversely proportional to the ash content.

Lactose has many aspects of significance in milk and milk products. It is a controlling factor of first importance in fermented and ripened dairy products, it contributes to the nutritive value of milk and milk products, it is related to the texture and solubility of certain stored dairy products, and it plays an essential role in the colour and flavour of highly heated (caramelized) dairy products. In essence, milk would not be milk in absence of lactose.

The structural formula of lactose is shown in Fig. 1.2.5. Lactose is a disaccharide composed of D-glucose and D-galactose. The aldehyde group on C_1 of galactose is linked to the C_4 of glucose through a β-1,4- glycosidic link. The aldehyde group of the glucose moiety makes lactose a reducing sugar with associated reativity. The individual sugars usually adopt a closed pyranose ring form that may be one of two anomeric types, called a and β-forms. The anomeric forms can interchange when open chain aldehyde form is adopted. This process is called mutarotation. The relative abundance of the different forms of lactose changes substantially when lactose is dissolved in water.

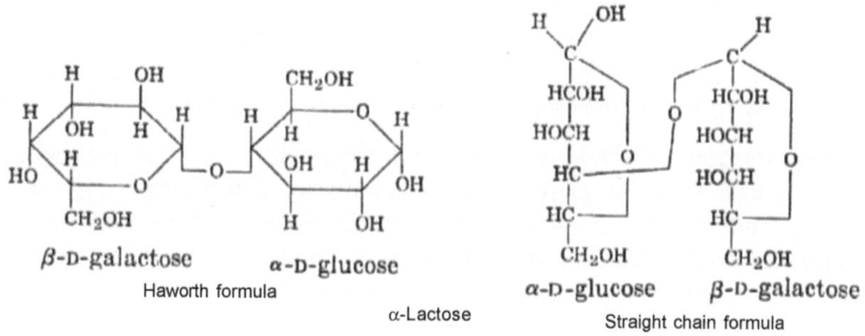

Fig. 1.2.5: Structural formula of lactose

Physical Properties: Lactose is normally found in nature or in dairy products in either of two crystalline forms, alpha hydrate and anhydrous beta or as an amorphous 'glass' mixture of alpha and beta lactose. Several other forms may be produced under special conditions. The designations a and b refer to the configuration of substituents on the number one carbon of the glucose moiety.

The β-form exhibits a specific rotation of$[a]^{20}_{D}$= +35.0° whereas the a-isomer shows a specific rotation of$[a]^{20}_{D}$ = +89.4°, both on the anhydrous weight basis. The a-form ordinarily is not met in the anhydrous state although it can be so prepared. It has a characteristic tendency to crystallize as the monohydrate, and in super saturated solutions crystallizing below 93.5 °C, it is this hydrate form of lactose which is deposited. Above 93.5° C, crystallization or drying of lactose solutions yields the b-anhydride, the other commonly encountered form of lactose. Careful drying of lactose monohydrate under vacuum above 65°C yields the a- anhydride, which form is stable indefinitely in the absence of water. Alpha lactose anhydride is converted to its hydrate below 93.5° C and to the β-anhydride above 93.5° C. All of these forms of lactose undergo mutarotation in aqueous solution, yielding a specific rotation of $[\alpha]_{D}^{20}$ = +55.4° (anhydrous basis) at equilibrium. The achievement of equilibrium at room temperature is a gradual process which in simple aqueous solution requires about 24 hours. This equilibrium is obtained instantaneously in the presence of a trace of ammonia (pH 9 or higher). At 20° C, and rotational equilibrium, a lactose solution will be composed of 62.25% β-form and 37.75% α-form. Thus, the equilibrium constant is 1.65 at this temperature. In all probability trace quantities of the free aldehyde form of lactose also exist in equilibrium solutions.

Depending on the temperature and conditions of drying the rapid removal from lactose solutions and from various dairy products can result in the formation of a lactose glass. These glasses are actually highly concentrated solutions containing various amounts of α- and β- lactose. The fact that such a glass has a vapour pressure which is not ordinarily in equilibrium with that of the air, tends to make it, and products containing it, very hygroscopic.

Solubility: An important difference lies in the solubility of α and β- forms of lactose. At 20° C the solubility of α-lactose is around 7.5 g/ 100g water, whilst that of β- lactose is around 48g/ 100g water. Thus, although in solutions of lactose under rotational equilibrium the β- form is present in the largest amount, the α- form, because of appreciably lower solubility, crystallizes out. Actually, this crystallization phenomenon involves a continuing shift; as the α- hydrate crystallizes out, some β-lactose shifts to the α-form in order to maintain equilibrium distribution. This process will continue indefinitely until crystallization ceases. As with most organic compounds, both α- and β- lactose exhibit increased solubility in water at elevated temperatures.

The relative insolubility of lactose in water, as compared with most other sugars, coupled with its capacity to form supersaturated solutions, is a matter of practical importance regarding certain dairy products. In water at 25° C the final solubility of lactose is approximately 18%. Thus, milk concentrated to 3:1 approaches saturation when held at room temperature. Cooling of such concentrated milk or the addition of substantial quantities of sucrose renders it supersaturated and susceptible to crystallization of α- lactose hydrate. Such crystals, which not uncommonly deposit in a characteristic tomahawk shape, are very hard and, when they are permitted to grow in an undisturbed manner, achieve sufficient size to impart a distinct gritty or sandy sensation in the mouth.

Crystallization of α-lactose monohydrate: Lactose crystallizes in two main forms. Alpha-lactose crystals are hard, slightly hygroscopic and slow to dissolve. In contrast, β- lactose crystals tend not to bind water and dissolve more readily. A third, amorphous, form of lactose can occur during spray drying. Amorphous lactose attracts water from the atmosphere and when the concentration of water reaches round 8%, lactose crystallizes in the α- monohydrate form. If this phenomenon is allowed to take place in milk or whey powder, caking can occur and the powder is then unfit for normal use. The poor solubility of α- lactose crystals can also have deleterious effects in other products like sweetened condensed milk or ice cream. The large crystals, usually significantly greater than 10 mm, or perceived as sandy, gritty or grainy. To a great extent, controlling crystal size can reduce this defect. The process of crystal formation begins with a process called nucleation. The nuclei form the starting-point for slow growth of lactose crystal. If there are few nuclei only, a comparatively small number of large crystals are formed slowly. However, by seeding the solution with numerous tiny crystals, crystallization is accelerated and the ultimate size is reduced.

Sweetness: Lactose is also characterized by a moderate, clean flavour with no aftertaste. In comparison to other sugars (Table 1.2.8), it is much less sweet. The relative sweetness of lactose is only 20-40% of that of sucrose. As a result lactose can be incorporated in foods or beverages at the relatively high concentrations without engendering excessive sweetness. This is one of the reasons why lactose is a suitable energy source in infant food formulae. Although lactose does not confer a high level of sweetness, it does confer 'body' or mouthfeel to products in which it is incorporated.

Table 1.2 8: Sweetness of some sugars relative to sucrose

Sugar	Relative Sweetness
Sucrose	1.0
Lactose	0.3
Glucose	0.7
Galactose	0.6
Maltose	0.5
Fructose	1.3

Chemical Reactions: In its chemical behaviour, lactose is like a number of similar carbohydrates and reacts according to the general rules of carbohydrate chemistry. Thus the reactions involve such groups as: (a) glycosidic linkage between the two monosaccharides; (b) the reducing group of the glucose; (c) the free hydroxyl groups; and (d) the carbon-carbon bonds.

Lactose is moderately reactive. However, it is not readily hydrolyzed to its monosaccharide units by acid. High temperature and low pH are required to achieve an appreciable degree of breakdown. Nevertheless, hydrolysis is readily catalyzed by the enzyme β-galactosidase (commonly referred to as lactase). Lactase is available in commercial quantities from several different sources and is used in number of important applications. Lactose may isomerize to lactulose on severe heating and the concentration of lactulose in heated milk is a fairly good indicator of the severity of heat treatment. For example, lactulose can be used to distinguish between sterilized and ultra-heat treated milk.

Lactose reacts readily with the a-amino group of amino acids and with the ε-group of lysine residues. The reaction is catalyzed by alkaline conditions and by severe heat treatment. The reaction sequence is very complex and results in browning, off-flavours and significant loss of nutritive value. In common with other sugars , lactose can be caramelized by heating. However, a complex mixture of reaction products is formed, including furfuryl alcohol, hydroxymethylfurfurol, aldehydes (formaldehyde) and organic acids (formic, acetic, pyruvic). The composition of caramel is greatly affected by lactose concentration, severity of heating and pH.

Lactose Intolerance: Some people are not capable of digesting milk. This is manifested by bloating, rumbling, and often diarrhoea and vomiting after milk ingestion. It has been established that this "milk intolerance" is mainly due to lactose content of milk and, therefore, this phenomenon is also called "lactose intolerance". When fed each molecule of lactose is degraded to one molecule each of glucose and galactose by enzyme lactase (β-galactosidase) present in intestinal juice. If this enzyme is deficient in certain individuals, they cannot digest lactose and consequently lactose intolerance results. This abnormality could be rectified by administering a lactose free diet. Generally malnourished infants and children develop lactose intolerance rapidly and family history in this regard plays vital role. A few children with persistent diarrhoea were rapidly cured when their diet of cow milk preparation were replaced with "soy milk". It is of interest that most of them when given cow milk after 19-27 days on soy-diet, tolerated them well.

Lactose provides energy for young mammals during the suckling period, thereafter lactase activity diminishes and so also does the intestine's lactose digestion capacity. This applies to all mammals, including humans. The age-related decline of intestinal mucosal lactase activity has been well documented in most human populations. Lactase activity may be low immediately after birth, increases rapidly independent of milk intake, but begins to decrease considerably soon after weaning. Lactose intolerance can develop in children after two years of age and progressively increase in frequency through childhood. Protein deficiency reduces lactase activity in infants and small children in developing countries where lactase deficiency may occur for several reasons at very young ages.

Adults with persistent lactase activity and correspondingly high lactose digestion capacity are common in only a few populations. Low or absent intestinal lactase activity is the normal state in adults in most ethnic groups, except in Caucacians, and this can be of great significance in countries with high milk consumption. It is general observation that population from low milk producing area exhibit more lactose intolerance as compared to population from high milk producing area. In developing countries, lactase deficiency due to low protein intake may occur at very young ages. However, to drink one or two glasses of milk (one glass equivalent to 250 ml or 12.5g lactose) may not cause this disease, especially when taken with meals, because this enzyme is rarely totally absent in the intestine. Therefore, it is not advisable to exclude milk totally from the diet of population with lactose intolerance.

Lactose is hydrolyzed to its components, glucose and galactose, by the disaccharidase enzyme lactase (-galactosidase) present in the microvillar membrane of columner epithelial cells in the middle and upper parts of the villi. The highest level of the enzyme activity is in the jejunum, with lower levels of the activity in the duodenum and ileum. The brush border membrane on the mucosal epithelial cells is responsible for the hydrolysis of dietary lactose. Only the brush border lactase is reduced in lactase deficiency.

The development of symptoms of lactose malabsorption, such as abdominal pain, cramps, headache, nausea, discomfort, bloating, diarrhoea and flatulence depends on several factors, including the amount of lactose consumed, gastric emptying rate, transit time, autodigestion by microbial β-galactosidases present, and the composition of meals in which lactose is one component.

Lactose intolerance refers to an inability to tolerate a standard or test dose of lactose without developing diagnostic biochemical changes, with or without clinical signs or symptoms, with gastrointestinal symptoms such as flatulence, bloating, abdominal cramps, or loose stools following the ingestion of lactose. It is commonly used for those with a low increase in blood sugar or high levels of hydrogen, following a lactose intolerance test, irrespective of symptoms.

Milk Salts: The salts of milk include those constituents except hydrogen ions and hydroxyl ions that are present as ions or in equilibrium with ions. A large part of the salt constituents of milk are mineral materials including metals and inorganic acid radicals. In addition, some organic acid radicals are present. A distinction is usually made between the major salt constituents of milk and the trace elements. The former category includes sodium, potassium, magnesium, calcium, phosphate, citrate, chloride, sulfate and bicarbonate. The latter group includes all other minerals and salt compounds. Obviously this distinction is made on the basis of concentration and not necessarily on the basis of importance in dairy processes and dairy problems.

Milk contains a number of minerals. The total concentration is less than 1%. Mineral salts occur in solution in milk serum or as casein compounds. The most important salts are those of calcium, sodium, potassium and magnesium. They occur as phosphates, chlorides, citrates and caseinates. Potassium and calcium salts are the most abundant in normal milk. The amounts of salts present in milk are not constant. Towards the end of lactation, and even more so in the case of udder diseases, the sodium chloride content increases and gives the milk a salty taste, while the amounts of other salts are correspondingly reduced.

Salt versus Ash: Ashing or incineration of milk destroys the organic compounds, leaving the mineral constituents behind. Most tabulations of the gross composition of milk include a figure for milk ash of approximately 0.7%. Actually, the ash does not truly represent the salt composition of milk for the following reasons: (1) organic radicals, such as citrate are destroyed by the incineration procedure, (2) phosphorus and sulfur of milk proteins and lipids appear in the ash. The organic sulfur is present in a non-salt form and the phosphorus occurs in a sort of "semi-salt" form having part of its potentially ionizable groups involved in ester linkage with hydroxyl groups of the proteins or lipids. (3) Carbohydrates appearing in the milk ash arise in part from carbon-di-oxide produced by decomposition of the organic materials. (4) Oxidation during incineration results in the formation of the oxides of the metals. (5) Some salt materials such as sodium chloride and carbonate may be lost by volatilization, but this complication can be avoided (at least for sodium and chloride) by properly regulating the temperature to not over 600^0 C. It is evident that the salt combinations and equilibria in milk cannot be deduced from a study of ash alone. The ash "content" gives a rough idea of the total mineral content and, of course, ashing is a useful technique for getting rid of organic matter as a prelude to analysis for many of the mineral elements.

Salt composition of milk: Average normal milk contains 0.70% ash, and this represents a salt content of about 0.9%. The percentage of salt and ash in milk varies with the breed, feed, season, and stage of lactation and disease. The white residue after incineration of a given weight of milk is used as a measure of the mineral content of milk. The concentration of major and trace elements found in bovine milk is shown in Table 1.2.9.

Table 1.2.9: Concentration of major minerals and trace elements in buffalo and cow milk.

Elements	Concentration (mg/100 ml)		
	Buffalo	Indian cow	Exotic cow
Major minerals	183.9	114.2	123.0
Calcium	19.02	11.0	12.0
Magnesium	44.75	50.0	58.0
Sodium	101.68	148.0	141.0
Potassium	8.74	84.8	95.0
Phosphate	177.6	166.0	160.0
Citrate Chloride	63.82	106.0	119.0
Trace elements	Concentration (mg/100 ml)		
Boron	50-145	27	
Cobalt	0.69-1.61	0.6	
Copper	7-21	13	
Iron	42-152	45	
Manganese	38.2-65.8	22	
Sulphur	15700-31400	30000	
Fluoride (ppm)	12.3-18.5	20-180	
Iodine (ppm)	8.5-19.4	5-50390	
Zinc	147-728		

Source: Aneja, *et al*., 2002

The mineral make-up of milk is crucial to the stability of the physicochemical equilibrium. Minerals in milk are present in complex equilibria such as colloidal, soluble: ionic and nonionic. Although their concentration is less than 1% in milk, minerals significantly affect the technological behaviour of milk, thus:

1. Heat stability and alcohol coagulation,
2. Preparation quality and storage stability of products like concentrated /heat desiccated milk products.
3. Clumping of fat globules upon homogenization of cream,
4. Firmness of curd during paneer / chhana and cheese manufacture,
5. Rennet coagulation of milk,
6. Flavour deterioration in milk and milk products due to oxidation catalyzed by copper and iron,
7. Nutritional importance, milk, an excellent source of calcium and phosphorus.

Buffalo milk contains more calcium and phosphorus (0.22 and 0.13%, respectively) than cow milk (0.12 and 0.09%, respectively). Moreover, the calcium / phosphorus ratio is higher in buffalo milk (2.26) than cow milk (1.96). Buffalo milk has low heat stability in concentrated form (2:1). Heat stability, expressed as heat coagulation time at 130° C is 31.82 min for buffalo milk, while it is 32.28 min for cow milk. However, when milk is concentrated 2 to 1, their corresponding heat coagulation times are 2.89 and 6.58 min, respectively. The soluble forms of calcium, magnesium and citrate are lower in buffalo milk than in cow milk.

Sodium, potassium and chloride are to a large extent (95-96%) present in true solution and in ionic form and therefore diffuse freely across the membrane during ultrafiltration, reverse osmosis and electrodialysis of milk and whey.

1.2.4. Minerals and nutritional significance

There are 20 minerals that are considered to be nutritionally essential for humans and these are sometimes classified into two groups, i.e. the macroelements (also known as the macrominerals) and trace elements. The macrominerals (sodium, potassium, chloride, calcium, magnesium, and phosphorus) are present in the body in amounts greater than about 0.01% by weight. The trace elements (the remaining 14 essential minerals) occur in the body at much lower levels and are required in the diet in amounts less than about 100 mg per day. The 14 trace elements that are considered essential in the human diet are iron, copper, zinc, manganese, selenium, iodine, chromium, cobalt, molybdenum, fluoride, arsenic, nickel, silicon and boron. While some of these, e.g. arsenic, nickel, silicon and boron have not been shown to be essential for humans, they are essential for experimental animals, and probably are also essential for humans. A number of other elements occur in milk, e.g. lithium, bromine, aluminium, strontium, silver, lead, tin, vanadium, mercury, cadmium, rubidium, and caesium. These are not nutritionally essential but many of them are toxic. However, their concentrations in milk are normally well below toxic levels.

Sodium, Potassium, Chloride: The mean values of sodium, potassium and chloride are shown in Table 1.2.10. Particularly high levels of sodium occur in colostrums followed by decrease within few days reaching to its normal values. The sodium content of milk is not influenced by dietary sodium intake within the normal range. Sodium concentration in milk tends to be higher at the end of lactation when milk yield is low. Removal of fat has little effect on milk sodium content. In contrast to most other minerals, the potassium concentration in colostrums is lower than that in mature milk, but increases to normal values within the first 2-3 days of lactation and is independent of potassium intake. The chloride concentration in milk decreases from colostrums to mature milk but increases sharply towards the end of lactation and is independent of dietary intake (Cashman, 2002).

Calcium, Phosphorus, Magnesium: The mean values of calcium, phosphorus and magnesium are shown in Table 1.2.10. The calcium concentration is slightly elevated in colostrums and at the end of lactation but varies little with feeding or season. There is little variation in the phosphorus content of milk throughout lactation. The mean concentration of magnesium in milk is unaffected by fat removal. Magnesium concentration in colostrums is two to three times that in mature milk and decreases to the level in mature milk within the first 1-3 days of lactation, remaining relatively constant thereafter. The concentration of magnesium in milk is unaffected by dietary magnesium intake.

Chemical Forms of Macrominerals: The chemical form of a mineral is important because it may influence intestinal absorption and utilization (the process of transport, cellular assimilation and conversion into a biologically active form) and thus bioavailability.

Sodium, Potassium, Chloride: Sodium, potassium and chloride are believed to be present in milk almost entirely as free ions. Practically all the sodium, potassium and chloride in milk is absorbed in the gastrointestinal tract, although much of what is absorbed is not retained.

Calcium, phosphorus, Magnesium: In cow milk 99% of calcium is in skim milk fraction, which explains why the calcium content is not affected by fat removal. Two-thirds of the total calcium occurs in colloidal form associated with the casein micelles, either in a calcium phosphate salt (about half of total milk calcium) or as calcium ions bound to phosphoserine residues (about one-sixth of total calcium); the remaining one-third is soluble. Ionized calcium in the soluble phase accounts for about 10% of the total calcium and most of the remaining soluble calcium occurs as calcium citrate. A small amount of calcium (0.15%) is bound to α-lactalbumin.

Of the total phosphorus in cow milk, 20% occurs as organic phosphate esterified to casein with the remaining as inorganic phosphate. About 44% of inorganic phosphate is associated with casein micelles as calcium phosphate and 56% is soluble, mainly as free phosphate ions.

In cow milk, 98-100% of the magnesium is in the skim milk phase, where 65% of the magnesium is in a soluble form (40% as magnesium citrate, 7% as magnesium phosphate and 16% as free magnesium ion), while the remainder is colloidal and is associated with the casein micelles (about half associated with colloidal calcium phosphate and half bound directly to phosphoserine residues in caseins).

Nutritional significance of macrominerals in milk and milk products

Sodium, Potassium, Chloride: Sodium is the principal cation in extracellular fluids and is the primary regulator of extracellular fluid volume. It is important in the regulation of osmolarity, acid-base balance and the membrane potential cells as well as in active transport across cell membranes. Chloride is the principal extracellular anion and is essential in the maintenance of fluid and electrolyte balance. Potassium is the principal intracellular cation, occurring in the cell at a concentration more than 30 times its concentration in extracellular fluid. Extracellular potassium contributes to the transmission of nerve impulses, to the control of skeletal muscle contraction and the maintenance of blood pressure.

Under normal circumstances, dietary deficiency of sodium, potassium or chloride does not occur, but the body can be depleted of sodium and chloride under extreme conditions, e.g. heavy perspiration, chronic diarrhoea or renal disease. Body depletion of potassium can occur under conditions where there are large alimentary or renal losses.

Minimum requirements for sodium, potassium and chloride (e.g. 500, 2000 and 750 mg per day, respectively, in adults) have been established. Actual intakes of sodium and chloride are considerably greater than minimum requirements in many populations and, given the evidence of a relationship of high salt intake to hypertension, it has been recommended that sodium intake be limited to 2.4 g per day. Similarly, considering the possible beneficial effect of potassium in hypertension, increasing potassium intake beyond the minimum requirement has been recommended.

Cow milk contributes little to dietary intakes of sodium (7% in U.K.), but some dairy products, such as cheese and butter, contain added salt and can be significant sources of sodium in some countries (e.g. about 13% of total sodium intake in the U.K.). It has been estimated that milk and dairy products provide 20% of total sodium and 24-29% of total potassium in the diet in Ireland and the U.K.

The concentration of sodium, potassium and chloride in milk are of physiological importance in the feeding of the young infant, and clinical problems may arise if there is an excessive intake of these nutrients. The kidney of the young infant, compared to that of adult, has limited capacity to concentrate solids and the renal solute load exerts a major effect on water balance. Renal solute load is determined mainly by sodium, potassium, chloride, phosphorus and protein (which give rise to urea). Cow milk has a much higher potential renal solute load (~300 mosmol/l) than human milk (93 mosmol/ l). The high renal solute load resulting from ingestion of cow milk may be of relatively little significance in most circumstances because the kidney merely excretes more concentrated urine. However, it does lead to a smaller margin of safety against dehydration which can occur in conditions of diarrhoea, fever and low water intake, and for this reason it is recommended that the upper limit of potential renal solute load in formulae for young infants should be about 220 mosmol/l. The recommended concentrations of sodium, potassium and chloride in infant formulae are in the ranges 133-403, 534-1338, and 369 -1360 mg/l, respectively. Cow milk-based infant formulae currently in use fall comfortably within these guidelines.

Calcium: The adult human body contains about 1200 g of calcium, which amounts to about 1.5-2.0% of body weight. Of this, 99% is found in bones and teeth where it is present as calcium phosphate, providing strength and structure. The remaining 1%, found in extra -cellular fluids and intracellular structures and cell membrane, is responsible for a number of regulatory functions such as maintenance of normal heart beat, blood coagulation, hormone secretion, integrity of intracellular cement substances and membranes, nerve conduction, muscle contraction and activation of enzymes.

Cow milk and milk products, such as cheese, yoghurt and dahi are very good sources of dietary calcium. The contribution of dairy products to total calcium intake has been estimated as 75% in the Netherlands, 55% (dietary intake data) to 72% (food disappearance data) in the U.S., 60% in U.K. and 52% in Ireland.

In the absence of milk and milk products in diet, calcium intakes in excess of 300 mg / day are difficult to achieve. This is far below typical recommended intakes for calcium. For example, the recently established Adequate Intake (AI) values for calcium in the U.S. are 1000 mg for adults, 1200 mg for older adults and 1300 mg for adolescents. On this basis, it might be considered that consumption of dairy products is very important in order to achieve an adequate calcium intake. However, there is still considerable disagreement on human calcium requirements, and this is reflected in the wide variation in adult recommended dietary intakes for calcium (400-1200 mg) which has been set by different authorities.

In recent years, considerable attention has been focused on the bioavailability of calcium in milk. Evidence from studies on experimental animals suggests that essentially all of the calcium in human milk, cow milk and cow milk-based infant formulae is potentially available for absorption in the gastrointestinal tract. In addition, it has often been suggested that the bioavailability of calcium in human milk is higher than in cow milk or cow milk-based formulae.

This arises from the findings that calcium was absorbed more efficiently by human infants from human milk than from cow milk or cow milk formula containing 738 mg Ca/ l. However, the absolute amount of calcium absorbed was greater from cow milk and formula with lower calcium contents (363-458 mg/l) was similar to that from human milk. Similarly, the efficiency of calcium absorption from human milk by weanling Rhesus monkeys has been reported as being significantly greater (72%) than from cow milk-based infant formulae (45-53%), but absolute absorption from human milk and formulae was similar due to the higher calcium concentration in the formulae. Moreover, bone mineralization in infants fed cow milk formula has been reported to be as good, if not slightly better, than in infants fed human milk.

Mean calcium absorption from cow milk by healthy human adults has been variably reported in the range 21-45%. Calcium absorption from cow milk has been reported as being higher (36.2% of dose) by β-galactosidase-deficient subjects than in β-galactosidase-sufficient group (25.7%) and it has been suggested that this reflected lower habitual calcium intake due to reduced milk consumption in the β- galactosidase- deficient subjects. It has been reported that calcium from different dairy products (including, whole milk, chocolate milk, yoghurt Cheddar cheese, processed cheese) is absorbed equally well.

Thus, while it appears that all of the calcium in human milk, cow milk and cow milk–based infant formulae is potentially available for absorption, the absolute amount of calcium absorbed by animals or humans is determined by physiological factors such as the efficiency of calcium absorption mechanism in the gastrointestinal tract, which may be influenced by calcium needs, vitamin D status and age, as well as by the calcium concentration in milk. In addition, some components of milk (lactose, phosphopeptides) may enhance calcium absorption.

There is strong evidence that lactose promotes intestinal absorption (particularly in the ileum) and body retention of calcium in rats. This effect of lactose is independent of vitamin D but the mechanism by which it occurs remains unresolved. It has been suggested that undigested lactose reaching the ileum interacts with the brush border membrane, increasing its permeability to calcium. Lactose also appears to increase calcium absorption by human infants. For example, calcium absorption has been reported to be significantly higher from a soy-based infant formula containing lactose (48%) than from a similar formula in which the carbohydrate source was a mixture of starch hydrolyzate and sucrose (33%). However, studies on the effect of lactose on calcium absorption by human adults are conflicting. One study found no significant difference between calcium absorption from milk and lactose-hydrolyzed milk by either β-galactosidase-deficient or β-galactosidase-sufficient subjects, while another study reported that calcium absorption was similar from milk (21.4%) and lactose-milk (lactose replaced by glucose) (26%) by healthy adult subjects, but lactose increased calcium absorption by β-galactosidase-deficient subjects. Overall, it is likely that lactose, at the levels normally present in milk, does not have a significant effect on calcium absorption by healthy adults consuming normal diets. It is possible that lactose affects the nonsaturable paracellular pathway for calcium absorption in the gut and its effect is most likely to occur in vitamin D deficiency, or when elevated levels of calcium are fed.

It has been suggested that phosphopeptides formed during the digestion of bovine casein may be involved in promoting calcium absorption. Such phosphopeptides have the capacity to chelate calcium and prevent the precipitation of calcium phosphate salts and may help to maintain a high concentration of soluble calcium in the intestinal lumen. There is evidence that phosphopeptides are present in the lumen of the small intestine of rats and pigs after a casein-containing meal; purified phosphopeptides have been shown to enhance the absorption of calcium by rats and chicks. The observation that calcium absorption by rats is enhanced by high casein meals is consistent with this. However, the nutritional significance of these phosphopeptides in humans consuming milk remains unclear.

Age-related osteoporosis, a common bone disease and a major cause of disability in Western countries, is characterized by reduced bone density resulting in increased bone fragility and susceptibility to fracture. The condition is particularly common in elderly women, particularly Caucasians. It has been estimated that osteoporosis afflicts 10 million Americans (half of the women over 45 years of age and 90% of the women 75 years of age).

Osteoporosis is a multifactorial disorder but there is increasing evidence that inadequate calcium intake, particularly throughout early life, is a contributory factor. Adequate calcium intake is required in early life in order to develop maximum bone mass at maturity (during the third decade of life) and there is evidence that the amount of bone mass present at maturity is an important factor influencing fracture susceptibility in the elderly. Peak bone mass at maturity appears to be related to the intake of calcium during the years of bone mineralization. Inadequate dietary calcium during the critical growth and building periods may result in failure to reach peak bone mass, causing osteopenia, osteoporosis, decreased skeletal integrity and increased risk of fracture in later life. Many believe that the most promising nutritional approach to reduce the risk of osteoporosis in later life is to ensure a calcium intake that allows the development of each individual's genetically programmed peak bone mass during the formative years, i.e. throughout childhood to age 25 years. In this regard, the prevalence of lower than recommended calcium intakes among adolescent and young adult females in many countries, e.g. in the U.S. and Europe, is of particular concern.

In recent years, evidence has been presented for a protective role of dietary calcium against hypertension, hypercholesterolaemia, diabetes mellitus, and colon and rectal cancer. However, consensus on the role of calcium in these conditions is lacking and further research is required.

Phosphorus: Phosphorus is an essential nutrient for humans and serves a number of important biological functions. Phosphorus occurs as organic and inorganic phosphates in all body tissues and fluids, is essential component of many biological molecules, including lipids, proteins, carbohydrates, and nucleic acids, and plays a central role in metabolism. As calcium phosphate, it is a major structural component of bones and teeth. Because almost all foods contain phosphorus, dietary phosphorus deficiency does not usually occur.

Cow milk and milk products, such as cheese, yoghurt and dahi, are good dietary sources of phosphorus and the contribution of milk and milk products to total phosphorus intake has been reported as 30-45% in Western countries. In the first few weeks of life, the infant's ability to regulate plasma calcium concentration has not developed fully and hypocalcaemia may result in neonatal tetany which used to occur more frequently in artificially fed than in breast fed infants. Excessive phosphorus intake contributes to this condition, and feeding unmodified cow milk, which has a high content of phosphorus, increases serum phosphorus and lowers serum (ionized) calcium in the newborn infant. For this reason, it is recommended that the calcium to phosphorus ratio in artificial infant food formulae should be greater than that in cow milk (~1.2:1) and more similar to that in human milk (2.2:1).

In experimental animals, a high intake of phosphorus or a low calcium to phosphorus ratio in the diet can lead to bone loss. However, it is generally agreed that wide variations in phosphorus intake or in the calcium to phosphorus ratio in the diet do not adversely affect bone in adult humans.

Magnesium: Magnesium has an essential role in a variety of physiological processes, including protein and nucleic acid metabolism, neuromuscular transmission and muscle contraction, bone growth and metabolism, and regulation of blood pressure and it acts as a cofactor for many enzymes.

There is little information on bioavailability of magnesium from milk in humans. Metabolic balance studies in infants showed that 16-43% magnesium is absorbed from cow milk-based infant formulae and that lactose enhances the absorption of magnesium. Cow milk and milk products contribute 16-21% of the total magnesium intakes in Western countries.

Dietary deficiency of magnesium is uncommon except in conditions of severe malnutrition and certain disease states. There is evidence that many young adults, especially women, in various European countries and in the United States fail to achieve the recommended intakes of magnesium and this raises the issue of possible adverse effects of lower than recommended intakes. Scientists have attempted to demonstrate that suboptimal intake of magnesium (i.e. below the RDA but not franc deficiency) is a contributor to the development of chronic maladies such as cardiovascular disease, hypertension, disorders of skeletal growth and osteoporosis, and diabetese mellitus. However, the results of studies in this area are ambiguous.

Content, Chemical Form and Nutritional Significance of Trace Elements in Milk and Milk Products: The trace element content of milk is not constant but is influenced by a number of factors such as stage of lactation, nutritional status of the animal, and environmental and genetic factors. Reported values in the literature for the concentration of many trace elements show a wide variation which is partly due to these factors, but also partly to analytical errors and contamination from milk collection and processing equipment and procedures. The average values of selected trace elements are shown in Table 1.2.9.

Iron, Copper, Zinc: Although several investigations have reported lack of a developmental pattern for iron in milk, at least one study has reported that iron concentration decreased by 35-50% during the first 3 days of lactation and remained relatively constant thereafter. The iron content of milk is relatively resistant to changes in dietary iron intake. Contact with metal containers can increase the concentration of iron in milk.

The iron is an essential trace element that acts as a catalytic center for a broad spectrum of metabolic functions. Iron as a component of haem in haemoglobin, myoglobin, cytochromes and other proteins, plays an essential role in the transport, storage and utilization of oxygen. It is also a cofactor for a number of enzymes. Deficiency of iron, resulting in anaemia, afflicts about 30% of the world population and occurs in both Western and developing countries (Cashman, 2003).

Milk and milk products are very poor sources of iron, and milk contributes little to total iron intake. Bioavailability of iron to the infant from human milk has been reported to be in the range 49-70%. Considerably lower absorption efficiency of iron from cow milk by human infants has been reported, usually about 10-34%. To compensate for the relatively low bioavailability of iron in cow milk, infant food formulae are often supplemented with iron. Iron absorption by infants from cow milk formula containing 12 mg/l iron as ferrous sulphate is about 4-7%, but because of the much higher concentration of iron in such formulae, the absolute amount of iron absorbed is considerably greater than from human milk.

Iron deficiency is one of the most common deficiencies in infancy and childhood due to a rapid growth and marginal supply of iron in the diet. It has been suggested that the iron stores of breastfed infant 4-6 months of age may become compromised if they are not replenished from dietary sources, and dietary iron supplementation has been recommended at not later than 4 months of age for full term infants and not later than 2 months of age for premature infants. Iron-fortified cow milk-based formulae are effective in preventing iron deficiency, which may be partly attributable to the fact that ascorbate is also added to formulae at levels which markedly enhance the absorption of added iron.

The concentration of copper in milk decreases by up to 50% during the first 3 days of lactation; it can be increased by dietary copper supplementation or by contact with metal containers and processing equipment.

Copper is an essential element for a wide range of animal species. It is required for iron utilization of iron and it is a cofactor for enzymes involved in the metabolism of glucose and synthesis of haemoglobin, connective tissues and phospholipids. Dietary deficiency of copper is uncommon except in conditions of severe malnutrition. Milk and milk products are considered poor sources of copper, and cow milk contributes little to the total dietary intake of copper.

Copper deficiency is rare in breastfed infants, but has been reported in formula-fed infants in some countries. Feeding infant formula containing 0.03- 0.40 mg/l copper has been shown to yield normal parameters of copper status similar to those of breastfed infants.

Mean zinc concentration in milk is 3.9 mg/l, but large variations in zinc content of milk (2-6 mg/l) have been reported. There is a large decrease (50%) in the concentration of zinc in cow colostrums during the first 3 days of lactation, with little change thereafter. Dietary zinc supplementation increases the zinc concentration in milk only slightly.

Zinc is essential for growth and development, sexual maturation and wound healing, and it may also be involved in normal functioning of the immune system and other physiological processes. It is a component of the hormone insulin and aids in the action of a number of hormones involved in reproduction, as well as being required for the synthesis of DNA, RNA and proteins and as a cofactor for many enzymes involved in most major metabolic processes. Zinc deficiency in humans was first reported in the Middle East in the early 1960s, giving rise dwarfism, impaired sexual development and anaemia. Mild deficiency of zinc, although difficult to detect, have been shown to occur in Western countries, particularly in infants and children, giving rise to low hair zinc levels, suboptimal growth, poor appetite and impaired taste acuity.

Dairy products such as milk, cheese and yoghurt are moderately good source of zinc, and it has been estimated that milk and dairy products contribute between 19 and 31% of the total zinc intake in Western countries.

It has been suggested that the bioavailability of zinc in human milk is greater than the cow milk. Human milk (but not cow milk) has a therapeutic value in the treatment of acrodermatitis enteropathica, a hereditary zinc malabsorption syndrome. The plasma zinc concentration of breast-fed infants has been reported to be significantly higher than that in infants fed a cow milk–based formula containing 1.8 mg / l zinc.

Manganese, Selenium, Iodine: The concentration of manganese is higher in colostrums (100-160 mg / l) than in mature milk (20-50mg / l) and a decrease of over 50% has been reported to occur during the first 3 days of lactation. Oral supplementation of manganese to cows can increase the manganese content of milk provided that large doses are administered over a long period.

Manganese is an essential element for every animal species studied. It is a specific cofactor for glycosyl transferases which are involved in mucopolysaccharide synthesis and a nonspecific cofactor for a wide variety of other enzymes. There are two known manganese metalloenzymes: pyruate carboxylase and super oxide dismutase. Manganese is widely distributed in foods, and dietary deficiency is not known to occur in humans.

Cow milk is a poor source of manganese and contributes little (1-3% in Western countries) to the total dietary intake of this mineral. Very little is known about the bioavailability of manganese in milk. One study reported that human milk (8.2±2.9%) was significantly higher than cow milk (2.4±1.7%), while absorption from cow milk-based infant formulae 1.7-5.9%. However, the absolute amount of manganese absorbed from cow milk and formulae was greater than from human milk due to the higher manganese concentration in these milks.

Mean selenium concentration in cow milk samples from fifteen countries was reported as 10 mg/l (range 3-40 mg / l). The concentration in milk depends on dietary intake and in areas such as New Zealand and Finland, where the selenium content of soil and plants is low, concentration as low as 3-5 mg/l has been reported. It has been shown that the selenium content of milk increased linearly from about 30-55 mg / l when dietary selenium was increased from about 2-6 mg / day.

Selenium is an essential component of the enzyme glutathione peroxidase which occurs in many human tissues where, together with vitamin E and the enzyme catalase and super oxide dismutase, it functions as an antioxidant, protecting cells against oxidative damage. In areas of China where the concentration of selenium in the soil is low, selenium deficiency causes Keshan disease, a cardiomyopathy that affects primarily young children and women of child bearing years.

The contribution of dairy products to daily dietary intake of selenium has been estimated as: 5mg (8% of the total intake) in the U.K., 13 mg (10%) in the U.S.

It has been reported that the average values for iodine content from various countries ranged from 100-770 mg / l with wide range of individual values from 20 to more than 4,000 mg / l. The concentration of iodine in milk is influenced by season and is closely related to dietary intake, and feeding winter rations containing mineral supplements results in considerable increase in iodine content.

The use of iodophors for teat disinfection increases the iodine content of milk. In addition, use of iodophors for the disinfection of containers, milking machines and processing equipment can also cause contamination of milk with iodine. The standardization of mineral feed supplements and supervised and restricted use of iodophor disinfectants have been recommended as measures to reduce the iodine content of milk.

Iodine is an essential component of thyroid hormones thyroxine and tri- iodothyronine, which are important in controlling the rate of basal metabolism and in reproduction. Dietary deficiency of iodine causes enlargement of the thyroid gland and goiter, while a large excess of iodine in the diet reduces the uptake of iodine by this gland and also produces signs of thyroid deficiency (thyrotoxicosis). Worldwide, 1.6 billion people (30% of the world population) are at risk of iodine deficiency. Of these, some 655million have goiter. While the highest prevalence of iodine deficiency is in less developed regions of the world, it persists in parts of the industrialized world, too, in countries such as Germany and Luxembourg.

The contribution of milk and milk products to the daily dietary intake of iodine has been estimated as: 37% of the total intake in the U.K. and only 6-7% in Germany.

1.2.5. Vitamins

Vitamins are organic substances which occur in very small concentrations in both plants and animals. They are essential to normal life processes. The chemical composition of vitamins is usually very complex, but that of most vitamins are known. The various vitamins are designated by capital letters, sometimes followed by numerical subscripts, e.g. A, B_1, and B_2.

Milk is a rich source of most of the vitamins except vitamin C. Almost all the vitamins are present in milk. Milk contains both fat and water soluble vitamins. The fat soluble vitamins are – A, D, E, K and water soluble vitamins are – B_1, B_2 group consisting of riboflavin, nicotinic acid, pyridoxine, pantothenic acid, biotin, vitamin B_{12}, folic acid and vitamin C or ascorbic acid. The approximate quantity of vitamins found in milk is shown in Table 1.2.10.

Table 1.2.10: Approximate quantities of vitamins found in milk

Vitamins	Quantity
Fat Soluble	
Vitamin A	20 IU/g fat
Carotene	5 μg/g fat
Vitamin D_3	1 IU/g fat
Vitamin E	28 μg/g fat
Vitamin K	
Water Soluble	**Traces**
Vitamin B_1	37 μg
Riboflavin	140 μg
Pantothenic Acid	400 μg
Nicotinic Acid	63 μg
Pyridoxine	37 μg
Biotin	1.6 μg
Vitamin B_{12}	0.3 μg
Folic Acid	0.3 μg
Ascorbic acid(Vitamin C)	2.0 μg

Source: Ling, E.R. (1956) Volume 1
Note: 1 μg= one millionth of a gram

Other constituents: Milk always contains white blood corpuscles (leucocytes). The content is low in milk from a healthy udder, but increases if the udder is diseased-usually in proportion to the severity of the disease.

Milk usually also contains dissolved gases. These consist mostly of carbon dioxide, nitrogen and oxygen. The proportions of these gases in milk change easily depending on the treatment given to the milk. The carbon dioxide content, which is high immediately after milking, decreases when exposed to air and agitation, while the oxygen and nitrogen content increase. Heating, cooling, aeration or vacuum treatment affect the gas content of milk in accordance with the gas laws governing the solubility of gases in liquids.

Dissolved nitrogen is an inert and passive component of milk. Carbon dioxide can exist in milk as carbonic acid or as bicarbonate. As carbonic acid it contributed to the acidity of milk. Milk exposed to the air after milking decreases in titratable acidity for a time due to loss of carbonic acid. Oxygen is known for its undesirable effect in milk, such as oxidized flavour development and the loss of ascorbic acid.

References

Aneja, R.P., Mathur, B.N., Chandan, R.C. and Banerjee, A.K. 2002. Technology of Indian Milk Products, 1st. Edn. Pub. Dairy India Yearbook, pp. 53.

Blanc, B. 1981. Biochemical aspects of human milk in comparison with bovine milk. *World Review of Nutrition and Dietetics*, 36:1-89.

Cashman, K.D. 2003. Trace elements, nutritional significance. *Encyclopedia of Dairy Sciences*, Vol.III, pp 2058.

Creamer, L.K. and MacGibbon, A.K.H. 1996. Some recent advances in the basic chemistry of milk proteins and lipids. *International Dairy Journal*, 6:539.

Epstein, H. 1974. Yak and chouri. *World Animal Review*, 9:8-12

FAO, 2004. http: // www.fao. org.

Fox, P.F., 2003. Milk. *Encyclopedia of Dairy Sciences*, Vol. III, pp 1805.

Gupta, N., Gupta, S.C., Pundir, R.K., Joshi, B.K. and Nivsarkar, A.E. !997. Characterization of Yak and Mithun, Annual Report (1996-97), pp 15, National Bureau of Animal Genetic Resources, Karnal.

Jahreis, G. Mockel, P. Shone, F. Moller, U. and Steinhart, H. 1999. The potential anticarcinogenic conjugated linolenic acid, cis-9 trans-11 $C_{18:2}$ in milk of different species.

Jenness, R. 1974. The composition of milk. In lactation, 3:3-107, (Eds) Larson, B.L. and Smith, V.R., Academic Press, New York. Dairy Chemistry, Wiley Eastern Pvt. Ltd., pp 2.

Marnila, P and Korhonen, H. 2003. Colostrum, *Encyclopedia of Dairy, Sciences*, Vol. I, pp 473.

Ohri, S.P. and Joshi, B.K. 1961. Composition of camel milk. *Indian Vet. J.* 38:514.

Sebedio, J.L. Gnaedig, S., Chardigny, J.M. 1999. Recent advances in conjugated linolenic acid research. *Current Opinion on Clinical Nutrition and Metabolism Care*, 2:499.

Walstra, P. and Jenness, R. 1984. Dairy Chemistry and Physics, New York, John Wiley.

Milk of Mammals other than Cow

The composition of the milk of all mammals, on the whole, is quite similar, the main constituents being water, fat, proteins, sugar, and minerals, there being, however, marked differences in the composition and quantities of these constituents. Broadly speaking, the milk of all mammals can be classified as follows:

a) Milk forming hard curds with rennet, e.g. milk of buffalo, cow goat and sheep.

b) Milk forming a very soft or no curd with rennet, e.g. milk of woman, ass and mare.

The milk can also be classified in two groups according to the type of β-casein present: A_1 and A_2 milk. A_2 milk is milk that contains the A_2 type of β-casein protein rather than the more prevalent A_1 protein. This milk is branded by A_2 Corporation and sold mostly in Australia, New Zealand and now in the United Kingdom. There is no consensus that A_2 milk has benefits over A_1 milk.

A_1 and A_2 α-casein are genetic variants of the beta-casein milk protein with different chemical structures. The A_1 α-casein type is the most common type found in cow's milk in Europe (excluding France), the USA, Australia and New Zealand.

A genetic test, developed by the A_2 Corporation, determines whether a cow produces the A_2 or A_1 type protein in its milk. The test uses hair from the cow's tail to determine this. The test allows the A_2 Corporation to give licenses to milk producers once these producers prove their cows produce A_2 β-casein protein in their milk.

1.3. Buffalo Milk

Buffalo milk is reputed for its richness and creaminess. It has higher proportion of fat, proteins, lactose and minerals as compared to cow milk. In general, buffalo milk contains on an average fat 7.0 %, proteins 3.8 %, lactose 5.1%, and ash 0.8%.

1.3.1. Fat

Buffalo milk is known for its high fat content. The size of buffalo fat globules varies from 4.15-4.60 mm which is significantly higher than that of cow milk (3.36-4.15 mm). About 99% of milk lipids are glycerides. Buffalo milk fat contains about 95% triglycerides, 4.1% diglycerides and 0.7% monoglycerides. Total concentration of glycerides in buffalo milk is higher than in cow milk. Buffalo milk fat contains higher proportion of C_4, C_{16}, C_{17} and C_{18} fatty acids than in cow milk fat (Arora, *et al.*, 1986). The proportion of C_4, C_8 C_{10}, C_{12}, C_{14}, $C_{14:1}$ in buffalo milk is, however, lower than cow milk fat.

The free fatty acid content of buffalo milk is significantly lower than that of cow milk. A similar observation has been made for clarified buffalo milk fat (ghee).

The average cholesterol level of buffalo milk is 20 mg/100 ml of milk. This value is significantly higher than cholesterol contents reported in cow milk. Since total fat percentage is much higher in buffalo milk than cow milk, the cholesterol content calculated as percent milk fat is significantly lower in buffalo than in cow milk fat. The total and free cholesterol estimated in buffalo milk fat is 275 and 212 mg/100 g, respectively which are significantly lower than 330 and 280 mg/100 g, respectively observed in cow milk fat.

The phospholipid content in Murrah buffalo milk varied between 32.4-41.4mg/100 g with an average value of 38.7 mg/100 g milk. The cow milk exhibited only a marginally higher average value of 39.2 mg/100 g (range 34.4-41.9 mg/100 g (Rama Murty and Narayanan, 1966). However, the phospholipid content of buffalo milk fat was much lower than in cow. Therefore, due to this inherent difference, butter and ghee made from buffalo milk were poor in phospholipid content.

1.3.2. Proteins

Buffalo milk is richer in total proteins, particularly the caseins and whey proteins than cow milk. The proportion of the various protein fractions, however, is similar in milk of both the species. Of the total proteins present, about 80% are caseins and the remaining 20 % are the whey proteins and other minor fractions. The primary polypeptide chains constituting buffalo milk proteins are αs1-caseins, αs2- caseins, β-casein, ϒ-casein, κ-casein, β-lactoglobulins, α-lactalbumins, blood serum albumins, lactoferrin, transferrin, fat globule membrane proteins and enzymes. In buffalo colostrums, the proportion of whey proteins is higher while the caseins are lower than in normal milk. The buffalo colostrum contains usually higher levels of immunoglobulins. Due to the unique properties of the milk immunoglobulins, their high levels in buffalo colostrum has generated considerable interest. Concentrations of these whey proteins, gradually decreases and tends to level off within a week of calving.

Almost all the buffalo milk casein is in the micellar form. The size of the buffalo casein micelles is large and varied from 80-250 nm, with majority falling between 110-160 nm in size (Hewdey *et al.*, 1989). In contrast, cow milk casein micelles are relatively smaller and vary from 70-110 nm in diameter. The proportion of α_ss1, αs2, β- and κ-caseins in Murrah buffalo milk is 40, 6.3, 35 and 12%, respectively.

Buffalo whey proteins were resolved in five fractions. The various fractions identified in whey proteins were β-lactoglobulin, α-lactalbumin, serum albumins and immunoglobulins. Of the total whey proteins β-lactoglobulin was 43.5%, α-lactalbumin 15.4%, serum albumins 3.2 and globulins 0.4%. The proportion of whey protein fractions in buffalo milk was markedly similar to that in cow milk. The amino acid composition of buffalo β-lactoglobulin is almost identical to that of cow. However, buffalo b-lactoglobulin did not exhibit genetic polymorphism (Sahai, 1996).

The physicochemical properties of buffalo and cow α-lactalbumin were apparently similar. No genetic polymorphism was observed. The cow lactalbumin variant A resembled the α-lactalbumin isolated from buffalo milk.

Buffalo colostrum has a very high concentration of immunoglobulins so that the immunity could be quickly transferred to the off-spring. Four classes of these protein - IgG, $IgA_{1,}$ $IgA_{2,}$ IgM have been identified in buffalo milk and colostrum. Immunoglobulins were apparently the largest molecules in buffalo colostrums. Their concentration in the first and the second milking were 43% and 32% of the total protein, respectively (Sahai, 1996).

Using immunoelectrophoresis and rabbit antibuffalo immunoglobulin serum, four antigenically distinct classes of immunoglobulins, IgG1, $IgA_{1,}$, IgA_2 and IgM were identified in colostral whey of Indian buffalo. The immunoelectrophoretical spectra of buffalo immunoglobulins was, however, markedly similar to that obtained in cow and sheep. IgG was the most predominant fraction of buffalo colostrum, while the dominant fraction in human milk colostrum was IgA.

IgG_1 was found to be predominant immunoglobulin in colostrum of zebu, comprising about 90% of total colostral immunoglobulins. The level of immunoglobulin secreted in colostrum rapidly decreased up to the second day postpartum and thereafter, it gradually declined to 2% of the early colostrum value within the first week.

The immunobiological role of buffalo immunoglobulins has generated considerable interest. Due to the high levels of the immunoglobulins in buffalo colostrum, efforts are being made to isolate and utilize them in infant foods as bioprotective additives.

Lactoferrin: The average lactoferrin content in buffalo milk is 0.320 mg/ml which is relatively higher than 0.05 mg/ml reported for cow milk. Buffalo colostrum is also rich source of lactoferrin with an average content of 0.75 mg/ml.

The unique biological role of lactoferrin, as a bacteriostatic agent against pathogenic microorganisms, has generated considerable interest. Therapeutic potential of lactoferrin against diseases such as leukemia are being actively explored. The high levels of this protein in buffalo milk and colostrum indicates new possibilities of its utilization as a rich source of lactoferrin for use in drugs.

1.3.3. Major minerals

Buffalo milk contains a high concentration of divalent cations of calcium and magnesium, however, the concentration of monovalent cations and anions such as sodium, potassium and chloride was lower than in cow milk. The concentration of polyvalent anions of phosphate and citrate were similar in the milk of both the species.

Salt Balance: Due to importance in heat stability, the balance between the cations of calcium and magnesium and the anions of phosphoric acid and citric acid in buffalo milk have been investigated in considerable detail. The distribution of these cations and anions between the colloidal and the dissolved phases, has also generated considerable interest.

Total divalent cations of calcium and magnesium were about 1.5 times higher in buffalo milk (about 200 mg/100 ml) as compared to 132 mg / 100 ml in cow milk. The amount of these cations in the colloidal phase of buffalo milk was also higher (~150 mg/100 ml), being almost double the amount in cow milk (~78 mg/100 ml milk). Levels of dissolved calcium and magnesium in buffalo milk were, however, almost similar to that of cow, due to the lower proportion of these cations in the dissolved phase of buffalo milk. About 21% of calcium and 46% of magnesium were in the dissolved state. The differences in the extent of partitioning of divalent minerals in milk of cow and buffalo have been attributed to the innate difference in concentration of casein in the milk of the two species.

Buffalo milk is richer in casein as compared to cow milk, and almost all (94.8%) the casein was in micellar form, whereas, around 10% of the cow milk casein was in the dissolved state. These divalent minerals are associated with micellar casein, therefore, a higher concentration of casein more so in micellar form in buffalo milk may be responsible for the higher proportion of these minerals in the colloidal phase, leaving lesser proportion in the dissolved phase.

The amount of total polyvalent anions of phosphorus and citrate in buffalo milk (241.6 mg / 100 ml) were almost similar to that in cow milk (246.8 mg / 100 ml). Proportion of these polyvalent anions in the colloidal phase was almost similar in the milk of two species. However, their proportion in the dissolved phase was relatively less in buffalo milk (140.9 mg / 100 ml) than in cow milk (186.4 mg / 100 ml).

The molar ratios of total cations and anions (Ca+Mg / P+Cit) was 0.8305 in buffalo milk, which was relatively higher than 0.5004 observed in cow milk.

Heat Stability: Since the first heat treatment of milk by Pasteur in 1860, thermal processing of milk has become an integral step in dairy processing and today the majority of milk, regardless of its ultimate use, is subjected to at least one heat treatment. The objective of the heat treatment of milk varies considerably, from being part of the manufacturing process for specific products, e.g. co-precipitates and yoghurt, to enabling the production of safe and stable products through the reduction or elimination of spoilage and pathogenic microbes. Accordingly, heat treatments vary considerably from mild (thermization at 65°C for 15 s), to very severe (in-container sterilization at 110-115°C for 10-15 min. Milk is extremely heat stable, owing principally to the ill-defined tertiary structure of the caseins, and can tolerate most processing conditions to which it is normally subjected: for example, it can be heated at 140°C for up to 20 min before it coagulates. However, problems may be encountered regarding the thermal processing and subsequent storage or processing of concentrated milk, homogenized milk products and cheese milk.

The ability of milk to resist heat coagulation for certain time is referred as heat stability of milk and the time required to cause coagulation at a given temperature is termed as heat coagulation time (HCT). The heat stability of milk is very commonly determined by placing a small amount of milk (1 to 2 ml) in a narrow sealed tube immersed in a thermostatically controlled oil bath maintained at 120, 130 or 140C. The length of time which elapses between placing of sample of milk in the oil bath at definite temperature and the onset of coagulation as indicated by flocculation, gelation or change in protein sedmentality is taken as the HCT. The HCT in such cases may be affected by quantity of milk taken in the tube, head space gas in the tube and the rate of agitation of milk tube during heating. The heat stability test for concentrated milk (approx. 20% TS.) is usually performed at 120C which is close to the in-container sterilization temperature. This test for heat stability of milk is commonly referred as 'Subjective method'.

The heat stability of milk is affected by a myriad of factors of which pH is the most significant. When pH of unconcentrated milk was artificially adjusted in the range of 6.5-7.0, there was a marked maximum in HCT/pH curve at pH 6.7 and a minimum at pH 6.9 and the stability was found to increase above pH 6.9. While one set of samples showed a very significant maximum and minimum, the stability of few other samples showed progressive increase with increased pH and showed no maximum or minimum. The former was referred as type A and the latter as type B milk. On concentration, not only does the heat stability decrease throughout the pH range 6.2 -7.2 but the shape of the heat stability-pH profile also changes. The heat stability in the region of the maximum (pH 6.7) decreases progressively with increasing concentration, and at 20% TS, the concentrated milk remains very unstable at pH values >6.8.

The majority of unconcentrated milk (~80-90% of milk from an individual cow and ~100% of bulk milk), exhibit a type A HCT- pH profile; stability at pH values < 6.3 is low at 140°C but increases progressively to a maximum at pH 6.7 (HCT~20 min); stability then decreases to a minimum at pH~6.9 (HCT~5min) with stability decreasing on the alkaline side of the minimum. For most of the year, the natural pH coincides with the pH of maximum stability. In type B milks, stability decreases as a function of pH, being less stable in the region of the maximum and more stable in the region of the minimum than type A milks. Concentrated milk (20% SNF) is relatively unstable and has a maximum stability at pH 6.4-6.6 (HCT~20 min at 120°C) with stability on either side of the maximum being very low. Coagulation of unconcentrated type B milk throughout the pH range 6.4-7.4 and Type A milk in the region of the maximum and on the alkaline side of the minimum is a single-stage process as determined by the objective heat stability assay. However, concentrated milk at its pH of maximum stability and type A milks in the region of the minimum coagulate by a two-stage.

The heat stability of milk is affected by the milk salts, although the natural variations in the milk salts are too small to account for the natural variation in the heat stability of milk. A reduction in the total mineral content of milk eliminates the minimum in the HCT- pH profile, whereas an increase in the total serum ion concentration destabilizes milk in the region of the minimum with little effect on maximum stability. A relatively small reduction (15%) in the concentration of divalent cations, Ca^{2+} or Mg^{2+}, in milk enhances stability throughout the pH range 6.5 - 7.5. Addition of phosphates to milk increases stability, presumably owing to their capacity to chelate calcium and also perhaps to their buffering ability, while the removal of indigenous phosphate shifts the HCT- pH profile to more alkaline values. Citrate which is present in milk at about 1800 mg kg^{-1}, is likely to be important for the heat stability of milk because of its ability to chelate calcium and its high solubility at high temperatures.

The macrocomponents present in milk also affect heat stability. Stability is unaffected by lipids *per se*. Removal of endogenous lactose from a type A milk results in a decrease in HCT_{max} and an increase in $HCT_{min,}$ while enzymatic hydrolysis of lactose to glucose and galactose enhances stability throughout the pH range. Of the milk proteins, β-lactoglobulin and k-casein have the greatest impact on the heat stability of milk. The addition of β-lactoglobulin to a serum protein-free casein micelle dispersion or to a type B milk results in the development of a type A HCT-pH profile, increasing and decreasing stability at pH 6.6 and 6.9, respectively. The addition of κ-casein to a Type A milk results in the elimination of the minimum in the HCT- pH profile. Of the other proteins, the addition of α_{s2}-casein to milk reduces stability, possibly because of its high sensitivity towards calcium. Urea, the major non-protein nitrogenous constituent in milk at 6 mMol per litre, stabilizes milk at HCT_{max} and at pH values on the alkaline side of the minimum and is thought to be responsible for up to 90% of the natural variation in the heat stability of milk (natural range for the concentration of urea in milk is ~ 190-450 mg per litre) The heat stability of unconcentrated type A milk in the region of the minimum is unaffected by urea and the stability of concentrated milk is unaffected by urea levels up to ~ 15 mMol per litre.

Effect of Processing Factors and Additives: In addition to variations in the heat stability of milk caused by compositional changes, several processing factors also affect stability. Preheating under ultrahigh temperature conditions (140°C for 2-14 min) increases the heat stability of type A milk and concentrates prepared from them, *while* the heat stability of type B milk is unaffected by preheating. It has been proposed that the stabilizing effect of preheat treatment is due to the denaturation of the whey proteins and precipitation of calcium phosphate under relatively mild conditions. Homogenization of milk prior to heat treatment markedly reduces the heat stability of milk. The destabilizing effect of homogenization is related to the adsorption of submicelles onto the interface of the newly formed fat globules, which then behave like κ-casein-depleted casein micelles. The deleterious effect of homogenization on the heat stability of milk may be offset by the preheat treatment, two-stage homogenization (rather than one-stage) or the addition of stabilizers, e.g. lecithin or sodium caseinate. Stability is unaffected by storage under refrigeration for up to 1 week but is reduced if the milk is stored at ambient temperature under controlled bacteriological conditions.

In an attempt to enhance the heat stability of milk proteins or determine the pH-dependence and coagulation mechanism of milk, the effect of numerous additives on the heat stability has been studied:

1. The effect of hydrocolloids varies considerably; starches stabilize milk while k-carrageenan, at low levels, has a stabilizing effect. Other plant-derived compounds that affect heat stability are polyphenols, which enhance stability, some very strongly.

2. Reagents that modify sulphydryl groups also affect stability. Oxidizing agents such as Cu^{2+}, $H_2O_{2,}$ $KBrO_{4,}$ KIO_3 and iodobenzoate convert a type A profile to a type B profile, while reducing agents, such as β-mercaptoethanol, markedly reduces stability.

3. Alcohols such as butanol, propanol, ethanol and methanol reduce the heat stability of milk proportionally to their ability to reduce the dielectric constant. It is thought that by reducing the dielectric constant these solvents collapse the protruding C-terminal of

κ-casein located on the surface of the micelle (hairy chains), making the micelles susceptible to calcium induced precipitation.

4. Reagents that react selectively with nucleophilic amino acid residues, e.g. formaldehyde with lysine and diketones with arginine residues, increase the heat stability of milk. The stabilizing mechanism appears to be related to their ability to crosslink proteins (thereby maintaining micellar integrity) or increase the net negative charge on proteins (thereby protecting against calcium- induced precipitation).

Heat Stability of Buffalo Milk: Maximum heat stability in buffalo milk was observed at its natural pH. Processes such as souring, addition of acid or alkali, which alter the pH, change the heat stability. Despite several contradictory reports, it has now been established that heat stability of fluid buffalo milk is comparable to that of cow milk.

Several innate physicochemical attributes and a number of processing variables influence the heat stability of buffalo milk. Alteration in salt balance by the addition of salts such as disodium phosphate, sodium citrate, sodium phosphate, dihydrogen sodium phosphate and urea changed the thermal stability of buffalo milk. It has also been suggested that casein might be the principal factor responsible for the heat stability characteristics of buffalo milk.

Proteins, total solids and fat contents of fluid milk do not appear to influence the heat stability of buffalo milk. However, when total solids in milk were increased by thermal concentration, the stability of concentrate was correlated with its fat and protein content.

There was a significant correlation between heat stability and non-protein nitrogen particularly urea in both buffalo and cow milk. Heat stability was also correlated with total and soluble calcium in milk of both the species. No correlation between heat stability of milk and its casein number, casein solvation and casein voluminosity was reported.

Rennet Stability and Curd Tension: The average rennet stability of buffalo milk was 25.6 minutes which was relatively lower than 28.2 minutes reported for cow milk. Rennet stability and curd tension were inversely proportional to the calcium content of the milk. Addition of sodium citrate or removal of calcium increased the rennet stability, whereas addition of calcium chloride decreased the curd formation time in buffalo milk.

Curd tension of buffalo milk has been extensively investigated due to its importance in digestion particularly in infants. The effect of various processing treatments on curd tension has also been investigated. The curd tension of buffalo milk varies between 32-85 g, which is higher than that of cow milk (28-54g). Heat treatment of milk resulted in considerable decrease in its curd tension. The decrease was 10-28% due to pasteurization, 58% due to boiling and 87% due to sterilization. The curd tension of milk was also reduced due to homogenization (28-73%). The addition of sodium citrate (0.1%), sodium hexametaphosphate (0.08%) or the mixture (0.10+0.08) of these two salts reduced the curd tension of buffalo milk by about 25.95 and 97%, respectively.

References

Arora, S.P., Singhal , K.K. and Chopra, R.C. 1986. Fatty acid composition of fat in milk and milk replacer diets. *Indian J. Dairy Sci.*, 39: 4, 495.

Hewdey, M.M., Nassib, T.A., El Din, M.M.Z., El Sokkary, E.S. Din, M.M.Z. El. Sokkary,E.S.El. 1989. Studies on buffalo casein. I. Composition of casein micelles. *Egyptian J. Dairy Sci.* 17:1, 87.

Rama Murty, M.K. and Naraynan, K.M. 1966. A method for the estimation of phospholipids in milk and milk products. *Indian J. Dairy Sci.*, 19: 1, 45.

Sahai, D. 1996. Buffalo Milk, Chemistry and Processing Technology. 1st ed. pp. 28, An SI Publication, 231, Old Housing Board Colony, Sector-13, Karnal, Haryana, India.

1.4. Goat Milk

Goats are found worldwide on all continents and are well adapted to tropical and temperate, arid and humid, cold and hot, and steep mountainous environments. The developing world is home to about 95% of the 700 million goats. They are valued for many different products and purposes in different part of the world: for meat, milk, cheese, yoghurt, mohair, cashmere, even for leather, manure, self-sufficiency in family food, *etc.* Goats' milk ranks fourth after cow, buffalo and sheep milk in terms of total world milk production. Although goat milk production (12.16 Mt,1999) accounts only for 2.16% of the total world milk production, goat keeping has a significant economic importance in countries where climatic conditions are not favourable for cattle keeping (Tziboula, 2003).

Generally, goat milk is considered inferior to cow or buffalo milk and used entirely for beverage purposes. In European countries the manufacture of goat's cheese is important.

Composition: Depending upon breed, feed, environmental stresses and stage of lactation of the goat, wide variations in the milk composition has been reported. On an average goat milk contains 14.8% TS, 5.6% fat, 3.80% protein, 4.8% lactose and 0.70% ash (Chandan *et al,* 1992). The amounts of fat, protein, sugar and ash are somewhat higher than those of cow milk. In general, proximate composition of goat milk resembles cow milk.

It has long been widely appreciated that goat milk is particularly well suited for consumption by the aged, the sick and convalescent and by young children. In number of cases where individuals are allergic to cow milk, the use of goat milk can not only induce relief from the distressing symptoms of this allergy but will also allow body growth to proceed at a normal rate. Goat milk has a similarity to human milk that is unmatched in bovine (cow) milk and also has several medicinal values. Goat milk differs from cow or human milk in having better digestibility, alkalinity, buffering capacity and certain therapeutic values in medicine and human nutrition (Coning, *et al.*1999).

1.4.1. Fat

Goat milk has smaller fat globule size, the average being of 3.5 μm in diameter than that of cow milk (4.5 μm) and on this account is more easily digestible by weak stomachs. Goat milk rarely forms a cream layer on account of small size of fat globules.

The composition of fat of goat milk is rather typical of that of other ruminants, having a relatively high content of saturated fatty acids with chain length of 4-12 atoms. Goat and ewe milk fat are characterized by higher content of C_6, C_8, C_{10}, C_{12} acids than those of cow and buffalo milk. The percent fatty acids reported in goat's fat are as follows:-butyric 2.1, caproic 1.9, caprylic 2.7, capric 7.9, lauric 3.9, myristic 10.2, palmitic 23.7, stearic 8.1, decanoic 0.2, tetradecenoic 0.4, hexadecenoic 2.1, and oleic 31.2.

It was found that phospholipid of goat milk was 0.037% as lecithin which is equivalent to 1.5 mg lipid P/100 ml. The cholesterol of goat milk was 17-39 mg/ 100 ml, which is higher than that of cow milk (7-16 mg/ 100 ml).

From technological standpoint, small globules and lack of their clustering ability impact adversely on cream and butter manufacturing processes. Also, the fat globule membrane of goat milk appears to be more fragile, resulting in vulnerability of fat to lipolysis and development of goat related flavours associated with volatile fatty acids.

1.4.2. Protein

The major proteins in cow milk are caseins and whey proteins. The composition of caseins of goat milk sets it apart from cow milk. Electrophoretic mobility under standard conditions shows that β-casein is the major component of casein fraction of goat milk, whereas αs1-casein is the major component of cow milk. Goat milk contains relatively higher level of $\alpha s\text{-}_2$ casein than cow milk, but the total $\alpha s\text{-}_1$ and $\alpha s\text{-}_2$ casein fractions are lower than αs1 fraction of cow milk. These differences may be related to the curd forming properties of goat milk during digestive processes and in the theological characteristics during cheese making as well as texture in fermented milks.

κ-casein content of goat milk and its cleavage by rennin specifically at positions 105 (phenylalanine) and 106 (methionine) resembles that of cow milk.

Because of differences in the ratio of αs_1-αs_2, β- and κ-casein in milk of cow and goat, the micelles and their behaviour during sedimentation, proteolysis and water binding capacity may be markedly different.

The primary whey proteins, α-lactalbumin and β-lactoglobulin exhibits some structural differences from their bovine counterparts. Certain immunological techniques permit distinction between the whey proteins of both species.

1.4.3. Minor proteins and enzymes

Lactoferrin, prolactin, transferrin, and immunoglobulin levels in goat milk are comparable to those in cow milk. Human milk contains 2 mg lactoferrin / ml, which is 10-100 times higher than goat milk. Goat milk does contain a folate binding protein, which results in much lower levels of folate in goat milk than in cow milk, the protease activity in fresh goat milk was higher than in cow milk.

Antigens derived from bacteria and viruses introduced via teat canal results in mammary gland secreting higher levels of immunoglobulins, especially IgG type, in both goats and cows. Goat milk contains relatively low levels of euglobulins or agglutinins. That is why goat milk creams poorly on cooling.

Distribution of enzymes in milks of goats and cows is quite different, the xanthine oxidase activity of goat milk is less than 10% of that of cow milk.

Lipolysis of goat milk differs markedly from that of cow milk. It has been reported that free fatty acid generation and resulting characteristic flavour of goat milk products was due to the distribution of lipoprotein lipase in various components of milk system. Cream, serum and casein phases of goat milk account for 46, 46 and 8% of total lipolytic activity, respectively. In contrast, in bovine milk 78% of lipase activity is associated with casein, and only 6% activity is related to cream and 17% to serum. The lipolytic system of caprine milk correlated with its susceptibility to spontaneous lipolysis triggered by cooling fresh milk. In human milk, 92% of lipase activity is in cream phase.

1.4.4. Minerals, salts and trace elements

Goat milk contains more chloride and potassium than cow milk (Table 1.4.1), the other minerals and salts appear to resemble cow milk composition. It has been reported that the trace minerals of milk are related to breed and lactation period. Mean levels of Mn, Cu and Fe in milk derived from French-alpine goats were 0.33, 5.0 and 1.7 mg/l.

Table 1.4.1. Minerals, salts and trace elements of goat and cow milk.

Mineral	Range (mg / 100 ml)	
	Caprine Milk	Cow Milk
Na	38-56	35.50
K	153-242	140-145
Ca	85-198	115.125
Mg	10-36	11.14
P	61-153	90-100
Cl	121-204	95-100
Citrate	70-180	150-210
Fe	0.043-0.246	0.03-0.11
Cu	0.013-0.314	0.01-0.12
Mn	0.005-0.020	0.003-0.037
Zn	0.192-1.411	0.222-190
I	0.0022-0.03197	0.005-0.07

Source: Jenness (1980); Rennar *et al,* (1989)

Selenium is an essential micronutrient, it prevents liver necrosis in rats. Selenium deficiency is correlated with abnormal cardiac function and fatal cardiomyopathy can be alleviated with sodium selenite supplementation in the diet.. The most vulnerable groups are lactating females and their young. Milk or milk formula for infant feeding provides an exclusive source of selenium in the first 6 months of life. The selenium content of milk is related to geographical location. Bioavailability of selenium is dependent upon form and distribution in the food. Goat and human milk contain higher levels of selenium (Table 1.4.2) than cow milk. Less than 3% of the total selenium is associated with the lipid fraction of the milk. Goat milk total peroxidase activity was 65% as opposed to 29% for human milk and 27% for cow milk. (Debski, *et al,* 1987)

Table 1.4.2: Selenium contents of milks of goat, cow and human.

Milk	Selenium content (mg/l)	
	Whole Milk	Skim Milk
Goat	13.3±0.4	13.1±0.5
Cow	9.6±0.4	9.5±0.3
Human	15.2±0.6	15.1±0.9

Source: Debski *et al*, (1987)

Vitamins and Other Constituents: Main vitamin contents of goat, cow and human milk is given in Table 1.4.3 In general, goat milk contains significantly lower amounts of folic acid and vitamin B_{12}.

Table 1.4.3: Vitamins and other constituents of goat, cow and human milk.

	Goat Milk	Cow Milk	Human Milk
Vitamin A (IU/100g)	185	126	241
Thiamin (mg/100g)	0.05	0.04	0.014
Riboflavin (mg/100g)	0.14	0.16	0.04
Pantothenic acid (mg/100g)	0.31	0.314	-
Niacin (mg/100g)	0.28	0.08	0.18
Vitamin B_6 (mg/100g)	0.05	0.04	0.01
Folic acid (mg/litre)	6	50	50
Vitamin B_{12} (mg/100g)	0.065	0.357	-
Vitamin C (mg/100g)	1.29	0.94	-
Orotic acid (mg/litre)	13	-	-
Carnitine (mg/litre)	16.4	-	-
ATP (mg/litre)	19	0.5	0.5
Phosphoserine (mg/litre)	1.6	-	-
Phosphoethanolamine (mg/litre)	54.6	-	-
Phosphoglyceroethalnoamine (mg/litre)	8.3	-	-
Free amino acids (mg/litre)	48	-	-
N-acetylneuraminic acid (mg/100ml)			
-Casein bound	0.28		
-Whey protein	0.23	-	-
Sialic acid in protease fraction (mg/litre)	13.89	27.94	-
Sialic acid in protease peptone fraction(mg/g)	9.60	20.59	-
Alkylglycerol (mg/g fat)	1.0	0.1	1.0

Source: Jenness (1980); Khatoon and Joshi (1987); Renner *et al*, (1989); Luke and Keith (1992).

It has been reported that High-temperature and short-time (HTST) pasteurization of goat milk was the best process to preserve various vitamins and for extending the shelf-life of milk. Losses of thiamine, riboflavin and vitamin C were lower when milk was processed by HTST, flash and UHT process than by LTLT and autoclave treatment.

References

Chandan, R.C., Attaie, R. and Sahani, K.M. 1992. Recent advances in goat production. Proceedings of papers presented at V Intr. Conf. on Goats, pp 1869.

Coni, E.; Bocca, B. and Caroli, S. 1999. Minor and trace element content of two typical Italian sheep dairy products. *J. Dairy Res.*, 66:589-598.

Debski, B., Picciano, M.F. and Milner, J.A. 1987. Selenium content and its distribution in human, cow and goat milk. *J. Nutr,* 117:1091-97.

Jenness, R. 1980. Composition and characteristics of goat milk. Review, 1968-1979. *J. Dairy Sci.* 63:1605-30.

Khatoon, J.A. and Joshi, V.K. 1987. Physicochemical characteristics of the proteose-peptone fraction of goat milk. 2. Amino acid composition, hexose and hexosamine contents. *Milchwissesnchaft,* 42(5):280-81.

Luke, B. and Keith, L.G. 1982. Calcium requirements and the diets of women and children. A review of dairy resources. *J. Reprod. Med.* (in press).

Renner, E., Schaafsma, G. and Scott, K.G. 1989. Micronutrients in milk. Micronutrients in milk and milk-based products, pp. 1-70 (Ed) Renner, E. Elsevier Appl. Science, New York.

Tziboula- Clarke, A. 2003. Goat milk. Encyclopedia of Dairy Science, Academic Press, pp: 1271.

1.5. Sheep Milk

On a world scale, the production of sheep milk, approximately 8 million tonnes, is of marginal importance compared to cow milk in quantitative terms (2% of the total); nevertheless, it is of major importance in Mediterranean and Middle Eastern countries where climatic conditions are not favourable for cattle raising. The numbers of sheep do not fully reflect the amount of milk produced, since sheep are often used for other purposes, such as meat and wool. In general, sheep milk is used essentially for cheese making, but in some countries part is made into yoghurt or whey cheeses.

Composition: Sheep milk is richer in all major constituents, than cow, buffalo and goat milk. On an average sheep milk contains 81.60% water (range 79.27-83.80), 18.4% TS (range 16.20-20.79), fat 7.09% (range 5.10-8.70), protein 5.72% (range 4.75-6.60), lactose 4.61& (range 4.10-4.95), ash 0.91% (range 0.70-1.10), the protein is made up of 4.44% casein, 0.98% whey protein and 0.047% ash (Ramos, and Juatez, 2003).

Milk is a mixture in equilibrium of proteins, fat, lactose and minerals in various different states of dispersion in water, such as emulsions, colloidal suspensions and true solutions. Sheep milk is more viscous than cow milk and is more resistant to the proliferation of bacteria during the first hours after milking, thanks to its greater immunological activity. It has a smell characteristic of the animal that produces it, and is an opaque white in colour. Sheep milk has a higher density, viscosity, refractive index, freezing point and measurable acidity than cow milk. Sheep milk is slightly more acidic than cow milk, possibly due to its higher protein content.

The variability in composition of sheep milk is due to genetic, physiological and environmental factors. The principal factor is breed; breeds selected for their high milk yield produce milk with lower total solids content than lower-yielding sheep. Fat shows more variation within breeds than proteins. Another factor to consider is the stage of lactation. Colostrum contains high levels of fat (10.7-17.2%) and protein (7.1-19.5%) and a low level of lactose (1.6-4.0%). The fat and protein contents of the milk decline during the first weeks postpartum, then increase gradually after the first month until lactation ends and the yield falls off. At the end of 7 months' lactation, fat values may be as high as 8.1-10% and protein as high as 6.8-8.9%. The lactose content falls slightly throughout lactation, and more sharply at the end (3.4-4.1%). Another factor having a notable influence on milk composition, especially on the fat content, is the feeding of the livestock. Other influencing factors include the age and health of the animal, the season, and milking times and procedures.

Table 1.5.1 shows the gross composition of sheep milk. Sheep milk contains higher concentrations of fat, protein, mineral salts and total solids than cow milk. The lactose content is comparable in the two species. Fat and protein are the principal components of the total solids constituting 69% in sheep milk compared to 56% in cow milk. The fat-to-protein ratio is higher in sheep than in cow milk and the cheese yield, expressed as kilograms of cheese per 100 litres of milk, is approximately 18 to 20 Kg, compared to 10 Kg for cow milk.

Table 1.5.1: Composition of sheep milk

Component	Average content (%)[a]	Range (%)
Water	81.60	79.27-83.80
Lactose	4.61	4.10-4.95
Fat	7.09	5.10-8.70
Crude protein(total nitrogen x 6.38)	5.72	4.75-6.60
Casein	4.44	
Whey protein	0.98	
Non-protein nitrogen	0.047	
Ash	0.91	0.70-1.10
Total solids	18.40	16.20-20.73
Solids nonfat	11.31	

[a]Average values calculated on the results reported by different authors.

1.5.1. Fat

Fat is one of the most important components of milk in terms of cost, nutrition and the physical and sensory characteristics that they impart to dairy products. They are present in the form of globules and are characteristically abundant in sizes of less than 4.5 μm. No appreciable differences have been found in the mechanism of fat globule secretion in sheep and cows; the structure and composition of the membrane are similar in both species. The phospholipid profile in both species is similar to that of the plasmatic membrane, which would tend to confirm their common origin. Along with triglycerides, the lipid composition of sheep's milk includes other simple lipids (diglycerides, monoglycerides, cholesterol esters), complex lipids (phospholipids) and liposoluble compounds (sterols, alcohols, hydrocarbons). Triglycerides constitute the principal group (nearly 98%), and include a large number of esterified fatty acids. The composition is, then, complex.

Fatty Acids: Fatty acids may be saturated or unsaturated (having from one to four double bonds). Most acids, from acetic to arachidonic acid, contain an even number of carbon atoms, while approximately 2% are saturated with an odd number of atoms, and roughly the same percentage of saturated fatty acids with branched methyl chains with an odd or even number of carbon atoms. Sheep's milk contains more caproic ($C_{6:0}$), caprylic ($C_{8:0}$), and capric ($C_{10:0}$) acid than does cows' milk. These fatty acids are associated with the characteristic flavour of sheep's milk cheeses and can also be used to detect mixtures of milk from different species (Table1.5.2).

Table 1.5.2: Fatty acid composition of sheep milk fat

Fatty acid	Percentage[a]
Butyric (C4:0)	3.0-5.8
Caproic (C6:0)	2.1-4.0
Caprylic (C8:0)	1.5-3.6
Capric (C10:0)	5.0-9.0
Decenoic (C10:1)	0.1-0.3
Lauric (C12:1)	2.9-5.2
Myristic (C14:1)	7.0-13.4
Myristoleic (C14:1)	0.4-1.0
Pentadecanoic (C15:0)	0.6-1.5
Pentadecenoic (C15:1)	0.2-0.6
Palmitic (C16:0)	20.0-28.5
Palmitoleic (C16:1)	1.0-2.8
Heptadecanoic (C17:0)	0. 2-1.0
Heptadecenoic(C17:1)	0.2-0.7
Stearic (C18:0)	6.2-13.1
Oleic (C18:1)	16.6-27.7
Linoleic(C18:2)	2.8-4.3
Linolenic (C18:3)	0.6-2.0

[a]Range based on the results given by different authors.

[b]All isomers.

The most important of the factors that affect fatty acid composition is the sheep's diet. The addition of animal fats causes a decrease of C_4- C_{14} acids and an increase of C_{16}, C_{18} and $C_{18:1}$ acids. If the forage intake is reduced, the proportion of C_4 to C_{16} fatty acids decreases accordingly.

Triglycerides: The triglyceride structure of the milk fat is responsible for the rheological properties of the fat and its behaviour during melting and crystallization. The triglyceride composition itself is of interest given that it can be used to verify the authenticity of milk fat.

Triglycerides are almost invariably accompanied by small amounts of di-and monoglycerides, mainly at position 1 and 2, which are therefore probably intermediates in the biosyntheses of triglycerides. The distribution of fatty acids in the triglyceride molecule, as determined by stereospecific analysis, differs slightly from cows' milk, but the distribution of acids in the molecule is not random. On the other hand, in both sheep and cow milk, butyric acid and other short-chain fatty acid (C_6–C_8) are esterified mainly at position $_{sn}$-3 of the glycerol molecule; the distribution of the other fatty acids (C_{10} or greater) exhibits no such marked specificity for position $_{sn}$-1 or $_{sn}$-2.

Unsaponifiable Lipids: The unsaponifiable fraction of the milk fat is composed largely of sterols, with a smaller proportion of hydrocarbons, basically squalene, and trace amounts of a number of normal and branched-chain hydrocarbons in the range C_{17}-C_{48} with odd and even number of carbon atoms, liposoluble vitamins and aliphatic alcohols. Ovine milk contains virtually no tocopherol or β-carotene.

Sterols are a minor fraction of total milk fat, the main component being cholesterol (270-350 mg / 100g of fat equivalent to approximately 20 mg / 100 ml of sheep milk), but small amounts of other sterols implicated in cholesterol biosynthesis have also been found in ovine milk: lanosterol (5-15mg / 100g fat) and, in still smaller proportions, dihydrolanosterol, desmosterol and lathosterol.

Phospholipids: The major phospholipids in both sheep and cow milk are phosphatidylserine, phosphatidylinositol and sphingomyeline. These account for roughly 0.8% of the total lipid fraction.

1.5.2. Proteins

Sheep milk contains 0.7-1.0% nitrogen. This is distributed in fractions the importance of which varies in terms of dairy technology and nutrition. Proteins account for approximately 95% of total nitrogen, while 5% is non-protein nitrogen. Milk proteins occur in two distinct phases; one is an unstable micelles phase composed of caseins, which exist as micelles, averaging about 190 nm in diameter, cemented by calcium phosphate and small amounts of magnesium, sodium, potassium and citrate, which scatter light and give the milk its opaque white appearance. The other is a soluble phase composed of whey proteins. The caseins precipitate at pH 4.6 at room temperature, whereas under the same conditions the whey proteins (β-lactoglobulin, α-lactalbumin and serum albumin) remain soluble.

Caseins: Caseins are the major proteins in sheep milk (76-83% of the total proteins) and are present in most types of cheeses. The denomination 'casein' embraces four types of polypeptide chain, as-$_1$casein, as-$_2$casein, β-casein and k-casein. The casein fraction also contains γ casein, a product of the breakdown of β-casein by plasmin.

Whey proteins: Whey proteins account for 17-22% of total proteins of sheep milk. The major proteins are β-lactoglobulin and α-lactalbumin. Beta-lactoglobulin, the principal protein in the whey consists of a polypeptide chain of 162 amino acids, Immunoglobulins, serum albumin and protease-peptones are present at smaller concentrations. The latter are products of the breakdown of β-casein by plasmin. Another soluble protein found in small amounts and possessing antibacterial properties is lactoferrin. In the case of rennet whey, casein macropeptides are also present, produced by the chymosin action on bond 105-106 of κ-casein. Serum albumin and immunoglobulins are not specific to milk and are considered to be the same as those found in the blood

Non-protein Nitrogen: Non-protein nitrogen accounts for between 5% and 6.8% of total nitrogen. Non-protein nitrogen compounds are: urea (45%), amino acids (16%), creatine (2.4%), creatinine (1.7%), ammonium (1%), uric acid (2.1%), and other uncharacterized compounds (32.3%). Sheep milk contains more urea and uric acid than cow milk.

1.5.3. Lactose

Lactose is the principal carbohydrate in milk. Chemically, it is a disaccharide consisting of D-glucose and D-galactose joined by a β-1-4 glycosidic linkage. Sheep milk contains 45-50 g of lactose / kg milk, and lactose accounts for 22-27% of dry matter versus 33-40% in cow milk. The lower lactose content does not present a problem in cheese making since enough lactose is available to ensure lactic fermentation.

1.5.4. Mineral Elements

Sheep milk contains mineral salts (around 0.9%). The most abundant elements are Ca, P, K, Na and Mg. Ca and P are the most important of the main constituents, both in nutritional terms and for their role in the stability of casein micelles and hence in the behaviour of the caseins during milk processing. The most abundant of the trace constituents are Zn, Fe, Cu and Mn. Table 1.5.3 shows the average concentration of macro and trace elements in sheep milk. With the exception of Na, the concentrations of these elements are higher than those found in cow milk. Sheep milk contains an average of 2 g of citrate / kg of milk, i.e. slightly more than cow milk.

The percentage of Ca and P in the soluble phase is, respectively, 20-25% and 35-40% of the total. These proportions are lower than in cow milk, but the absolute concentrations in the soluble phase are comparable for the two species. Therefore, the concentration of both elements in the colloidal phase are much higher than in cows' milk, given the higher levels of casein found in sheep's milk. Na and K are the principal elements in the soluble phase. Of the trace elements mentioned, Zn, Mn, Fe and Cu, the first two are associated mainly (around 90%) with colloidal fraction of the milk, while Fe and Cu are associated to a lesser extent (70% and 65%, respectively).

Table 1.5.3: Mean values and ranges of mineral of sheep milk[a]

	Na	K	Ca	P	Mg	Fe	Cu	Zn	Mn
			(g / l)			(mg / l)			
Mean	0.50	1.20	1.98	1.30	0.18	0.76	0.41	7.50	0.07
Minimum	0.27	0.96	1.80	1.17	0.10	0.34	0.32	4.75	0.04
Maximum	0.81	1.96	2.39	1.70	0.22	1.40	0.95	8.50	0.14

[a] Data calculated on the results reported by different authors.

1.5.5. Vitamins

Vitamin content is generally higher in sheep than in cow milk. The average values and the ranges of variation are shown in Table 1.5.4.

Table 1.5.4: Vitamin content of sheep milk /100 g.

Vitamins	Mean	Range
A (mg)	50	-
Carotene (mg)	5	2-7
B_1 (mg)	48	28-70
B_2 (mg)	0.23	0.16-0.30
Nicotinamide (mg)	0.45	0.40-0.50
Pantothenic acid (mg)	0.35	-
Biotin (mg)	9.0	-
B_{12} (mg)	0.51	0.30-0.71
C (mg)	4.25	3.00-6.00

Source: From Souci S-W, Fachmaun W and Krant H (eds.) (1986) Food Composition and Nutrition Tables, 3rd edn. Stuttgart, Germany: Wissenschaftliche Verlaggesellschaft.

Enzymes: Enzymes are constituents of the mammary gland, which pass into the milk during the secretion process. The enzymes found in milk are highly specific and are chiefly oxidoreductases, transferases and hydrolases. Particularly important for technological purposes are proteinases and lipases. Lipase, lysozyme, ribonuclease and xanthineoxidase are less active in sheep's milk, whereas alkaline phosphatase, despite possessing the same molecular weight and the same properties, is more active than in cow's milk. The most abundant enzymes is lactoperoxidase, which has proved impossible to distinguish from the bovine form but appears to be more thermolabile.

The native proteinases include aminopeptidases, thermolabile acid proteinases and serine proteinases, which are heat resistant. Serine proteinase, also known as alkaline proteinase or plasmin, is heat stable and hydrolyses Lys-X and Arg-X bonds. It becomes more active after thermal treatment.

Renneting Properties: Renneting properties of sheep milk are affected by a number of factors such as pH, physicochemical composition, micellar system, salts equilibria, calcium concentration, and temperature and time of heating. Sheep milk coagulates well and is very suitable for making high-quality cheeses. Coagulation is faster than for cow milk, and less rennet is needed to coagulate in the same time as with cow milk. Curd formation is also faster than in cow milk, but syneresis takes longer. The reason for this difference may be that sheep milk contains more casein, ionic calcium and colloidal calcium than cow milk. Renneting time and rate of firming is practically unaffected by the addition of calcium.

The coagulation properties of sheep milk are less affected than cow milk by storage at 4°C or by heat treatment. In fact, although severe heat treatment (90°C, 10 min) delays the coagulation in sheep milk, gelation does take place. In cow milk, on the other hand, heating for 1 min at 90°C prevents gelation. The reason for this difference in the behaviour of cow and sheep milk could be that in the latter the micelles grow considerably in size, attaining 1.75 times the size of micelles in fresh milk when heated to 85 or 90°C.

References

Alichanidis, E and Poshroniadou, A. 1996. Special features of dairy products from sheep and goat milk from the physicochemical and organoleptic point of view. In: *Production and Utilization of Sheep and Goat Milk,* pp. 21-43. Brussels: International Dairy Federation.

Anifantakis, E.M. 1986. Comparison of the physicochemical properties of sheep's and cows' milk. *International Dairy Federation Bulletin* 202: 42-53.

Fuente, M.A. Olano, A. and Juarez, M. 1997. Distribution of calcium, magnesium, phosphorus, zinc, manganese, copper and iron between the soluble and colloidal phases of sheep's and goats' milk. *Lait* 77: 515-520

Rainal, K. and Remeuf, F. 1998. The effect of heating on Physicochemical and renneting properties of milk: a comparison between caprine, ovine and bovine milk. *International Dairy Journal* 10: 135-149.

Ramos, M. and Juarez, M. 1981. The composition of sheep's and goats' milk. *International Dairy Federation Bulletin* 140: 1-19.

Ramos, M. and Juarez, M. 2003. Sheep Milk. *Encyclopedia of Dairy Sci.,* Academic Press, pp:2539-45

1.6. Yak Milk

The yak is one of the world's most remarkable bovines, adapted to living on 'the roof of the world in conditions so harsh that few other domestic animals can survive. Yak has many uses, milk production being one of them. The milk production of yak milk is relatively low, averaging only 100-300 kg / lactation, yet its milk is one of the richest sources of fat with range of 5.8-7.9% (Jain and Yadav, 1985).

Yak milk is a popular food item in countries where it is domesticated. Yak milk provides an excellent supplement of animal proteins, vitamins, minerals and other nutritionally valuable constituents, as well as calories to diets. Yak milk is probably the only source of milk and milk products for human population living in one of the most hostile climates on the globe.

Yak milk is dense, golden yellow in colour and sweetish in taste. It is very much liked by local people due to its peculiar flavour. It is sparingly used and drunk as raw milk. The common practice is to boil it before using for drinking.

Composition: Milk is a complex mixture of lipids, carbohydrates, proteins and many other organic and inorganic salts dissolved or dispersed in water phase. It is not uniform mixture. In yak milk every constituent without exception has a range of variation, smaller for some and large for others. The range depends on a wide variety of factors. The major milk components studied most extensively are fat, protein, lactose and minerals. The minerals are usually grouped collectively as ash. Table 1.1.1 shows some analytical figures from several sources for the major constituents of mid- lactation milk of yak cows in comparison to other animal species.

Jain and Yadav (1985) and Gupta *et al* (1997) reported that the mean value of yak milk consists of 17.93% total solids, 6.43% fat, 5.94% protein, 4.68% lactose, 0.87% ash, 0.30% calcium, 0.29 mg / 100 ml phosphorus, 0.74 mg / 100 ml iron, 122.50 mg / 100 ml potassium, 70.50 mg / 100ml sodium along with pH 6.64, titratable acidity 0.17% and specific gravity 1.04, respectively.

It is clear that yak milk is comparable to that of buffalo but appears far superior in the relative proportion of the major constituents than in the milk of *Bos taurus* or *Bos indicus* cow. The minor constituents include minerals, vitamins, non-protein nitrogenous compounds, pigments, enzymes and other substances which are present in relatively small amounts. However, from nutritional point of view the minor components may not be less important than the major ones, e.g., calcium, phosphorus and some of the vitamins are just as essential as protein to yak calves as to human beings.

1.6.1. Fat

Fats in milk are in the form of small globules which have a protecting membrane. Because of globules milk fat is not a simple oil-in-water emulsion, but is complex mixture of different components such as cholesterol, vitamins A, D and L- tocopherol. The fat globule size ranges from 1-10 μm in diameter with average of 5-6 μm. The importance of large fat globules in yak milk is considered in terms of firmness and ultimately the keeping quality of butter. The qualitative profile of saturated and unsaturated fatty acids in yak butter is similar to that reported for cows, buffaloes and other ruminants.

1.6.2. Proteins

The yak milk contains relatively higher level of total proteins, the average being 5.4%. The two major groups of proteins are casein and whey proteins. Albumins and globulins are the two most important whey proteins which remain in the whey or milk serum after the precipitation of casein. The other constituent is the proteose peptone. The α-lactalbumin is a low molecular weight protein (14,200) and is required in the formation of lactose synthetase, a lactose producing enzyme. The α-lactalbumin in yak milk is significantly less than in cattle and buffaloes. This may be the reason why yak milk has comparatively lesser lactose content than cattle and buffaloes. The proportion of β-lactoglobulin among whey proteins is largest in yak milk, like other mammalian species. The percentage of β-lactoglobulin in yak milk varies from 35.2± 5.7 to 44.7±7.1 in different stages of lactation and is higher than in buffalo and cattle milk. Immunoglobulins (Ig) are glycoproteins of high molecular weight (15,000-1, 00,000). They possess specific antibody activities. There are three types of immunoglobulins, *viz.*, IgA, IgGM and IgGI, in milk of bovine species including yak. In yak milk their level ranges 30.7±6.4 to 39.2±9.0% of total whey proteins which is marginally higher than that of cattle. Like blood serum, a milk serum albumin or whey albumin has also been detected and isolated. This protein has the molecular weight of around 66,000. Its fraction in yak milk has been reported to be low (7.0±3.1%) in the beginning of lactation, but increases as the lactation progresses. Interestingly, the level of albumin showed a marked decline near the fag end of lactation. Lactoferrin, an iron-binding protein is also found in yak milk.

Non-protein Nitrogen Fraction: Certain nitrogenous compounds which usually form a minor component are related to proteins. In milk, like in cow or buffalo milk, there is small fraction of the total nitrogenous compounds in the form of substrates which are not true proteins, but give some of the protein reactions. This is known as proteose-peptone fraction. It is more in colostrum than in routine milk.

The total nitrogen was 0.582% in milk from Ladakhi yak and 0.630% in milk from Himachali yak. The non-casein nitrogen levels were 0.132% in Ladakhi and 0.216% in Kinnauri yaks.

1.6.3. Minerals

The principal minerals in yak milk, like in other bovine milk, include sodium, potassium, calcium, iron, phosphorus and chlorides. It is considered that milk rich in lactose would have lesser salts. This concept holds true for yak milk as it is low in lactose but rich in salts. In yak milk sodium, potassium and chloride are present as free ions, some parts of calcium and magnesium are also present as free ions. Most of the trace elements are present as complex compounds involving casein and other molecules

1.6.4. Utilization

Traditional Uses: The milk of yak like other bovine milk besides being consumed as liquid, is also used for preparing a variety of palatable products of much better quality than the original milk by relatively simple and traditional methods. In fact, more than yak milk, its products are considered indispensable by the highlanders. Milk fat in the form of butter or ghee is the most important component in the socioeconomic life of yak herders. Churpi (a kind of cheese) is the other component of the diet of the local people.

The countries like Mangolia and in some parts of People's Republic of China, yak milk is processed in factories for making industrial products of commercial use. In Nepal, small- scale Swiss cheese factories have been established in yak herding areas, and several kind of cheeses are becoming popular among local people and tourists coming to the picturesque Himalayan Kingdom.

Tokita, *et al*. (1981) reported that milk is an important component of Sherpa diet. Besides butter, milk- tea, traditional dairy products such as *shoshim* and naturally fermented milk *sho* (yoghurt) are prepared from butter milk after churning out butter and thera (yoghurt, butter milk). The buttermilk is heated to coagulate and the curd (serkam) is made into churpi (a type of cheese), chursife and shomaar containing curry by addition of milk fermentation. Churshife is the basis for a number of products, e.g. shopka and churshife- maar (a sweetmeat containing butter, milk and sugar). Joshi and Lund (1994) also reported that in Nepal yak milk is used for preparing cheese and butter. These products are processed by traditional methods.

Milk-Tea: Milk-tea is a mixture of tea and milk and is a staple part of the diet. In the warm season, when there is a plenty of milk available, or when given to guests, the brew will contain 20% milk or even more; the colour of the drink is yellow. Herd's men and their families more usually drink a lighter coloured tea with only 5% milk added. The milk-tea is brewed from tea leaves added to water and boiled for a few minutes; milk is added as required and boiling continued for few more minutes. Sometimes a little salt is added. Also, mostly among Tibetan people, zanba may be added to the brew, making it both a food and a drink. Zanba is the staple food of Tibet. It consists of a roasted oat or barley flour, or a mixture of the two made into a paste with yak butter and, for eating usually rolled into balls. While whole milk is normally used in the tea, skim milk is also used so that an increased amount of butter can be produced.

Milk boiled up with mushrooms and added salt is regarded as a delicacy by the herd people. Raw milk is also sold to milk powder plants, built in recent years to produce milk powder and, to a very limited extent, also butter and other products. Only little milk is sold for direct consumption in towns and villages in the upland areas.

Butter: Butter is the main product from yak milk and represents one of the staple foods of the local people. The raw butter contains 12-15% water, 1% protein and the rest fat. (Butter after long storage contains about 3% water).

Method of preparation: The traditional method in China is to squeeze the butter in a bag made of hide, or to make it in a churn. Milk separators are coming into use in some areas and cream separated in this way before churning produces better butter with lower water content and longer storage life than the older methods.

When butter is made by churning, the milk is allowed to stand for a day to ferment and then heated to about 20°C. The warm milk is poured into a churn up to 80 cm high and 60 cm in diameter. A stick for stirring is held in the center of the churn by the lid. The herdsmen (or, usually, the women) rotate the stick until the fat solidifies and further churning becomes difficult after between 1 and 4 h, depending on the size of the churn and quantity of milk. The lump of the fat floating on the surface are then removed by hand and washed with water. Next, water is squeezed out and the butter is made into cylindrical or cube-shaped blocks by using a plank of wood. Lastly, the butter is stored in a bag of calf hide or yak rumen. Each bag weighs approximately 50 kg. The butter will keep for 1-2 years without going mouldy.

When butter is made in hide bag, the milk is first heated, as before, and poured into a bag of calf or goat hide. The herdsman inflates the bag by blowing into it and closes the opening. The bag is then shaken until the fat solidifies into globules, after which the content is emptied into another container. Thereafter the procedure is as already described.

If using a milk separator to make butter, the milk is first heated to 30-35 °C and then filtered. The separator is operated by turning a handle, the fat separates. The fat and skim milk are put in separate containers, and the rest of the butter making process is as before.

Sometimes a little sour milk is added as a starter to the raw milk to increase the amount of butter that can be made.

Uses of Butter: Butter is used for number of foods including zanba, pancakes and dishes fried in butter. It is also added to milk -tea and consumed salted or unsalted according to the area. In some areas, butter is used in tea when milk is not available, but butter-tea is also drunk from choice.

In another use of butter it is melted and mixed in equal quantities, with roasted flour. The mixture is kneaded and stored. When required, this dough is melted into salted or sugared water and eaten in that way, or further mixed with seeds such as peanut, sesame, walnut or soybean, or mixed with Chinese dates. These ingredients provide extra flavour and make the food favourite among Tibtan people especially for their guests.

Butter is used also for many purposes other than food, including its use for tanning and for polishing fur coats. It is used as a fuel in domestic lamps and by lamas in sacred lamps and on family altars. Women also use butter on their skin and as hair grease and as a lubricant to assist in hand-milking. Butter is a component of some Tibatan medicine. When mixed with different colouring materials, butter is also used to make moulded sculptures-some very large-for religious ceremonies and New Year celebrations.

Toffee: A product of consistency of toffee (korani, in sherpa) is made by boiling milk very slowly to evaporate the water.

Milk Residue: Products called 'milk residue' by herdsman in China come in more than one form. They are made mostly from skim milk after the preliminary separation of fat to make butter, but can also be made from whole milk. Milk residue can come in both hard and semi-soft form.

To make the milk residue, milk is heated to 50-60°C and sour milk is added for curdling. The mixture is then poured into a wicker basket or gauze bag and the whey strained off. The remaining curds are spread on a cloth to dry. Milk residue from skimmed milk is white and hard, and that made from whole milk yellow and brittle. The protein content is around 55% and the lactose content around 21%.

A softer form of milk residue sometimes has a little sugar added to develop fermentation and is akin to a fermented cottage –type cheese, but drier than the western variety. It is served as a snack on its own or mixed with butter zanba.

Milk Cake: This is usually made from whole milk from which between one-third and two-third of the water has been evaporated during natural drying, but it remains relatively soft. Starch is sometimes added to give cake consistency. It is usually eaten with butter and sugar and is one of the dishes offered to guests.

Sour Milk (yoghurt): Sour milk is a favourite among the herds people throughout the year but more available during the summer season when most milk is produced. A little sour milk is added to freshly boiled milk that has been poured into a pail when the temperature has dropped to 50°C. The mixture is allowed to cool to 40°C. The pail is then covered and wrapped in wool to maintain its warmth. After 5-6 h in summer, or longer in winter, milk has soured. Either whole or skim milk can be used to make this product, with the whole milk product having more colour and taste. The sour milk is drunk or eaten alone or sometimes mixed with zanba. The product is similar to natural yoghurt made from cow milk in the West. Fruit or other flavours are not added.

Manufacturing Products

Dried Milk: Factories for the production of dried milk exist in proximity to yak rearing areas in several of the provinces of China, as well as in Nepal and possibly elsewhere. The dried milk is widely available in the towns of the region.

Cheese: Local production of cheese from yak milk has been traditional in remote northern parts of Nepal and northwest India. This is a hard casein product called churpi, special to the Himalayan region, made by drying the soft cheese produced first. The yield of churpi is about 4.5%, containing 8-10% moisture, 8-9% fat and 80% protein on dry matter (DM) basis.

Churpi is usually made from skim or whole milk. The milk is heated to 50-60^0 C and mixed with curdled or sour milk. The mixture is filtered, dried and cut into small pieces. It contains about 55% protein and 21% lactose (Cai L. and Wiener, 1995). It is also used as vegetable cheese and mixed with other vegetables by the local people in the yak-herding areas of India, Nepal and Bhutan.

Wada and Kakaoka (1991) reported that the Nepal Dairy Development Corporation (NDDC) operates seasonal dairies in summer for processing of milk of Yak and cattle. Cheese is made from this milk. Three types of Nepali yak milk cheese (soft, hard and processed) bought at NDDC were assayed for general composition and distribution of nitrogenous compounds. These were compared with two types of Japanese commercial cheese (Gouda and Cream cheese). In general, composition of Nepali cheese made from yak milk resembled the Gouda cheese.

Since the 1950s production of a Swiss- style cheese has been developed in Nepal. There are now 11 cheese factories run by the Nepalese Dairy Development Corporation and a number of privately run cottage factories producing, in 1998/99, 150 tonnes of yak cheese.

Processing: The standard procedure of cheese manufacture is followed with slight modification. The procedure includes standardizing the fat content of milk, pasteurizing, adding culture and rennet, coagulation, cutting, cooking followed by moulding and pressing. The cheese blocks are brined and stored for ripening. After about 5 months of ripening a good flavour develops. The yield of cheese is about 10%. The composition of 3- month old Nepalese yak cheese is: total solids 68.2%, fat 49.4% on dry matter basis, and salt 1.37%. The pH is 5.75.

Dahi: A process has been standardized to prepare good quality dahi from pure yak milk and mixed milk (Sharma, 2003). The average composition of dahi was 13.8% total solids, 3.5% fat, 0.8% titratable acidity and 5.0 pH. To prepare dahi a lactococcal culture was inoculated in boiled and cooled milk at 25°C and incubated for 14-16 h. The keeping quality of dahi obtained using this culture was more than 3 weeks at refrigeration temperature.

Paneer: The process for manufacture of good quality paneer (unripened cheese) from yak milk and mixed milk has been standardized. It was observed that the quality of yak milk paneer was better than that of cow milk. This may be due to higher casein content in yak milk. The yak milk paneer consisted of about 17% fat, 25% protein, 2.5% lactose, 1.2% ash and 54% moisture.

Sweets - Yak milk and mixed milk were also utilized for making sweets, viz Gulabjamun and Burfi. The procedures for preparation of good quality, hygienic and relatively long life sweets have been standardized. On an average, the Gulabjamun consisted of about 71% total solids, 7% fat, 4% protein, 58% carbohydrate and 2.5% ash. Similarly Burfi consisted of about 71% TS, 13% fat, 4% protein, 52% carbohydrate and 1.7% ash. Organoleptic qualities, *viz*. colour, smell, taste and texture of yak milk sweets were distinctly different from that of cow milk sweets. Gulabjamun was more granular and coarse and the body was slightly harder after cooling. The texture of Burfi was *danedar and* coarse. It was a little hard and rough.

References

Blanc, B. 1981. Biochemical aspects of human milk in comparison with bovine milk. *World Review of Nutrition and Dietetics*, 36:1-89.

Epstein, H. 1974. Yak and chouri. *World Animal Review*, 9:8-12.

Jain, Y.C. Yadav, R. S. 1985. Yield and composition of milk of Himachali yak, yak hybrid and hill cow. *Indian J. Animal Sci.*, 55:223-224.

Jenness, R. 1974. The composition of milk. In lactation, 3:3-107, (Eds) Larson, B.L. and Smith,V. R., Academic Press, New York.

Nivasarkar, A.E., Gupta, S.C. and Gupta, N. 1997. Yak Production, an, ICAR Pub., National Bureau of Animal Genetic Resources, Karnal, 1st. Ed., p 274.

Tokita, F., Hosono, A., Takahashi, Fi, Ishida, T. and Otami, H. 1981. Animal Products in Nepal. III. The Sherpas and their livestock farming. *Japanese J. Dairy and Food Sci.*, 30:55-60.

Wada, H. and Kataoka, K. 1991. Study on composition of Nepalese cheese made from yak milk. *Japanese J. Dairy and Food Sci.*, 40: 1-4.

1.7. Camel Milk

In the extremely hot arid areas of Arabia and all the drought-stricken areas of the world, where continuous drought decimates the cattle, sheep and goat populations, only the camels survive and continue producing calves and milk. Camels can produce an adequate amount of milk to sustain their calves and even human being. Of prime importance for the young camel, and especially for man, who drinks the milk, is the composition. Cows exposed to heat, especially when drinking water is scarce, produce milk that has much higher dry matter content than normal (Bianca, 1965). The fat content is especially high. This milk would certainly not provide suitable diet for man or animal exposed to the same climatic and water stresses. Data concerning the composition of milk vary greatly. This can be partly attributed to the inherited capabilities of the animals, but the stage of lactation, age and the number of calvings also play a role. Of special significance to the quality of the produced milk are the feed and water quantity and quality.

Most camel milk is drunk fresh. It is also consumed when slightly sour or strongly soured. Camel milk is generally opaque white. Normally it has sweet and sharp taste, but sometimes it is salty. At times the milk tastes watery. In certain countries there are prejudices among the urban population concerning camel milk. It is considered as having unpleasant taste. The changes in taste are caused by the type of fodder and the availability of water.

The specific gravity of camel milk is less than that of cow, sheep and buffalo (Shalash, 1979). Fresh camel milk has a relatively high pH (6.5-6.7). This is similar to the pH of sheep milk. When camel milk is left to stand, the acidity rapidly increases, the increase being from 0.03% to 0.014% after 2h of storage.

Camel milk is very similar to goat milk and c ompares very favourably with human milk (Davis and McDonald, 1953). This again stresses the importance of camel milk for human nutrition. Camel herders living only on milk in Kenya (Fields, 1979) and in the Ahaggar region of the Sahara (Gast *et al.*, 1969) are healthy and vigorous. Camel milk is renowned in its health giving qualities, which includes good bone growth.

The most important factor in camel milk is water content. Young camels and especially the humans living in drought areas, are in need of fluid to maintain homeostasis and thermoneutrality. The water content of camel milk fluctuates from 84-90%. When examining only the effects of the lack of drinking water on camel milk, the diet remaining unchanged throughout the year, great changes in the water content of milk were found (Yagil and Etxion, 1980). The camels were allowed ad libidum drinking water only during the winter. From spring until the summer end the mothers and calves were allowed to drink only once a week for one hour. With water freely accessible, the water content of the milk was 86%, but when water was restricted the water content of milk rose to 91%. These changes reflect the range presented in the literature and thus makes it important as to when the milk was sampled by the various investigators. Water content of fodder would also affect water content of milk. Thus, it would appear that the lactating camel loses water to the milk in times of drought. This could be a natural adaptation in order to provide not only nutrients but also necessary fluid to the dehydrated calf. Whatever the explanation, the diluted milk at times of water deprivation makes an excellent food for man.

With the increase in water content of milk produced by thirsty camels, there was a decrease in the fat content from 4.3to 1.1% (Yagil and Etxion, 1980). In the literature, the percentage of milk fat of camels varies from 2.6 to 5.5. Again, the hydration status of the animals as well as the type of forage eaten would determine the fat content of milk.

The milk fat is also different from that of other animals. When left standing, fat is distributed as small globules throughout the milk. The fat globules are very small, 1.2-4.2 microns in diameter (Dong Wei, 1981). The ratio of fat to total solids averages 31.6% (Shalash, 1979). This is much lower than that of the buffalo, which is 40.9%. The fat appears to be bound to protein. This would explain why it is difficult to extract the fat by usual method of churning sour milk (Rao, *et al.*, 1970). Camel milk fat has a low Reichert value of 16.4 (Dhingra, 1934). The fatty acid composition of camel milk fat was found to be as follows (wt. percentage):

Butyric, 2.1; Caproic, 0.9; Caprylic, 0.6; Capric,1.4; Lauric, 4.6; Myristic, 7.3; Palmitic,29.3; Stearic,11.1; Oleic, 38.9; Linoleic, 3.8.

Compared to cow, buffalo and sheep milk fat, camel milk fat contains less short chain fatty acids, but the same long chain fatty acids can be found. Gast *et al.* (1969) claimed that the value of camel milk is to be found in the high concentration of essential fatty acids such as linoleic and other polyunsaturated fatty acids. The total saturated acids in whole fat were 62.6% mole percent.

The distribution of phospholipids in camel milk (expressed in mole percent) was reported (Morrison, 1968) to be as follows: Phosphatidyl ethanolamine, 35.9; phosphatidyl choline, 24.0; Phosphtidyl serine, 4.9; phosphatidyl inositol, 5.9; sphingomyelin, 28.3.

The milk protein content of camel milk ranges from 2.0-5.5% (Yasin and Wahid, 1957). The total protein in camel milk is similar to that of cow milk. Dilanyan (1959) reported the casein content of dromedary and Bactrian milk as 2.7 and 0.89%, respectively and that of albumin as 3.8 and 0.97%, respectively. Camel milk casein and their fractions were found to be poor in crude protein when compared with cow milk.

Milk from dehydrated camel has a severely decreased protein percentage (Yagil and Etzion, 1980). Again this demonstrates the direct effect of drinking water on the composition of milk. It must be stressed that protein content of feed will also directly affect that of milk.

Sestuwheva (1958) found that the lactose content of camel milk remained unchanged from the first month up to the end of lactation. The concentration in milk vary from 2.8-5.8% (Yasin and Wahid, 1957). These were approximately the same range as found between the hydrated and dehydrated animals. The changes in lactose concentration would account for the milk being described as sometimes sweet and sometimes bitter.

The mineral content of milk is expressed as total ash in Table 1.1. The total ash content of camel milk varies greatly, and the lowest percentage of ash was found in the milk produced by dehydrated animal (Yagil and Etzion, 1980). Camel milk is rich in chloride. Although milk from the dehydrated camel showed decrease of fat, protein and lactose content, that of sodium and chloride increased. This would account for the salty taste. Both concentration of calcium and magnesium phosphate declined in the milk of dehydrated camel. However, these concentrations are still adequate for human nutrition.

Camel milk is rich in vitamin C (Knoess, 1979). This is important from the nutritional standpoint in areas where fruits and vegetables containing vitamin C are scarce. Kheraskov (1961) found the vitamin C content of camel milk to vary between 5.7 and 9.8 mg percent. As lactation progresses, the vitamin C content decreases. The vitamin C levels are three times that of cow milk and one-and- a-half times that of human milk. Vitamin B12 in camel milk declined from 3.9 mg/ l at 1.5 months lactation to 2.3 mg / l at the fourth month lactation. Vitamin B1 and B2 concentrations are adequate. Carotene concentrations in the milk declined from 0.46 mg / kg at 1.5 months lactation to 0.16 mg / kg at four months lactation. The vitamin A content has been reported as being as little as 0.037 mg percent (Kheraskov, 1961).

From all the data presented, it is clear that the camel produces nutritious milk for human consumption. It is also evident that the taste and quality of milk is directly affected by the amount of water drunk, and the amount and quality of feed eaten. The fluctuations in fat, protein, fat and salt are determined by the amount of water drunk.

References

Bianca, W. 1965. Cattle in a hot environment. Reviews of the progress of dairy science, Section A, Physiology, *J. Dairy Res*, 32: 291-345.

Davis, J.O. and MackDonald, S.J. 1952. Richmond's Dairy Chemistry, Ed. 2, Charles Griffen & Co. Ltd., London, 101.

Dhingra, D.R. 1934. Fatty acids and glycerides of the milk fat of camels, *Biochem. J.* 28:73-78.

Dilanyan, S.H. 1959. Utilization of mare's, ewes', camels and yak's milk in the USSR, Report Int. Comm. Dairying in warm countries, Dairy Fed Brussels.

Field, C.R. 1979. Ecology and management of camels, sheep and goats in Northern Kenya, Unesco/IPAL. Report Nairobi.

Kheraskov, S.G. 1961. Composition, properties and nutritive value of camel milk, *Vop, Pitan*, 20: 69-72.

Knoess, K.H. 1979. Milk production of the dromedary, In: IFS Symposium, Camels, Sudan, 201-214.

Morrison, W. R. 1968. Fatty acid composition of milk phospholipids, III Camel, pig and ass milks. Lipids, 3(2): 107-110.

Rao, M.B., Gupta, R.C. and Dustur, N.N. 1970. Camels' milk and milk products. *Indian J. Dairy Sci.*, 23:71-78.

Shalash, M.R. 1979. Utilization of camel meat and milk in human nourishment. In: IFS Symposium, Camels, Sudan, 285-306.

Yagil, R. and Etzion, Z. 1980. The effect of drought conditions on the quality of camel milk. *J. Dairy Res*, 47:159-166.

1.8. Human Milk

Human milk is a unique, species-specific, complex nutritive fluid with immunologic and growth properties. The primary function of mammalian milk is to nourish the neonate in the most efficient manner possible from the dam's perspective, while providing the neonate with additional benefits from enhanced immune protection and a source of non-nutrient growth promoters, hormones, and other bioactive components that serve as biochemical messengers within the body. In addition, several components in human milk help to maintain mammary tissue integrity, optimizing milk output and composition. This unique fluid actually evolves to meet the changing needs of the baby growth and maturation.

Human milk, a biologically complex fluid containing many hundreds of different constituents, is ideally suited to meet the term infant's nutritional needs during the first 4- 6 months of life, provided that the mother is also healthy and well nourished. For this reason, infant formula manufacturers often refer to the gross composition of human milk as the 'gold standard'. However, it is important to remember that, unlike infant formula, the composition of human milk is not uniform. Significant changes in the composition of breast milk occur not only between individual women, but also within a single feed, between feeds, throughout the day, throughout the lactation period, with changing maternal diet and as a result of other external factors such as exercise or metabolic illness. Implicit in these findings is the understanding that a single description of human milk is somewhat erroneous. Nevertheless, it is important to establish data on the composition of human milk at various key stages of lactation.

Gross Nutrient Composition: There are three stages in human lactation that are clearly identified by changes in specific components in the milk., such as the whey proteins and lactose. These compositional changes appear uniquely to match the changing physiological needs of the infant, and can be defined based on the following time periods: 1-5 days postpartum, colostrum; 5-21 days postpartum, transitional milk; and >21 days postpartum, mature milk. Nutrient information relating to human milk at the predominant stages of lactation is given in Table 1.8.1.

Table 1.8.1. Gross nutrient content of human milk at different stages in lactation (g/100ml)

Nutrient	Colostrum (1-5 days)	Transitional Milk (5-21 days)	Mature Milk (21 days)
Protein	1.5-1.7	0.9	0.8-0.9
Non-protein nitrogen	0.5	-	0.45
Lactose	4.1-5.8	5.4	6.8
Glucose	0.2-1.0	-	0.2-0.3
Oligosaccharides	2.4	-	1.3
Lipid	2-3	3-4	3-5
Ash	0.25	-	0.20

Human milk differs markedly from cow milk. It is chalky-white in colour and somewhat watery in appearance. The reaction to litmus is alkaline. The human milk is more variable in composition than the cow milk, which is probably due to the relatively irregular life of the woman against the regular and ordered life of a cow. Moreover, cow milk is usually the mixed milk of at least a few cows, while human milk is normally milk of a single woman. The average composition of human and cow milk is given in Table 1.8.2.

Table 1.8.2: Average composition of human and cow milk

Constituents	Human Milk	Cow Milk
Water (%)	87.10	87.30
Fat (%)	3.75	3.70
Protein (%)	1.10	3.30
Casein	0.44	2.71
Whey Protein	0.66	0.59
Lactose	6.80	4.70
Ash (%)	0.21	072
Calcium (mg / l)	340	1250
Phosphorus (mg / l)	140	960
Iron (mg / l)	1.20	0.80
Copper (mg / l)	0.60	0.16
Vitamins / l		
Vit. A (IU)	1898	1025
Vit. B_1	160	440
Vit. B_2	360	1750
Niacin	1470	940
Vit. C (mg)	43	11

Human colostrums differ from mature milk in both the types and amounts of individual components. Colostrum has much higher protein content and lower lactose content than mature milk. The specific gravity of colostrum is 1.040 compared with 1.060 for mature milk. Although the fat and ash content of colostrum and mature milk do not differ significantly, variations in specific micronutrients are apparent, with the concentrations of sodium, chloride and magnesium being higher, and potassium and calcium lower, in colostrum.

1.8.1. Composition

Human milk contains hundreds of different constituents some of which are shown in Table 1.8.2. The water-soluble constituents found in the aqueous phase account for 87% of milk volume, and include some salts, vitamins and trace elements, lactose, oligosaccharides, whey proteins and nonprotein nitrogen (NPN) components. Complementing the aqueous phase is a colloidal dispersion (0.3% of volume) containing casein held in micellar form, which contributes to the white colour of milk. Calcium phosphate and some membrane fragments, called lipoproteins, are also linked to the casein micelles. A further 6% of milk volume is made up of an emulsion containing fat globules, fat globule membranes, triglycerides and other lipid components, including the fat-soluble vitamins. The remainder consists of cellular components, nonpeptide hormones and other minor fractions.

Three-dimensional Structure of Human Milk: Under a microscope, the appearance of human milk is truly amazing. While a fluid, human milk shows a substantial structure in the form of compartmentation. Within the various compartments hundreds of nutrients and bioactive substances are sequestered. The most elegant example of this structure are lipids. Lipids are enveloped at the time of secretion from the apical mammary epithelial with plasma membrane, becoming the milk-fat globule. Certain proteins, growth factors, and vitamins become sequestered within this milk-fat globule and are embedded within the membrane itself.

The membrane acts as a stabilizing interface between the aqueous milk components and compartmentalized fat. This interface allows controlled release of the products of lipolysis and polar materials into milk serum (aqueous phase). The bipolar characteristics of the membrane necessary for the emulsion stability of the globules themselves; thus, the structure of human milk provides readily available fatty acids and cholesterol for micellar absorption in the small intestine.

Proteins, carbohydrates and designer fats for optimal brain development: Human milk provides appropriate amounts of proteins (the major components of which are alpha-lactalbumin and other whey proteins), carbohydrates (lactose), minerals, vitamins and fats for the growing infant. The fats are comprised of cholesterol, triglycerides, short-chain fatty acids and long-chain polyunsaturated (LCP) fatty acids. The LCP fatty acids (18-22 carbon) are needed for retinal development. Large amounts of omega-6 and omega-3 LCP fatty acids, predominantly, 20-carbon arachidonic acid (AA) and the 22-carbon docosahexaenoic acids (DHAs) are required for developing brain and retina during prenatal and during early postnatal growth.

An infant, particularly a preterm infant, may have limited ability to synthesize optimum levels of DHA from linoleic and linolenic acids. These two fatty acids may be essential. Recently, some infant formulas in the U.S. have added AA or DHA. Increasing evidence suggests that breast fed infants have better visual acuity at 4 months and slightly enhanced cognitive development than bottle fed infants, even when socioeconomic factors are taken into account. These differences are more pronounced in premature infants.

Proteins: Human milk contains more whey proteins and less casein, therefore, human milk will not form a firm clot with rennet as cow milk does. This is fundamentally the reason why infants digest cow milk less easily than human milk.

Many of the functional properties of human milk are delivered via the milk proteins. Provision of essential amino acids for growth is the most obvious roles for milk proteins. Determining the gross amino acid composition of human milk will accurately describe amino acid content, and in the past this figure has been used to define the amount of protein available to the infant for growth and development. However, milk proteins also provide the infant with immune protection, increased digestive capacity, and enhanced micronutrient availability, and, as many bioactive component of human milk are of protein origin, implicit in their functionality is a resistance to digestion. Investigation of the nutritive value of human milk protein reveals that although most (~95%) milk protein is available, a proportion does not contribute significantly to amino acid nutrition. To determine accurately the amounts of amino acids, and therefore protein, used for nutrition by the breastfed infant, a correction needs to be made for bioavailability.

The total protein content of human milk consists of two major groups, caseins and whey proteins as well as some minor components and proteins present in the milk fat globule membrane. The ratio of whey to casein changes during the initial stages of lactation, from 90:10 immediately postpartum, to 60:40 in mature milk and 50:50 in late lactation. These ratios directly reflect a decrease in the content of immune proteins in line with the development of the infant's own immune system.

Casein: Human milk contains two (b and K) caseins, and is devoid of a- casein, the predominant casein found in bovine milk. The casein pattern differs depending on the stage of lactation, with κ-casein detectable in human milk only from day 3-4 postpartum onwards. A unique feature of human milk is the high degree of glycosylation of k-casein (40-60 % glycosylated) and other milk proteins (e.g. Immunoglobulins (Igs) and lactoferrin). Glycosylated proteins exhibit anti-infective properties and enhance the absorption of some micronutrients. As part of the normal digestive process, the caseins in human milk release smaller peptide into the gut lumen. These casein fragments are thought to enhance the absorption of calcium by keeping it in solution in the gut lumen. Other casein derived peptides have been linked to the regulation of intestinal motility and to the growth promotion of beneficial bacteria in the infant's gut.

Whey Proteins: α-lactalbumin, lactoferrin, serum albumin and secretory IgA (sIgA) are the main whey proteins found in human milk. β-lactoglobulin, prominent in bovine milk, does not occur in human milk. The predominant sources of amino acids for nutrition amongst the whey proteins are α-lactalbumin and serum albumin. The other whey proteins, while contributing to nutrition to some extent, have primary function in other roles. Lactoferrin, an iron binding protein, has bacteriostatic properties that may impact on infant and mammary gland. Lysozyme is capable of cleaving proteoglycans in the cell wall of certain bacteria, providing an antibacterial effect. The immunoglobulins in human milk are distinct from those found in blood serum, indicating selective synthesis in mammary gland. SIgA, formed by linking of two serum IgA molecules by disulphide bonds, is present in very high concentrations in colostrums, but the sIgA content declines rapidly to a much lower level within 14 days of lactation. SIgA protects the infant by blocking the attachment of pathogenic bacteria to the gut epithelium. Other immunoglobulins in human milk provide immune protection through activation of the complement system, or by promoting phagocytosis.

Other Protein - containing Compounds: In addition to casein and whey proteins, human milk contains other proteins, most of which are in aqueous phase. These minor proteins contribute in many ways to the health and well-being of the infant, for example, by facilitating transport of certain vitamins and minerals. Milk-borne peptide hormones and enzymes assist in the digestion of other milk components (e.g. bile-salt stimulated lipase and amylase).

According to an American research, breast milk contains a protein that could reduce the risk of obesity. It was reported that high levels of the protein, adiponectin, in breast milk helps in processing of sugar and fat in the blood. Low levels of this protein have been linked to obesity, type 2 diabetes, insulin resistance and coronary artery diseases. Another protein found in breast milk called 'leptin 'also helps to regulate body fat but the levels of adiponectin is more significant than leptin. The longer they are breast-fed the better it is.

Non-protein Nitrogen: Compared with the milk of other mammalian species, human milk is notably different with regard to the NPN fraction. In human milk, the NPN fraction represents a very high percentage (20-25%) of total nitrogen (N). Urea N accounts for almost 50% of the NPN in human milk, with more than 200 compounds, including free amino acids, carnitine, taurine, amino sugars, nucleic acids, nucleotides and polyamines, making up the remainder. In general, the total NPN of human milk remains constant throughout the lactation period, although there may be some variation in individual NPN components.

Given that the total protein content of human milk is low compared to other species, yet supports adequate growth of the breastfed infants, the suggestion has been made that the urea found in the NPN fraction of human milk is used by the infant for protein synthesis. This would have major implications for infant formula manufacturers, necessitating a total re-evaluation of infants' protein requirements.

Taurine and glutamine, two predominant free amino acids in human milk, are considered conditionally essential, as the infant appears to have a requirement for these amino acids above what the body can synthesize. Taurine plays an important role in fat digestion by conjugating with bile acids to form bile salts. Although no direct link has been established between a deficiency in taurine and abnormal development of retinal and brain tissue in infants, the addition of taurine to infant formulae is now routine. Glutamine is involved in cellular metabolism of enterocytes and in the immune response associated with inflammation and sepsis.

During periods of rapid growth or tissue repair, a dietary source of nucleotides may be beneficial, as *de novo* synthesis of nucleotides can be a limiting factor. The infant is in a state of rapid growth and cellular development, and human milk is rich in nucleotides. To date, however, no link between nucleotides in human milk and enhanced cellular function in the infant has been made. Despite this lack of direct evidence, some regulatory authorities have approved the inclusion of nucleotides in infant formula.

Carbohydrate: Lactose constitutes the largest component of human milk besides water. Lactose concentration decreases as lactation progresses, in line with the decline in milk volume.

Oligosaccharides constitute the next greatest fraction of carbohydrate in human milk, representing more than 27% of the carbohydrate in colostrum. This gradually decreases to 15-16% of carbohydrate as oligosaccharides in mature human milk. Most oligosaccharides found in human milk contain lactose at the reducing end, and may contain fucose or sialic acid at the nonreducing end. Human milk is unique compared to other mammalian milks due to its content of complex oligosaccharides. Milk oligosaccharides provide a low osmolar source of calories for the infant, and have been classed as 'soluble' fibre because they appear to remain largely undigested in infant's gut. Human milk oligosaccharides contain significant quantities of sialic acid, which is essential for brain development, and they are also thought to stimulate the growth of bifidus bacteria, and to inhibit the adhesion of pathogenic bacteria to the epithelial surfaces. Approximately, 130 oligosaccharides have been identified in human milk. Glucose and galactose are present in much smaller quantities in human milk, as are other carbohydrates such as monosaccharides, and peptide bound and protein bound carbohydrates.

Lipids: Human milk contains less fat than cow milk. The fat globules, on the whole, are smaller than those of cow milk. The lipids in human milk occur in globular form, emulsified in the globular phase, and provide the infant with a major proportion (45-55%) of the energy needed to support growth. They also contain bioactive components important to the infant's the retinal and neural tissue development.

The triglycerols (TAG) account for 98% of total fat, and 90% of this is fatty acids (FA). Phospholipids (0.8%), cholesterol (0.5%) and other minor lipid components make up the remainder of the fat, which includes fat-soluble vitamins and some protein fractions.

In the first few weeks of lactation, total lipid content increases from around 2 to 3.5-5%. As the fat content increases, so too does the average size of the milk fat globules, which in turn results in the reduction in the ratio of phospholipids and cholesterol to a TAG.

The TAG composition in human milk is determined by the types and quantities of the FA incorporated in the glycerol molecule. Human milk contains 8 major FAs in amount greater than 1% and is an excellent source of the essential FAs. Human milk contains higher level of linoleic acid than cow milk. Linoleic acid is an essential fatty acid and prevents heart disease, atherosclerosis. The structure of the triglycerides in human milk is such that the absorption and utilization of human milk lipid is more efficient. It has been reported that triglycerides are broken down to diglycerides and then to monoglycerides. Monoglycerides with the fatty acids in the 2- position are absorbed as such. In human milk, palmitic acid is mainly in the 2- position, in cow milk (or in most vegetable oils), it is more often in 1- or 3- position. The splitting of fatty acids from triglycerides is an enzymatic reaction under the influence of lipase present in intestinal secretion. However, in contrast with cow milk, human milk in itself is rich in lipase which even at the refrigeration temperature of 4°C or in deep freeze liberates free fatty acids from triglycerides preferentially from 1- and 3-position. As the fat of human milk contains a high proportion of palmitic acid in 2- position, it will be absorbed as 2- monoglycerides from the intestine, whereas from cow milk fat lipase liberates palmitic acid in the 1- or 3-position and sets it free. This free palmitic acid is precipitated by calcium in the intestinal lumen and is excreted as calcium palmitate soap. This leads to loss of fat and calcium.

It has been reported that free fatty acids (FFA) are the most important source of energy for the infants. The lipase in human milk makes FAA available in large proportion even before the digestive phase in the intestine, thus improving the supply of necessary energy for the infant. Lipid digestion and absorption are enhanced further by four enzyme systems. These are, in order of utilization: the gastric phase with lingual lipase and gastric lipase; and the intestinal phase with pancreatic lipase and bile salt- stimulated lipase BSSL). The gastric phase is important because the milk fat globule would otherwise resist the action of pancreatic lipase and BSSL. Unlike the other lipases, which are endogenous, BSSL is secreted in human milk specifically to assist the infants with milk fat digestion.

Of all the components in human milk, the lipid fraction is the most variable. Changes in fat content occur not only during the first few weeks of lactation, but also in milk secretions throughout the day, and even within a single feed, with the hind milk being significantly higher in fat content than the foremilk. Variations also exist in the fat content of milk from individual women, although by far the greatest variation occurs and in the types and amounts of FAs. The fatty acid composition of human and cow milk is shown in Table 1.8.3.

Table 1.8.3: Fatty acid composition of human and cow milk

Fatty acids (Mole %)	Human Milk	Cow Milk
Butyric (C_4)	0.26	2.7
Caproic (C_6)	0.10	2.0
Caprylic (C_8)	0.10	2.0
Capric (C_{10})	0.80	3.2
Lauric (C_{12})	4.70	3.6
Myristic ($C_{14:0}$)($C_{14:1}$)	7.90	11.8
Palmitic (C_{16})	26.70	36.8
Stearic (C_{18})	8.30	8.1
Oleic ($C_{18:1}$)	37.40	17.7
Linoleic ($C_{18:2}$)	10.6	2.10
Linlenic ($C_{18:3}$)	Trace	-

It is apparent from the above table that human milk fat contains very low level of volatile fatty acids resulting in R.M. value 1.4–3.4, Polenske value 1.9–2.2 and Kirschner value 1.9–2.0. Human milk is richer in copper and iron than others, but very poor in calcium and phosphorus.

Micronutrients

Vitamins: Most vitamins found in human milk increase in concentration when it proceeds from colostrum to a mature secretion (Table 1.5), with the exception of carotenoids (α-carotene, β-carotene, lutin, cryptoxanthin and lycopene), retinal and vitamin E content, which decrease. Reduction in the concentration of some vitamins may not alter the total amount available to the infant, however, as any reduction is offset by an increase in the quantity of breast milk consumed.

The milk from healthy, well nourished woman usually contains sufficient quantities of most of the vitamins required by the infants. Deficiencies in vitamin D, with consequent development of rickets; have been reported in breast fed infants, directly linked to the mother's diet, and the infants lack of exposure to sunlight. To meet physiological requirements, vitamin K is routinely given to newly born babies because transplacental transfer is limited, and the level in milk is low.

Minerals: In general the macromineral content of human milk remains stable during the lactation period after an initial decrease in the concentration of chloride, potassium, sodium and sulphur (Table 1.8.2). Most of the sulphur in human milk is found in sulphur-containing amino acids, methionine and cysteine, with only a small fraction (10%) existing in salt form. The sulphur amino acids predominate in the whey proteins, so a reduction in whey protein content during the first few days of lactation is matched by a similar reduction in sulphur content.

Human milk has a higher calcium to phosphorus ratio (2:1) than that in milk from other mammalian species (e.g. bovine milk calcium phosphorus ratio is 1.1:1), although the absolute amount of calcium and phosphorus are lower. A low phosphorus content suits the infant's limited renal capacity. In addition, the contribution of phosphate to the buffering capacity of human milk is such that a low pH results, promoting the growth of beneficial gut bacteria.

Human milk contains what would initially appear to be an inadequate level of iron, yet breastfed infants rarely deplete their iron stores until after 4-6 months of age. Maximum utilization of iron in human milk is achieved with the assistance of lactoferrin, most likely via specific protein receptors in the gut that link with lactoferrin and therefore facilitate iron absorption.

1.8.2. Anti-infective properties

Breast milk is commonly known as the best form of nutrition for neonates and infants. Human milk has bioactive properties that facilitate the transition of life from in utero to ex utero. This dynamic fluid provides a dynamic array of bioactive substances to the developing infant during critical period of brain, immune, and gut development.

Paediatricians hold a common opinion that breastfed infants experience less infectious disease than those artificially fed. The greater resistance of breastfed infant is especially evident in gastrointestinal disorders, but it extends to a wide variety of other acute and chronic infections. In a survey it was observed that wholly bottle fed infants had greater morbidity rates for gastrointestinal disorders, respiratory infections, and otitis media. Infections tended to be of longer duration and mortality and case fatality were notably greater. Breastfed babies, compared with bottle fed, have less diarrhea, urinary tract infections, pneumonia, vomiting, asthma, earaches, allergies, cot death, various viral and bacterial infections, cancers, learning disabilities and psychological problems. Milk's living cocktail of antibodies and cells provide protection in a number of ways (Newman, 1995, Russell, 1995).

Helpful molecules: Helpful molecules in milk include antibodies, e.g. immunoglobulin A, which is abundant in human breast milk, perfectly compensates for the baby not producing this until several weeks after birth. These antibodies contain a secretary region to shield them from degradation by digestive enzymes. When the mother is exposed to pathogens in the immediate environment, within hours the next milk contains antibody highly targeted against those pathogens. Thus the baby receives protection against the infections it is most likely to confront. Interestingly, these antibodies ignore' good' bacteria in the gut which crowd out pathogenic ones. Milk *oligosaccharides* mimic the binding sites whereby bacteria gain entry into the cells lining the baby's gut (mucosal lining). Milk also contains *lactoferrin,* which binds to iron, thus inhibiting bacterial metabolism by rendering iron, which they much need, unavailable to them. Other milk molecules include *Bifidus* factor to promote growth of good bacteria, specifically *Lactobacillus bifidus*; free fatty acids which damage the membranes surrounding enveloped viruses; and *fibronectin* to boost cellular defenses and aid repair of inflammation-damaged tissues.

Another distinctive biochemical difference between human milk and cow milk concerns the important group of neucleotides. Although both human and cow colostrums are rich in a great variety of neucleotides, normal cow milk contains only a small total amount represented chiefly by orotic acid. Neucleotides are required indirectly for protein synthesis, with the intermediary of the large molecule ribonucleic acid (RNA). It can be assumed that the synthesis of the protein in the newborn infant will be improved by the dietary supply of neucleotide.

The ratio of calcium to phosphorus is 2.2 times higher in human milk than in cow milk. Infants that are fed cow milk during their first two weeks of life may develop a tetany due to a low calcium content of their blood serum. This is caused by the inability of the infant's kidneys to excrete the excess of phosphorus absorbed from the cow milk, so the phosphorus accumulates in the serum, combines with calcium and thus lowers the calcium content of serum.

Cellular Defenses: White blood cells in milk have various functions. They engulf bacteria, produce enzyme lysozyme, which disrupts bacterial cell walls, manufacture antibodies, mobilize other parts of the immune system, and produce chemicals (such as gamma interferon, monocyte inhibition factor) to stimulate the infant's own immune response. The infant response matures more quickly (than in bottle fed babies) under the influence of other breast milk factors such as cortisol, epidermal and nerve growth factor, insulin-like growth factor and somatomedin C. These close up the newborn's leaky mucosal lining, rendering it impermeable to pathogens. Other compounds stimulate the baby's own production of IgA, lactoferrin and lysozyme. These are found in the urine in larger amounts compared with bottle feeders, indicating that breast feeding induces local immunity in the urinary tract.

Further Benefits: The macronutrients in milk (carbohydrates, lipids and proteins) are perfectly balanced, and radically change in concentration according to the infant's stage of development. This even includes compensating for the special nutritional state of premature birth. Milk also contains vitamins and minerals, and also hundreds of other micronutrients, most of whose functions yet remain to be discovered. Some micronutrients enhance the bioavailability of other micronutrients. Earlier research concluded wrongly that human breast milk was lacking in vitamin D, and so supplements were recommended. Then a form of vitamin D unique to breast milk was discovered which totally meets the infant's needs.

Even today's formula milk falls far short of such optimum design. Also formula milk contains cow milk proteins, which are preferably avoided in the first 6 months, after which ordinary cow milk is an acceptable supplement, rendering expensive formula milk unnecessary. But formula milk is a big business, mothers face advertising, cultural and work pressures. However, to provide immunity, 4 breastfeeds every 24 hours need not impede a reasonable working day. Now it is well recognized that God has designed the baby to feed at the breast. This brings the motivation, peace and assurance that substitutes are inferior to God's best. The recent findings on breast milk's provision of immunity should reinforce our motivation.

Intestinal Flora: A further distinctive feature regarding infants fed human milk as compared with those fed on cow milk concerns the intestinal flora. Unlike the mixed intestinal flora of infants fed on cow milk formulae, the intestinal flora of healthy breast fed infants is characterized by the prevalence of a particular species of Lactobacillus, namely *L. bifidus*. This is because this organism needs a growth factor called bifidus factor which is found in large quantities in human milk (40:1, human milk: cow milk)

Human milk is known to contain a non-specific antimicrobial factor, lysozyme, in concentrations as great as 0.2 mg/ml. This enzyme is bacteriolytic against Enterobacteriaceae and gram positive bacteria. The lysozyme from breast milk is thermostable (100 °C) at acid pH and twice as active as the lysozyme of egg white. Lysozyme is found in large concentrations in faeces of breastfed infants but not in those fed cow milk formula. It is then possible that lysozyme contributes to the development and maintenance of the special intestinal flora of breastfed infants.

References

Beaudry M, Dufour R., Marcoux S. 1995. Relation between infant feeding and infections during months of life, *J. Pediatr*, 126 (2): 191-7(Medline).

Committee on Drugs. 1994. The transfer of drugs and other chemicals into human milk. *Pediatrics* 93:137-150.

Crawford, M.A. 1993. The role of essential fatty acids in neural development: implications pediatr nutrition, *AM. J. Clin Nutr*, 57L5 suppl): 703S-709S (Medline).

Darragh, A. 2003. Human Milk, *Encyclopedia of Dairy Science*, Academic Press, pp 1350-59.

Goldman, A.S. 1993. The immune system of human milk: antimicrobial, anti-inflammatory and immunomodulating properties. *Pediatr Infect Dis J*, 12(8):664-71 (Medline).

Jensen, R. 1999. Lipids in human milk. *Lipids*, 34: 1243-71.

Lawrence, R.M. and Lawrence, R.A. 1999. Biochemistry of human milk. In: Breastfeeding, A Guide for the Medical Profession, 5th m Ed., pp 95-155.

Newman, J.1995. How breast milk protects newborns, *Scientific American*, 273 (6): 58-61.

Russell, R.D. 1995. Design in infant nutrition, Impact NO. 259, ICR.

Wagner, C.L., Andrson, D.M ,Pittard, W.B. 3rd, 1996. Special properties of human milk, *Clin Pediatr*, 35(6): 283-93 (Medline).

2

Nutritive Value of Milk

"Tell me what you eat and I will tell you what you are. The destiny of people depends on the nature of its diet."

A. Brillat-Savarin

Milk is the only product which is considered nature's almost perfect food. It is treasure house of unlimited nutrients. It is considered best and ideal food by virtue of possessing almost all the nutritional factors, *viz.*, fats, proteins, carbohydrates, minerals and vitamins. They are not only of higher quality but are present in milk in such form and proportion that their digestion and assimilation in the body is very efficient. Milk also plays a supplementary role in our nutrition. If it is included in our diet it enhances digestion and assimilation of nutrients of other food products. This is the reason that it is kept in high esteem as a food and is called the nectar for living beings.

Milk is the first taste of food for whole mankind. It establishes the mother-infant bond and is a life promoter. Of the many fluids that biology offers milk is perhaps the most versatile in terms of its use– as food, as a growth stimulant and as a defense package to the user. To the infant mammal – be it a mouse, calf or a human child, mother's milk is more than a source of energy and nutrients. It contains a wide variety of substances that defend the growing infant against infections.

Milk, a perfect blend of nutrition and palatability, plays an important role in preserving mental and physical health. Milk has long been recognized as the most wholesome and complete single food available in nature for health and as a medicine, both preventive as well as curative. Ancient chronicles as recorded in the *Upnishads, Puranas* and *Vedas* extol the beneficial and therapeutic properties of milk and milk products. It has been stated that cow milk, dahi and ghee impart knowledge and radiance, cure heart trouble and anaemia besides other bodily diseases.

Milk occupies a special position among foods in being an animal food that has a vegetarian connotation. Breast milk is the sole source of subsistence for newly born infants. For children, adolescent, elderly people, pregnant and nursing mothers, milk plays an important role in meeting the requirements of many essential nutrients (Table 2.1), and hence milk is considered as a protective food. Milk helps to balance human diet by supplementing good quality protein, calcium and vitamins particularly, vitamin A and riboflavin. Milk is not only an excellent source of good quality protein but also of calcium and vitamin B_2 besides other nutrients. However, it is deficient in iron and vitamin C. Despite this limitation, milk is considered an ideal food for infants and children and a good supplementary food for adults. In addition, milk contains several bio-protective molecules that ensure health security to humans.

"Every person, young and old, should drink milk. Milk contains a large variety of nutritional constituents and considering its cost per pound, more food for the money than any other food material available"

— Charles H. Mayo, M.D.

It often has been said that milk is the only natural substance created solely for use as food. Milk's value as a whole is greater than just the sum of its known components. Not only do the components of milk complement each other in their digestion and assimilation, but also they supplement other foods, especially the cereals. Clinical reports have established that there exists a close relationship between the type of food intake, microbial ecological system of the gut and human health. Thus lot of interest has been generated in recent past in manufacture of probiotic and other health foods. Milk and milk products serve as an ideal vehicle to deliver functional ingredients such as probiotics, prebiotics, fibres, phytosterols, stanols, micronutrients, *etc.*

Milk and dairy products are major dietary items in Europe and North America; they contribute 20-30% of dietary protein, ~15% of dietary lipids and ~ 80% of calcium. An adequate intake of calcium, especially in childhood, is critical for bone development and the prevention of osteoporosis in later life, especially in older women; hence milk and calcium-rich dairy products, e.g. rennet coagulated cheeses, are very important. While human milk is probably the best for human infants, they survive and grow very well on bovine milk. Although bovine milk was probably fed to human infants in medieval and even ancient times, the first formulated infant food was produced by Justus von Liebig in 1856. The development of sweetened condensed milk and sterilized evaporated milk in the mid nineteenth century was a major factor in reducing infant mortality during the early ears of twentieth century. The production of modified (humanized) formula is now a wide spread, important and profitable sector of the dairy industry. Today's consumer is increasingly interested in the quality and health benefits of what he or she eats. Milk and milk products generally enjoy a positive image both in terms of quality and health benefits.

2.1. Nutritional Quality of Milk Proteins

Proteins form the important component of muscle and other tissues. Almost all enzymes and some hormones are also proteins. Milk proteins are said to be of 'high biological value' as they contain all essential amino acids in amounts and proportions required to support growth and perform numerous functions within the body. Proteins contribute to building and repair of body tissues, participating in muscular contraction, acting as antibodies, as body's immunological defense mechanism and supplying energy. Caseins make up approximately 80% of milk proteins, the remaining being whey proteins. The properties of caseins, leading to the formation of micelles by entrapping calcium and phosphate ions, are of physiological significance. Casein micelles are good carriers of these two important elements as well as a good source of amino acids by themselves.

Whey is a pure, natural high quality protein complex derived from milk. It is not a single protein but consists of individual protein components including lactoferrin, β-lactalbumin, glycomacropeptide and immunoglobulin offering a number of health benefits. The major whey proteins of bovine milk are β-lactoglobulin and α-lactalbumin, the former representing half the total whey proteins. It functions as binder and transporter of retinol and significantly enhances retinol uptake. It also is a carrier of antibodies, hence possessing immunological properties. Alpha-lactalbumin is important from the nutritional point of view, as it is readily digestible. Whey proteins especially are of higher nutritional quality, containing 51% essential amino acids, as compared to 45% in casein. The sulphur amino acids are higher in whey proteins than in casein. The protein efficiency ratio (3.1), Biological Value (91) and Net Protein Utilization (82) of milk proteins are very close to that of egg proteins (3.8, 100 and 94, respectively). Lactalbumin is superior to casein having Biological Value (BV), Net Protein Utilization (NPU) and Protein Efficiency Ratio (PER) 100, 92 and 3.6, respectively. The corresponding values for casein are 77, 76 and 2.5, respectively. Lysine, one of the essential amino acids, which is found in the cereals in limited quantity, is abundant in milk proteins. Tryptophan, another essential amino acid, content in milk is also high. This amino acid is converted to niacin, an important vitamin in the body at the ratio of 60:1. Therefore, despite milk being a poor source of niacin, it is very effective in prevention of pellagra, the deficiency disease of niacin. Only 14.5 g of lactalbumin or 28.5 g milk proteins are enough to meet the daily requirement of essential amino acids for adult humans, opposed to 50-60 g proteins required from mixed vegetarian diet (Kansal, 1992a). Whey protein contains the highest concentration of branched chain amino acids (BCAA) of any single protein source. The BCAA content is important to athletes because BCAAs are integral part of muscle metabolism and are the first amines sacrificed during intense exercise and muscle catabolism.

The amino acid composition of whey protein is very similar to human skeletal muscle protein, providing almost all the amino acids in equal proportion. Virtually every amino acid present in whey exceeds FAO/WHO nutritional intake recommendations, both for children aged 2 to 5 and for adults. Whey protein has been known for some time to have a biological value superior to that of other naturally occurring protein (e.g. egg, soya, beef, and casein). Whey protein is an ideal protein having the highest Protein Digested Corrected Amino Acid Score (PDCAAS score) of 1.14, having no limiting essential amino acid to detract from quality-whey actually having excess of them.

Table 2.1: Nutrient content in milk (per 100g)*

Nutrients	Cow	Buffalo	Human
Protein (g)	3.4	3.8	1.0
Fat (g)	3.7	7.0	3.8
Lactose (g)	4.6	5.1	7.0
Calcium (mg)	120	210	31
Vit.C (mg)	1.8	2.2	4.7
Vit.A (IU)	126	178	274
Vit. E (μg)	110	180	540
Thiamine (μg)	42	90	15
Riboflavin (μg)	172	157	37
Pyridoxine (μg)	48	50	10
Folic acid (μg)	5.0	6.0	4.3
Vit. B_{12} (μg)	0.45	0.42	0.003

*(Kansal, 2004)

Supplementary Value and Digestibility: The BV of vegetable proteins can be raised by including milk proteins which contain a surplus of certain essential amino acids (lysine and threonine). Milk proteins can be added to cereal based products to increase their lysine and threonine contents. A breakfast consisting of milk, egg and bread has an excellent NPU value, and provides balanced amount of minerals and vitamins. Whey proteins have even better supplementary value. The digestibility of milk proteins is rated higher (96%) than that of plant proteins (74-78%). Because of their high BV, the milk proteins are useful in the diet of patients suffering from liver and gall bladder diseases, hyperlipidaemia and diabetes.

More than other protein supplements, whey protein powder is commonly used by body builders and other athletes to accelerate muscle development and aid in recovery. Whey protein has the highest value in providing branched-chain amino acids, which result in building and retaining muscle tissue. Some individuals with suppressed or otherwise abnormal immune systems or degenerative diseases use undenatured bioactive whey proteins to increase their antioxidant levels. These native whey proteins are good source of cysteine, a conditionally essential amino acid, which is the rate -limiting factor for the body's production of glutathione, an important antioxidant. In a study, it was found that whey supplements may prevent blood sugar spikes after high carbohydrate meals, which is useful for diabetics.

2.2. Nutritional Benefits of Milk Fat

Fats are significant in diet in a wide variety of ways. They contribute to the palability of foods by influencing taste, texture and mouthfeel. They provide a concentrated source of energy (9 Kcal/g). Lipids, when deposited as body fat, help protect vital body organs and provide a store of energy for long-term exertion. Food lipids are a source of fat-soluble vitamins (A,D,E,K) and essential fatty acids (linoleic and α-linolenic).

Compared to other fats and oils, milk fat is easily digestible. The digestibility of milk fat is 99%, while that of natural palm oil 91%. The excellent digestibility of milk fat is due to dispersion of fat globules in the aqueous phase of milk forming an emulsion. These are absorbed directly unlike other dietary fats that have to be emulsified by bile, pancreatic enzymes and intestinal lipases before they can pass through intestinal wall. Also, milk fat is rich in short and medium-chain fatty acids. The ester bonds involving short-chain fatty acids are more easily cleaved by lipases. The easy digestibility of milk fat makes it a valuable dietary constituent in diseases of stomach, intestine, liver, gall bladder, kidney and disorders of fat digestion (Kansal, 1994).

In infant and child nutrition, milk fat is of immense benefits. It helps them in meeting their energy requirements by increasing energy density of the diet. A sufficient fat supply is essential for thriving babies, a rosy and smooth skin and also resistance to bacterial infections. Mother's milk contains lipase, which plays an important role in digestion of fat in infants, particularly so since the glands responsible for digestion of fat are not fully developed in infant (Kansal, 1995).

Of the fatty acids 62% is saturated (mainly butyric, caproic, myristic, palmitic, stearic acid) and 37% unsaturated (mainly oleic acid). In the unsaturated fatty acids, 3.8% is PUFA (2.1% linoleic acid, 0.5% linolenic acid). Conjugated linolenic acid is present only in the milk of grass fed cows. Milk fat has a low content of essential fatty acids (EFA), linoleic and linolenic. The EFA requirement is only 3% of total calories, two-third of which is met from invisible fat present in dietary cereals, pulses and vegetables. Therefore, there is no justification to replace milk fat with another fat having higher linoleic content. Mother's milk contains relatively higher EFA content than cow or buffalo milk. The babies fed purely on cow or buffalo milk do not receive sufficient amount of EFA, even then the risk of a deficiency of linoleic acid is not likely, provided this diet is not given for too long without supplementation with vegetable foods (Kansal, 1995).

2.3. Minerals

Minerals usually exert their biological effects through enzyme systems. The roles they play in the body are many and diverse, with each mineral having specific functions. In general, mineral function as components of skeletal tissues, as constituents of organic compounds of soft tissues, as activators and components of enzymes, as acid –base regulators, as osmotic pressure regulators, as promoters of neurotransmission and cell transformation and division and as controllers of muscle excitability. All the minerals now known to be needed for nutrition of human beings and which must be supplied by diet are present in milk in varying quantities.

Milk, Richest Natural Source of Calcium: Recent research has shown that poor nutritional status with respect to calcium is related to diseases like osteoporosis, hypertension, and colon cancer. The hypertensive patients have shown significant reduction in blood pressure in response to increased calcium intake. The effect of calcium on blood pressure is mediated by 1) increase in urinary excretion of sodium, 2) preventing the rise in vitamin D hormone, which increases blood vessel resistance, 3) relaxing smooth muscle cells which lines the blood vessels, 4) suppressing the rennin-angiotensin system and 5) increasing production of endothelial relaxing factors (IDFA, 1995).

Milk is an excellent source of calcium and good source of phosphorus, two major bone-building minerals, but is relatively poor in iron and magnesium. The calcium in milk is well utilized in human body. Lactose, present in milk helps in absorption of calcium. The amino acids, lysine and arginine increase the intestinal absorption of calcium, both are present in milk in generous amounts. Citric acid and vitamin A also encourage calcium uptake and are present in milk. Fortification of milk with vitamin D is helpful in increasing calcium utilization. It is an established fact that calcium is solubilized in acidic environments and also that calcium as present in milk is highly absorbable in the intestine, although the pH of the intestinal contents is near neutral or slightly alkaline. It has been suggested that moderate and exchangeable binding of calcium to caseinphosphopeptides (breakdown peptide of casein) present in the intestine is responsible for the high absorbability of calcium in milk. Moreover, milk does not contain phytate and its oxalic acid content is negligible (2 mg/100 g). These substances are naturally found in cereals and vegetables and inhibit calcium absorption. It is difficult to meet the requirement for the vulnerable groups at risk of calcium deficiency without consuming milk and milk products.

In western countries milk and dairy products provide up to 75% of total calcium intake. A 250 ml serving of cow milk contains calcium equivalent to 60% of ICMR's recommended Dietary Allowance (RDA) for adults. Equal amount of buffalo milk contains 95% of calcium RDA for adults. Calcium in all forms of milk is equally well utilized. Incorporation of milk in diet also improves the bioavailability of calcium from vegetable foods (Kansal, 1998). In essence, to obtain an optimum dose of calcium, a wide range of factors have to participate, including a balanced diet, which is not easy to achieve, without milk and milk products.

Milk is rich in phosphorus that reduces urinary calcium excretion, and counter balances, at least in part, the calciuric effect of dietary proteins. Milk and most dairy products, except some processed cheese, have a near 1:1 calcium to phosphorus ratio considered to be ideal for retention of calcium in the body (Kansal, 1998).

The calcium content of human milk is considerably lower than that of cow milk, but calcium from human milk is better utilized by infants. This could be due to nature of fatty acids, the higher calcium to phosphorus ratio and the higher concentration of lactose in human milk.

Iron plays a vital role in human nutrition as a component of several metalloproteins such as haemoglobin, myoglobin and cytochrome. It serves as a carrier of oxygen and as an activator of vital cell functions. Although the quantity of iron is less, it is present in a readily soluble form and, therefore, is completely absorbed from the intestine than is iron from other iron-rich foods.

2.4. Milk, A Rich Source of Vitamins

Vitamins are potent organic substances which occur in minute quantities in natural foods. They act as biochemical regulators and coenzymes involving control and coordination of specific chemical reactions in the body. Milk is a rich source of vitamins not only in terms of their contents but also their better bioavailability. The water soluble B vitamin content of milk is fairly constant. Milk is a good source of thiamin which is required for normal appetite and digestion. It also keeps the nervous system healthy and in the release of energy from food. Milk is one of the richest natural sources of riboflavin (Vit. B_2). It aids in oxygen uptake and helps in adapting the eye to light. Optimum amount of riboflavin is also necessary to keep the skin, tongue and lips normal. Although, milk contains only small amounts of preformed niacin (Vit B_3), nevertheless, it is a very good source of this vitamin. Niacin can be synthesized in the body from tryptophan, which is present in milk proteins in good amount (480 mg / l). Indeed, milk is used as a dietary ingredient for patients suffering from pellagra, a niacin deficiency disease. Niacin aids in keeping the nervous and digestive system healthy. For vegetarian, milk is a sole natural source of vitamin B_{12}, as the vitamin is present in only animal foods. Milk is also a good source of folic acid, a haematopoitic vitamin present in free or bound form. This vitamin is also sensitive to light but is stable even in alkali under anaerobic condition. Breakdown of the acid is catalyzed by riboflavin and FMN (Flavin mononucleotide). Susceptibility of folic acid to oxidation varies with the form of the acid and the form dominant in milk (monoglutamate 5- methyltetrahydrofolic acid) believed to be easily oxidized. Therefore, milk is an unsuitable milieu for folic acid as the dominant form is very sensitive to oxidation in presence of both oxygen and riboflavin.

Milk is a good source of fat-soluble vitamins. Milk is an outstanding source of vitamin A and its precursor β-carotenoids. Bovine milk, particularly colostrum, has high level of vitamin A activity as retinol which is heat stable. Vitamin A or carotene initiates vision from light energy and it is essential for the growth and maintenance epithelial tissue of the eye. Hence, it has an indirect influence in preventing ocular diseases. It aids in keeping the skin clear and smooth and is involved in corticosterone synthesis. Vitamin A deficiency is a major cause of widespread blindness among children in India. A 250 ml serving of cow milk contains vitamin A sufficient to meet 75% daily vitamin A requirement of preschool child (Kansal, 1999). Vitamin E functions as an antioxidant preventing the oxidation of carotenoids, vitamin A and PUFA and as an aid in preventing nutritional muscular dystrophy. Although low in concentration but the daily intake of 280 ml of milk supplies adequate quantities of this fat soluble vitamin. Milk also contains vitamin K that is required for the synthesis of pro-thrombin and hence is useful in normal blood clotting.

2.5. Therapeutic Properties and Extra-nutritional Role of Milk Constituents

Proteins: Milk proteins have high buffering power, therefore, it is useful in the treatment of inflammation of mucous lining of stomach and of stomach ulcers, preventing hyperacidity. Milk and milk products are used as a source of proteins in hyperuricaemia and goat disease. In contrast to other foods, these do not contain purines which are precursors in the synthesis of uric acid that causes gout when deposited in the joints or may lead to formation of urinary calculi (Kansal, 1992a).

Milk and milk products such as milk concentrates, powders and cheeses are known to be anticariogenic. This anticariogenic effect has been attributed to the multiphosphoseryl–containing sequences of casein and their ability to stabilize calcium phosphate. These sequences can be released as casein phosphopeptides (CPP) from an enzymatic digest of casein. The CPP have remarkable ability to stabilize calcium phosphate in solution as amorphous calcium phosphate (ACP). Through their multiple phosphoseryl residues, the CPP bind to ACP nanoclusters in metastable solution preventing their growth to the critical size required for nucleation and phase transformation to an insoluble crystalline calcium phosphate. The casein phosphoseryl residues are essential for ACP interaction. The casein phosphopeptide-amorphous calcium phosphate complexes (CPP-ACP) have been shown to localize at the tooth surface and prevent demineralization and promote remineralization of enamel subsurface lesions. The proposed anticariogenic mechanism for dairy products therefore is the localization of ACP at the tooth surface which buffers the free calcium and phosphate ion activities, thereby helping to maintain a state of supersaturation with respect to tooth enamel, preventing demineralization and promoting remineralization.

Milk also contains minor protein fractions that have gained interest because of their physiological functions. Prominent among these proteins are lactoferrin, lactoperoxidase and lysozyme which exert bacteriostatic and bactericidal effect. Lactoferrin is an iron-binding glycoprotein capable of retarding the growth of many bacterial species *in vitro*. This is an effect attributed to its ability to chelate iron, which is essential for bacterial growth. However, besides its bacteriostatic properties, lactoferrin has bacteriocidal activity towards a number of other organisms. It damages the outer membrane of enteric Gram-negative bacilli, causing the release of lipo-polysaccharide from the bacterial cell wall, thereby sensitizing the cell for antibacterial action.

Lactoperoxidase is the most prominent enzyme in bovine milk, where it in concentrations of around 30 mg / l. A wide range of bacterial species is affected by the LP system. Gram-negative organisms may be inhibited or killed. Gram-positive bacteria are more resistant and are generally only inhibited in their growth.

Antimicrobial components of milk such as immunoglobulins which are present in high concentration in colostrum and lower concentration in milk are high molecular weight glycoproteins that provide passive immunity against enteric and respiratory bacteria and viruses. Their bio-protective actions include complement fixation and phagocytosis of the microorganisms by ingestion as well as agglutination and cytolytic action against antigens. They also protect against invading pathogens by binding to their antigenic sites to block their attachment to epithelial tissues. Colostrum has a very high concentration of immunoglobulins, facilitating quick transfer of immunity to the young born calf. These high levels decrease rapidly up to the second day post partum and thereafter decrease gradually. In concert with other bio-protective factors, immunoglobulins offer protection primarily by binding and neutralizing toxins of viruses and preventing contact between entero-pathogenic microorganisms and epithelial cells, thus hindering infections.

Lysozyme is a low molecular weight enzyme present in milk as well as in colostrum. In view of the antibacterial effect and possibly the impact on the general immune system of the neonate, there has been considerable interest in developing food applications of lysozyme. Although lysozyme from egg white had found more industrial applications in the past, it has now been recognized that the enzyme isolated from human or bovine milk has far greater lytic activity compared to egg lysozyme. The enzyme has also anti-inflammatory properties.

It has also been reported that milk is capable of killing tumor cells and immature cells, while sparing (indeed nutritionally helping) normal cells. The molecule that confers this selective and beneficial ability on milk is the protein called α-lactalbumin. This protein in conjunction with calcium leads to the apoptosis (programmed cell suicide) of cancer cells.

Lipids: The fatty acids present tear open bacteria and viruses. Special molecules in milk, glycoconjugates, prevent bacteria from adhering to cells in the surface of internal organs. And then there are antibody molecules in milk that prime and prepare the infants to face many antigens and thus make the child immunologically competent. Milk thus not only nourishes and helps body growth but also aids in the infant's immunity against infection and invasion

Short and medium-chain fatty acids with 4-12 carbon atoms, which occur in a relatively high concentration in milk fat, are reported to have antibacterial and fungicidal activity against gram-negative bacteria and certain moulds. Milk fat has a protective effect against human tooth decay. This effect has been ascribed in part to adsorption of milk fat on to the enamel surface and in part to antimicrobial effect of fatty acids (Kansal, 1995).

Recently, much attention has been directed towards an unusual fatty acid, conjugated linoleic acid (CLA), which is naturally present in milk and dairy products. Since the first report of Pariza's research group of CLA antimutagenic activity (Ha *et al.*, 1990), there has been an explosion of interest to discover several other biological activities in different experimental models. As on today several bio-protective properties of CLA have been demonstrated such as anticarcinogenic activity in mouse fore-stomach (Ha *et al*, 1990), mammary cancer prevention in rats (Ip *et al* 1991), anti-carcinogenic activity in rat colon (Liew, *et al*, 1995), anti-diabetic activity in rats (Houseknecht, *et al*, 1998), reduction in body fat and anti-atherogenic activity in rabbits (Pariza *et al*, 1996) and immunomodulation in rats (Sugano, *et al*, 1996). CLA is a milk fat molecule considered good for everything.

Milk fat has several other bioprotective molecules e.g., sphingomyleins, butyric acid, myristic acid, b-caroteines and fat soluble vitamins that have potential to inhibit the process of carcinogenesis and athergenesis and stimulate immune systems. While butyric acid has anti-cancer properties, myristic acid helps body fight infection by activating macrophages (Parodi, 1996).

Functional Peptides: Many milk-derived peptides possess functional properties. Several peptides with opium like (sleep inducing) activity have been extracted from the degradation products of milk proteins. These include β-casomorphins (from β-casein), exorphin (from a_{s1} casein), β-lactostensin (from lactoglobulin) and serorphin (from serum albumin). These opium like peptides have been shown to prolong gastrointestinal transit time exerting anti-diarrhoeal effect. They also stimulate secretion of insulin and somatostatin (Flat *et al*, 1993).

Glycomacro peptide (GMP) derived from k-casein induces production of cholesystokinin, a hormone associated with satiety. GMP and other fractions of k-casein digest inhibit the adhesion of oral actinomycetes and streptococci to erythrocytes, and binding of cholera toxins to its receptors (Beucher, *et al*, 1994).

Several immunostimulatory peptides have been identified from both bovine and human casein and whey proteins. These peptides have been shown to stimulate the phagocytic activities of murine and human macrophages and enhance resistance against certain bacteria. Certain peptides from casein stimulate the production of immunoglobulins (Parker, *et al*, 1984).

Low molecular weight peptides generated as a result of cleavage of lactoferrin by pepsin exhibit broad spectrum antibacterial activity inhibiting the growth of a number of gram-negative and gram-positive species including strains that are resistant to native lactoferrin. Lactoferrin B, a potentbactericidal fraction derived from bovine lactoferrin, stops the proliferation of clostridial species in the gut of mice fed on bovine milk. Lactoferricin, a more recently isolated antimicrobial peptide derived from bovine lactoferrin, is similar in its antibacterial effectiveness to many clinically proven antibiotics, causing complete inhibition of *Listeria monocytogenes*. Trials conducted with buffalo lactoferrin have indicated that its antimicrobial activity is comparable to that of its bovine counterpart. Small amounts of protein isolated from buffalo milk whey can effectively inhibit *E. coli* and *Staphylococcus aureus.*

2.6. Milk, A Cholesterol Lowering Food

Several studies have shown that milk reduces serum cholesterol levels of the consumers. Experiments with volunteers have shown that cholesterol levels do not rise when as much as two litres of milk is consumed daily. On the contrary, the cholesterol level is reduced. Experiments with animals have shown that even buffalo milk, containing 7% fat, lowers plasma cholesterol levels. Both decreased formation and increased breakdown of cholesterol are responsible for the cholesterol lowering effect of milk. Orotic acid and another necleotide associated with proteose-peptone fraction of milk proteins and calcium are suggested to have cholesterol reducing properties. Milk slows down the biochemical process leading to atherogenesis in rabbits fed on atherogenic diet (Aggarwal and Kansal, 1991a, 1991b). It has been suggested that the regular intake of milk keeps blood vessels healthy (Kansal, 1991).

Therapeutic Role of Milk Sugar: Lactose, the principal milk sugar, is slowly metabolized and therefore, a considerable portion of it passes into the large intestine where it promotes the growth of lactic acid producing bacteria. Lactic acid creates a desirable condition that inhibits the growth of proteolytic and putrefying bacteria in the intestine and replaces them gradually with acidophilic bacteria. Lactulose, a disachharide, originally not present in milk, is produced from lactose during heating or long storage. It is not hydrolysed by intestinal lactase, and hence passes almost completely into large intestine where it is fermented by. *L. bifidus* and *L. acidophilus* to produce lactic acid. Thus, lactose very effectively favours the growth of acidophilus bacteria. Microbial flora in the intestine of infant fed on mother's milk consists almost entirely of anaerobic lactobacilli, e.g., *L. bifidus*. Glycoproteins and oligosacchrides, present in mother's milk in high concentration, promote the growth of bifidus bacteria and thus provide baby resistance against intestinal infection (Kansal, 1992b).

Several investigations have shown that lactose promotes the utilization of calcium, magnesium and phosphorus. The acidic condition created by fermentation of lactose by intestinal bacteria may increase the solubilization and absorption of calcium. Part of the effect may also be due to the ability of lactose to form soluble complex with calcium. The lactose effect on calcium absorption has been observed in human infants and rats, but not in human adults. Lactose promotes the diffusion of calcium across the intestinal wall, which is the only route of calcium transport in human infants, since the active transport system is not developed at the time of birth. In adults, the calcium transport is predominantly via calcium carrier protein, induced by vitamin D- hormone, which is not influenced by lactose (Kansal, 2002).

Since lactose is slowly absorbed, it has slight laxative effect. It is due to lowering of the pH that increases the peristalsis of the intestine. The blood glucose does not rise rapidly on glucose diet. Milk consumption, therefore, enables the diabetic person to obtain the biologically highly valuable milk proteins without running the risk of rise in blood glucose levels (Kansal, 1992b).

Lactose may have some role in slimming diets, owing to its less rapid absorption compared to the more soluble carbohydrates and its property to discourage fat deposition in the body. The low solubility of lactose also makes it less irritating to the stomach and intestinal mucosa than the highly soluble sugars. Thus, milk is valuable in diets during treatment of ulcers of the stomach and duodenum.

In general, these properties of lactose are primarily important in the nourishment of the young. That is why lactose is said to be the excellent food to the babies, providing much firmer flesh than other kind of sugars. It has been reported that the growth of certain species is more satisfactory when butterfat and lactose are fed together than when the butterfat alone is fed as a part of the diet. Lactose may have some value in reducing diets because of its less efficient utilization compared to other carbohydrates, its tendency to encourage gastrointestinal motility, and its property of discouraging fat deposition in the body. In the young galactose derived from lactose, may be utilized in the synthesis of cerebrosides, important structural units in the brain and medullary sheaths of the nerves.

Based on the known nutritional contribution of milk to man, we conclude this chapter by stating that man's diet throughout life should include a generous amount of milk and milk products, thereby minimizing the possibility that nutrition will be a limiting factor in the quality and length of man's life.

References

Aggarwal, R.A.K. and Kansal,V.K. 1991. The influence of skim milk on plasma lipids, lipoproteins and lecithin: cholesterol acyltransferase activity in cholesterol fed rabbits. *Milchwissenschaft*, 46: 335-337.

Beucher, S. W., Levenez, F., Yvon.,M. and Corring, T. 1994. Effects of gastric digestive products from casein on CCK release by intestinal cells in rats. *J Nutr. Biochem.*, 12:578-584.

Fiat, A.M., Migliore, S.D. Jolles,P. Drouet,I., Bal, D.S.C. and Caen, J. 1993. Biologically active peptides from milk proteins with emphasis on two examples concerning immunomodulating activities. *J.Dairy Sci.*, 76:301310.

Ha, Y.L.,Storkson,,J. and Pariza, M.W. 199o. Inhibition of benzo (a) pyrene induced mouse forestomach neoplasia by conjugated dienoic derivatives of linoleic acid., *Cancer Res.* 50:1097-101.

IDFA, 1995. International Dairy Food Association. Health claims concerning the role of adequate dietary intake of calcium in reducing the risk of hypertension. (Prepared by The Weinberg Group Inc.). 16 October.

Kansal, V.K. 1992a. Essentialities of milk proteins in human diet. *Indian Dairyman*, 44:328-331.

Kansal, V.K.. Lactose in human health, *Indian Dairyman*, 44:497-500.

Kansal, V.K., 2004. Milk: A nutritious and protective food, good for every body-A rejoinder to anti-milk campaign, *Indian Dairyman*, 56: 39-47.

Pariza, M.W., Park, Y.,Cook, M.E., Albright, K.J. and Liu. W. 1996. Conjugated linoleic acid (CLA) reduces body fat. *FASEB. J.*: A 3227.

Parker, F, Migliore- Samour, D.,Floch, F., Zerial, A., Werner, G.H., Jones, P. 1984. Immunostimulating hexapeptide from human casein: amino acid sequence, synthesis and biological properties. *Eur. J. Biochem.*, 145: 677.

Parodi, P.W. 1996. Milk fat components: Possible chemo preventive agents for cancer and other diseases. *Aust. J.Dairy Technol.*, 51:24-32.

3

Physical and Physicochemical Properties of Milk

Milk is a complex colloidal dispersion, the physical and physicochemical properties of which depend on intrinsic compositional and structural factors, extrinsic factors such as temperature, and post-milking treatment.

There is no clear dividing line between physical properties and physicochemical properties. However, physical properties may be thought of as the measure of the bulk behaviour of milk and of how milk interacts with energy, while physicochemical properties are measures of how bulk behaviour and energy interactions depend on the constituent colloidal particles, molecules, atoms and ions in milk.

Knowledge of physical properties is of importance particularly in the technological and engineering design and control of milk processes and processing equipment. Knowledge of physicochemical properties provides the basis for the design of modern methods of milk analysis, determination of milk microstructures and elucidation of the complex chemical reactions that occur in milk.

In the dairy industry measurements of the physical properties of milk and milk products are made to secure data necessary for the design of dairy equipment (e.g., heat conductivity and viscosity) to determine the concentration of a component (e.g., specific gravity to estimate solids-not-fat or freezing point to determine added water), or to assess the extent of a physical or chemical change (e.g., titratable acidity to follow bacterial action or viscosity to assess aggregation of protein micelles or fat globules). The great advantage of physical measurements for such purposes is their speed and simplicity as well as their potentialities for automation.

Use of physical property to measure concentrations or changes in degree of dispersion demands knowledge of the contribution of the several components to that property. Furthermore, the natural range of variation of the property in milks or products is of major interest. The precision and suitability of possible methods of measurement are also of prime importance.

Some of the physical and physicochemical properties of particular significance in fluid milk processing will be discussed in relation to (a) general physical principle involved, (b) contribution of milk components, (c) normal range of values and variations, (d) major processing effects, (e) objectives of study in dairy field, and (f) methods of measurements

Colour: The colour of the fluid dairy foods is caused by the scattering of light by the fat globules, casein micelles, colloidal calcium phosphate and to some extent by the pigments carotene and riboflavin. The milk colour varies from white to yellow according to the coloration (carotein content) of the fat. Colour of buffalo milk is richer than that of cow milk due to larger number of fat particles as well as large size of casein micelles / colloidal calcium phosphate complex. The white colour of whole milk is due to the scattering of the entire light spectra, the fat globules being the most significant factor. Relatively small fat globules will scatter more light and make the product whiter, whereas clumping or clustering of the fat globules will decrease the whiteness. This is particularly true for creams. Homogenization increases the number and total volume of fat globules. This results in whiter colour of homogenized products than their unhomogenized counterparts. Lack of fat globules and water soluble pigment, riboflavin produces yellowish or bluish green tint in skim milk. After removal of casein particles from skim milk, the resultant whey has a distinct green fluorescence. The yellow colour of cow milk fat- both butter and ghee is due to the presence of fat soluble pigments, carotene and xanthophylls. Butter with no added colour is light yellow as a result of its carotene content. Because of variability in the carotene content of milk, derivatives of the annatto seed are used to colour butter and cheese. Synthetic coffee whiteners are also artificially coloured. The smaller the particles that scatter light, the bluish is the colour of the material. The addition of solids provides more particles to scatter light and thus gives more desired whiteness to the product, whey, from which most of the casein and colloidal calcium phosphate have been removed, is greenish in colour because of the riboflavin.

Flavour: Milk is such a bland tasting food that it is difficult to describe its taste attributes. While processed milk of good flavour quality has a bland taste, it does, nonetheless, have a characteristic flavour, described as a slight sweet taste. To some degree, this flvour quality can probably be attributed to milk salts and lactose. But the reason for milk's characteristic taste is far more complicated than this.

The sensory perception of milk is significantly impacted by its pleasant mouthfeel, which is primarily due to emulsion of fat globules in an aqueous colloidal protein phase. But the volatile constituents in milk make the strongest contribution to its aroma and flavour. Dimethyl sulphide was one of the first important aroma-contributing chemicals identified in milk. Significant improvements in analytical techniques and instrumentation have occurred since then, and dozens of other odoriferous chemicals have been identified in milk, including aldehydes, ketones, alcohols, fatty acids, lactones, esters, sulphur compounds, nitrogen compounds and aromatic hydrocarbons. Complicating the understanding of what odorants are most important to good milk flavour are three factors: a) the large number of volatiles present in milk, b) their low concentration level, and c) in some cases, their low odour detection theshold levels.

Milk has a clean, pleasantly sweet flavour. The buffalo milk has a smooth, pleasant, slightly sweeter and richer flavour than cow milk apparently due to the higher fat, protein and lactose. However, any off-flavours are readily discernible. They develop when balance of flavour compounds is disturbed due to the microbiological activity or processing treatments or chemical or biochemical reactions during milk production, processing and storage. A common cause of off-flavour development is tainted feed.

Density: Density is the physical property used to compare masses of different substances or of a given substance under different conditions. Density is weight per unit volume:

Density = weight / volume

The numerical value of density depends on the units of weight and volume used in calculation. Thus it has been found convenient to express density in reference to some standard substance. Water is commonly used as the reference substance. The dimensionless constant thus obtained is called specific gravity:

Specific gravity = Density of substance / density of water

Since the density of any substance including water varies with the temperature, it is necessary to specify the temperature when reporting densities or specific gravities. Any temperature can be used, but in practice certain standard temperatures have become established long usage. In the metric system the density of water is 0.999973 g / cm^3 at 3.98 °C. For most purposes, it can be said 1.0000 at 4° C. When the specific gravity of a substance is referred to water at 4°C, it is numerically equal to the density of that substance in the metric system. In dairy parlance the specific gravity of milk has usually been reported at 60° F / 60° F, (meaning density at 60° F divided by that of water at 60° F) or at 20° C/20° C.

The density of fluid milk products is the weight per unit volume and is the average of the densities of the individual milk components. Thus it will be dependent upon the concentration of the individual components, the degree of hydration of the proteins and the specific volume of the milk fat system at a particular temperature.

The density of milk products previously has been reported generally in terms of specific gravity (density of product / density of water) with average values at 15.5°C being given as 1.032 and 1.036 for whole milk and skim milk, respectively.

The effect of changes in fat and solids-not-fat (SNF) content on density was found by Betscher (1960) to be linear; fat decreases specific gravity about 0.010 / 10% changes in fat content and SNF increases specific gravity about 0.035 / 10% changes in SNF content.

Specific gravity = 1.0+ (0.0035 x % SNF – 0.001 x % fat)

The dependence of density on temperature is understood, although the effect of temperature on water and milk differ, primarily because of the protein and lipid systems. The maximum density of fresh whole milk is at – 5.2°C as compared to 4°C for water. In the temperature range of 10 - 40°C the density of milk changes linearly with temperature change, but at a rate different from water, which may reflect changes in protein hydration.

The density of milk decreases from a maximum at –5.2°C to a minimum at 40°C. Above 40 °C, change in density is erratic. The specific gravity of milk, which is the ratio of density of milk to that of water at that temperature, is reported at 15.5°C. The specific gravity of fresh whole milk lies in the range of 1.030- 1.035, with an average of 1.032. Milk fat and SNF at 15.5°C have specific gravity of 0.93 and 1.614, respectively. Although buffalo milk contains more fat than cow milk, it has higher specific gravity because of higher SNF content.

The percentage of total solids or SNF in milk is calculated using the following formula:

$\% TS = 0.25D + 1.22F + 0.72$

$\% SNF = 0.25D+0.22F + 0.72$

where, $D = 1000 (d-1)$

d = density of sample of milk at 20° C

F = fat percentage of sample

The density and the specific gravity of milk may be determined by either measuring the weight of a known volume or the volume of a known weight. The weight of a known volume may be determined either with a pycnometer or with a hydrostatic balance. A pycnometer is a vessel that can be filled with liquid at a given temperature and weighed. The volume contained at any temperature can be calculated by dividing the weight of water contained by the density of water at that temperature, Then:

$$\text{Density of milk at } t° = \frac{\text{weight of milk contained at } t°}{\text{volume of pycnometer}}$$

If specific gravity is sought, it can be calculated simply as follows:

Specific gravity of milk at t°

$$\text{Relative to water at } t° = \frac{\text{weight of milk contained at } t°}{\text{weight of water contained at } t°}$$

In the measurement of density and specific gravity by the determination of volume of a known weight, float called lactometer is employed. The principle involved is that a floating object sinks until it has displaced a weight of fluid equal to its own weight. The volume of displaced fluid is greater the smaller the density of the fluid. Lactometers are constructed of a large glass float with a slender glass stem carrying a scale on which small increments of displaced volume can be read. The scale is actually calibrated, not in terms of volume but in a function of either density or specific gravity. The two principal types of lactometers are the Quevenne and the New York Board of Health. The Quevenne is calibrated in degrees which bear the following relation to specific gravity:

°Q = 1000S – 1000

Where °Q = Quevenne degrees,

S = specific gravity at 60° F / 60° F.

Thus, a specific gravity of 1.032 is equivalent to 32° Q.

Acidity and pH: The freshly drawn milk is amphoteric to litmus, i.e. it turns red litmus blue and blue litmus red. Milk is slightly acidic, normally ranging in pH from 6.3 to 6.9, the greatest number of samples falling between 6.4 and 6.8. Mixed herd milk commonly shows a pH range of 6.5 to 6.7 with an average of pH 6.6. Colostrum is somewhat more acidic than normal milk, ranging from 6.1 to 6.4, but becomes normal within about 5 days after parturition and remains constant over the major portion of the lactation period. At the end of lactation the pH of milk generally rises and may be about 6.8. Udder infections cause an increase in the pH of milk, values not infrequently falling above 7.5 for milk from cows with severe mastitis. Milk with pH values above 6.8 is generally considered to be abnormal, and may relate to mastitis or to very advanced lactation. Except in cases of extensive bacterial growth, pH does not provide a useful index of the quality of the modern milk supply. Organoleptically detectable microbial souring will generally be related to as slight a pH change as 0.01 to 0.05. The titratable acidity of fresh buffalo milk is reported to be 0.16% which is relatively higher than that of cow milk (0.15%). The pH of fresh buffalo milk varies between 6.63-6.80 which is apparently higher than 6.5-6.7 reported for cow milk. Pasteurization, boiling or sterilization of buffalo milk did not result in a significant change of milk acidity. The buffering capacity of buffalo milk is higher than cow milk due to higher proteins, phosphates and citrates.

Since the pH of milk lies below the end-point of phenolphthalein (pH 8.3), base is consumed in changing the pH of milk from 6.6 to the phenolphthalein end point, the titer being proportional to the buffering capacity of the components of milk. The titratable acidity thus obtained has been used as an index of the quality of fluid milk. The titration value is expressed in terms of percent lactic acid (=0.09 x meq/100ml). Titration of fresh milk generally requires from 13-18 ml of 0.1N NaOH/100ml, or 0.13 to 0.18% acidity expressed as lactic acid, most samples falling within the range of 0.14 to 0.17%. The components which contribute to the titratable acidity of fresh milk are as follows:

Components	Acidity (%)
Citrates	0.01
Whey proteins (albumin)	0.01
Carbon dioxide	0.01 to 0.02
Caseins	0.05 to 0.08
Phosphates	Remainder (0.04-0.10)

The primary contributors to the titratable acidity of milk are caseins and phosphates. The titratable acidity of cream can be calculated from the formula: -

$$\frac{\%\text{ Serum in cream}}{\%\text{ Serum in milk}} \times \text{acidity of milk}$$

Heavy cream generally has as titratable acidity of 0.09 to 0.11%. Any process, which concentrates the non-fat solids of milk will increase the titratable acidity and should not be confused with the titratable acidity increase due to souring.

Cultured products normally have pH levels between 4.2 and 5.2 in the finished product and titratable acidity between 0.70 and 1.30, depending upon the product and fermentation.

Viscosity: Viscosity is a property of all fluids. It can be expressed only in relative terms, and, for convenience, the relative viscosity of any fluid is compared with water. Water flows with ease. Syrup pours much more slowly than water and posses a greater viscosity. Milk is slightly more viscous than water, approximately 1.5 to 1.7 times more viscous, owing to the presence of solids in milk, some of which are in solution, others in suspension and still others in the form of emulsion. All liquids appear more viscous at low than high temperatures. Milk is no exception to this rule. Milk is quite different, however, from most fluids in that its original viscosity is partially destroyed under certain conditions, while under others it may be increased. The original viscosity of milk is reduced when milk is heated to temperatures commonly used in pasteurization. On the other hand, when milk is subjected to temperatures such as those reached under pressure, an increase in the viscosity of milk results. When milk is subjected to prolonged agitation the viscosity is reduced. Aging, souring and the development of certain types of bacteria in milk are responsible for an increase in viscosity. It is conceded, generally, that the increase in viscosity is due to the changes taking place in the proteins of milk, primarily casein, which has hydrophilic properties similar to other proteins.

Viscosity is the resistance of a liquid to flow or deformation, arbitrarily defined by the general equation:

$$\eta = (F/A) / (dV/dx)$$

Where h is the coefficient of viscosity, F = Force in dynes cm^{-2} required to maintain a unit velocity gradient between two parallel plates with the planes separated by a unit distance (x), A = area in cm^2, and dV/ dx = velocity gradient in sec^{-1} perpendicular to the plane. The unit of h = poise = dynes cm^{-2} to maintain a velocity of 1cm per sec between parallel planes 1cm apart, considered to be nearly Newtonian. Cream, chocolate milk, cultured buttermilk, sour cream, yoghurt, ice cream mix and evaporated milk exhibit varying degrees of non-Newtonian behaviour. Dairy products such as yoghurt and sour cream or products containing hydrocolloid stabilizers (gums) are pseudoplastic and simultaneously sensitive to the time of shear at a given shear rate, which is termed thixotropy.

The viscosity of milk and cream gives an impression of "richness" to the consumer. From an organoleptic standpoint, viscosity contributes to the mouth feel and flavour. Viscosity of milk and milk products depends on temperature, concentration, and state of casein micelles and fat globules. Since the content of total solids is more in buffalo milk, its viscosity is also more.

Viscosity has a marked effect on the body and mouth-feel of fluid products and is a significant factor in most equations relating to engineering processes of fluid milk products (such as Reynolds number describing flow characteristics and Grashoff and Prandtl number for heat transfer).

Viscosity values of 1.2, 1.45 and 2.0 centipoises at low rates of shear in a capillary viscometer and at 20°C have been given for whey, skim milk and whole milk, respectively. The average viscosity of buffalo milk was reported to be 2.245 centipoise at 20°C. It is reported that the casein system and the fat-globule system contribute significantly to the viscosity of fluid milk products.

The viscosity of fluid dairy products can be related to the following: -

a) Serum – lactose content, proteins content, casein micelle structure, hydration of protein, hydrocolloid stabilizers.

b) Fat – fat content, fat globule size, fat globule clustering, emulsifiers.

The viscous behaviour of milk products is affected by concentration, temperature and the state of dispersion of the solid components. Conditions and treatments that affect the stability of casein are very significant in the viscosity of milk. Some such factors are acidity, salt balance, heat treatment and the action of various enzymes and bacteria.

Specific heat: To raise or lower the temperature of any substance a given number of degrees, a certain amount of heat must be added to or taken from the material. All substances vary in the amount of heat required, because they differ in their chemical nature and their physical state. The ratio between the amount of heat required to raise a given weight of substance to a given temperature and the amount of heat required to raise the same amount of water to the same temperature is termed as specific heat. The unit of heat is known as the "calorie" and is the amount of heat required to raise 1 gram of water from 15-16° C, that is, 1° C. Since water remains the standard, however, the specific heat of a substance is the number of calories required to raise a definite amount of substance through 1° C in temperature. It is commonly stated that the specific heat of a substance is the number of calories required to raise 1 gram of substance through 1° C.

It is exceedingly important, however, to bear in mind that the amount of heat required to raise the temperature of a fluid is affected by the specific gravity or density. Water has its greatest specific gravity at 3.9° C and it is at this temperature, therefore, that the specific heat of water is taken as standard with which other substances can be compared. It is important, however, to note the specific heat of a substance at various temperatures. Milk has a specific heat of 0.938 at15° C, of 0.920 at 0° C, of 0.930 at 40° C and of 0.918 at 60° C. At 15° C the specific heat of whey is 0.976; of skim milk; 0.943; 15% cream, 0.923; 20% cream, 0.940; 30% cream, 0.983; 45% cream, 1.016; 60% cream, 1.053; butter, 0.527; and butter fat, 0.467. In this case it is interesting to note that as the fat content of cream is increased the specific heat increases. With skim milk and whole milk, skim milk of low fat content has a higher specific heat than whole milk. The heat capacity of buffalo milk ranges between 0.84 to 0.86 cal/g/C at 30° C. It is of further interest to observe that butter and butter fat containing a small amount of other constituents of milk have a very low specific heat.

The specific heat and heat capacity are used interchangeably. The quantity of heat required to raise the temperature of a unit amount of material through a unit temperature range is defined as the heat capacity of that material.

$$\text{Heat capacity (Cp)} = \frac{Q}{m\,(t_1 - t_2)}$$

Where Q is the amount of heat to raise a mass (m in grams) from temperature $t_1 - t_2$. The average specific heat is utilized in heat transfer calculations. At 15°C, the specific heat of water is 1. The specific heats of various fluid-milk products are given in Table 3.1.

Table 3.1: Specific heat of various fluid milk products (BTU per LB-F)

Product	Fat (%)	SNF (%)	Specific heat
Skim milk	-	8.8	0.944
Whole milk	4.0	8.7	0.93
Cream	25.0	6.7	0.83
Heavy cream	40.0	5.6	0.77
Butter oil	99.7	-	0.50
Fortified skim milk	-	12.5	0.93
Fortified skim milk	-	20.0	0.89

Source: Peoples (1962)

Surface tension: At an interface between liquid and gas, such as water and air, the molecules of liquid in the surface are subject to forces of attraction side ways and downward but not upward. Molecules in the interior of the liquid are acted on by mutual attractive forces in all directions. The cohesion or tension of molecules in the surface, resulting from the imbalance of forces acting on them, causes the surface to act as though covered with a film or skin. This phenomenon is called surface tension. Surface tension often is classically demonstrated by carefully placing a needle on the surface of water. Although the needle is of much greater density than the water and will rapidly sink to the bottom once it has penetrated through the surface at any point, careful horizontal positioning will enable the force of surface tension to keep the needle afloat. Surface tension is usually expressed in dynes per centimeter (dynes / cm), which is an expression of the force acting along a linear component of surface.

The stability of the milk-fat emulsion, foaming and cleaning of equipment surfaces are but several examples of the significance of the properties of interfaces to the dairy food industry. The surface tension of milk, most commonly measured by pulling a ring from the surface at 0°C, is from 55 to 60 dynes / cm, decreasing to 40 to 45 dynes / cm at 40° C. At 20° C the surface tension of water is 72.75 dynes / cm and whole milk averages 50 dynes / cm. Milk proteins, milk fat, phospholipids and free fatty acids are the principal surface-active components contributing to the surface tension of milk. No significant difference has been reported in the surface tension of buffalo and cow milk.

Various investigators have shown that caseinate, b-lactoglobulin, α-lactalbumin and bovine serum are surface-tension depressants, whereas the immune globulins have little effect. The protein and phospholipid complex from the surface of the milk fat globule may be the most significant factor in depressing the surface tension of milk / air and plasma / fat interfaces. Fatty acids, released by lipolysis of milk-fat have a marked depressing effect on surface tension.

In measuring surface tension or interfacial tension aging of emulsions and colloidal suspensions causes changes in surface and interfacial tension relationships. Materials that aggregate at surfaces relieve stress relationships and reduce surface tension.

Surface properties are relevant to creaming, fat globule function, foaming, and emulsifier used in dairy products. Surface tension increases as milk temperature rises. Processing treatments such as heating, sterilization, homogenization and shear tend to increase surface tension. However, homogenization of imperfectly pasteurized milk or contamination of homogenized pasteurized milk with raw milk causes partial hydrolysis of milk fat, resulting in low surface tension, bitter flavour and rancidity of milk.

Refractive index: When light passes at an oblique angle from a less dense medium such as air into a more dense medium such as water, it is bent or refracted. The magnitude of the bending, expressed as a ratio of the sines of the angles of incidence and refraction of the light, is the refractive index. It is designated by the letter n.

$$n = \frac{\sin i}{\sin r}$$

where i = angle of incidence

r = angle of refraction

The refractive index of a pure liquid is a characteristic constant for that liquid, under specified conditions of temperature and wavelength of light. The refractive index of water at 20° C with the D line of the sodium spectrum (589.3mu) is $n^{20}_{D} = 1.33299$. The refractive index of liquids containing dissolved solids, such as milk is increased over that of water to an extent determined by the number and kind of molecules of dissolved material. Thus it is evident that measurement of refractive index can be useful in determining the total solids content of foods. Since the food components that are not in solution have little or no effect on refractive index, the term "total soluble solids" is frequently used in the food industry to denote the type of food solids that can be measured by refractive index. One of the most important uses of refractometry in this connection is in the analysis of syrups, jams and jellies for sugar content.

Since milk contains material, which ranges in dispersion from that truly dissolved to colloidal material, which is opaque to the transmission of light, a problem is posed in the determination of refractive index. Therefore, the fat at least must be removed. Observations on the non-fat phase of milk yield values for refractive index generally falling within the range $n^{20}_{D} = 1.3340$ to 1.3480. The components of milk contributing to its refractive index in descending order of importance are: water, proteins, lactose and minor constituents.

Freezing point: Certain properties of solutions depend upon the number of solute particles (molecules or ions) present. These are known as colligative properties in contrast to constitutive properties, which depend on the nature of the solute molecules. Important colligative properties of solutions are the depression of the vapour pressure and freezing point of the solvent, the elevation of the boiling point and osmotic pressure. Measurement of any of these properties can be used for determining the concentration of solutes in a solution, but in so far as milk is concerned the depression of freezing point is by far of most interest and usefulness.

The freezing point of water is the temperature at which ice and water exist in equilibrium with each other, it is the temperature at which they have the same vapour pressure. The addition of a solute to water lowers the vapour pressure because it hinders the ability of the water molecule to escape from the surface. Thus it happens that ice and solution will be in equilibrium (i.e, have the same vapour pressure) at a lower temperature than pure water and ice. The amount of depression of the freezing point is proportional to the fraction of the total number of molecules, which are solute molecules. Thus

$$\Delta T = T^0 - T = K \frac{N_2}{N_1 + N_2}$$

Where ΔT = freezing point depression

T_0 = freezing point of water

T = freezing point of solution

K = constant related to vapor pressure

N_2 = number of solute molecules

N_1 = number of solvent (water) molecules

In dilute solutions N2 is very small compared to N1, and consequently

$$\Delta T = K^1 \frac{N_2}{N_1} = K^1 \frac{W_2/M_2}{W_1/M_1} = K^1 \frac{M_1/W_2}{M_2/W_1}$$

Where W_1 and M_1 stand respectively for weight and molecular weight of solvent and W_2 and M_2 for weight and molecular weight of solute. In dilute aqueous solutions freezing point of water is lowered by 1.86° C for each molecule of solute added to 1000g of water.

Thus,

$$\Delta T = \frac{1.86 \times 1000 \times W_2}{M_2/W_1}$$

In chemistry, the freezing point depression "T is often determined to calculate the molecular weight of the solute M_2. In dairy chemistry, its principal use is to detect additions of water and to compute its concentration.

The freezing point of milk is its most constant physical property, the secretary process of the mammary gland are such that the osmotic pressure of milk is kept in equilibrium with that in blood. Any depression of the synthesis of lactose is compensated by increases in the concentration of sodium and chloride. It must not be thought, however, that the freezing point of milk is absolutely invariant. It varies somewhat but within very narrow limits. The vast majority of individual cow samples fall between –0.525°C and –0.565°C. Actually few fall outside the range of –0.530°C and –0.550°C. The average is close to –0.540°C. Herd and bulk milk will exhibit an even narrower range of variation, unless water has been added either intentionally or accidentally.

The nutrition and environment of the milch animal and stage of lactation have but little influence on the freezing point of milk. Colostrum has a slightly lower freezing point than normal milk of the order of –0.570° to –0.580°C. Lactose is the major component responsible for the freezing point depression of fluid milk followed by the soluble salts. Materials of high molecular weight, such as fat, protein or colloidal calcium phosphate, have negligible effect on the freezing point because of the relatively small number of molecules per gram. Processing operations that do not involve either dilution or concentration of milk have a negligible influence on freezing point. Even rather severe heat treatment is without effect. Souring, which involves a net increase in the number of molecules in solution as lactose (and sometimes citrate) is degraded, naturally results in a lowering of a freezing point. The freezing point is determined principally by the concentration of small molecules and ions in solution. Materials of high molecular weight contribute a negligible amount because they contain few molecules per gram. Thus, a gram of lactose has about 1000 times the effect of a gram of β-lactoglobulin because its molecular weight is only about 1/1000 as great.

Oxidation-Reduction Potential: Ordinarily oxidation may be defined as the uptake of oxygen or the loss of hydrogen. In the same manner, reduction may be defined as the process of losing oxygen or gaining hydrogen. However, in a broader sense the processes of oxidation and reduction are not necessarily limited to the gain or loss of oxygen and hydrogen. In ionic systems it can be demonstrated that the phenomenon may involve simply the loss or gain of electrons. The following equation involving ferric chloride and hydrogen sulfide demonstrates this point:

+2e

$$2Fe^{+++} + 6Cl^{-} + H_2S \qquad\qquad 2Fe^{++} + 6Cl^{-} + 2H^{+} + S$$

-2e

In this equation two electrons are gained by the ferric ion in being reduced to ferrous ions, whereas the hydrogen sulfide loses two electrons in being oxidized to elemental sulfur. Therefore, oxidation can be defined as the loss of electrons and reduction as the gain in electrons. An associated fact, which can be deduced in this connection is that every oxidation is accompanied by a reduction and vice versa.

In the field of chemistry, compounds frequently are characterized as oxidizing agents or reducing agents. It will be clear from the above that this refers (depending upon whether an ionic or organic substrate is involved) to the relative ease with which the compound gains or loses electrons, gains or loses oxygen, and gains or loses hydrogen.

The relative tendency of a substance in solution to yield or take on electrons can be measured if a standard substance that will donate or accept electrons can be inserted in the system to establish a difference in potential. In practice, the potential difference created by a platinum electrode in a solution of an oxidant or reductant is measured by completing a circuit through a calomel half-cell and a potentiometer. The voltage measured under these conditions reflects the oxidizing or reducing capacity of the solution. The potential is called the oxidation reduction potential of the redox potential. It is designated by the symbol "Eh". Positive potential, which involves loss of electrons from the platinum electrodes is indicative of oxidizing properties, whereas negative potential, which involves gain of electrons at the platinum electrode, reveals reducing property.

In addition to potential, oxidation reduction systems also have a quality known as poise. This term, which is closely analogous to buffer capacity in pH and acidity equilibria, refers to the resistance that a system offers to change in oxidation reduction potential when treated with oxidizing or reducing agents.

Oxidation-Reduction Potential of Milk: The Eh of milk normally falls within the range of + 0.2 to + 0.3 volt. The values are more commonly found between + 0.23 and + 0.25 volt. The Eh of fresh unheated milk is largely the result of its oxygen content. The average redox potential (Eh) of fresh Indian buffalo milk is + 0.312 (range being + 0.3077 to + 0.3163), which was relatively higher than + 0.234 reported for Indian cattle. Pasteurization of buffalo milk resulted in an increase in Eh, however, boiling or sterilization of buffalo milk significantly decreased the Eh values. The principal poising material under normal oxygen tension may be ascorbic acid. In addition to heat treatment, bacterial activity and contamination with trace metals, particularly copper influence the Eh of milk. In all probability bacteria accomplish a lowering of the potential through use of available oxygen in the medium as well as by elaborating reducing substances in the course of their metabolism. The well known methylene blue reduction test of milk is based on this phenomenon.

References

Betscher, J.J. 1960. Friction characteristics of fluid milk products. Ph. D. Dissertation, Ohio State University, Columbus.

Harper, W.J. and Hall, C.W. 1976. Physical properties of milk. Dairy Technology and Engineering. AVI Publication, pp: 39.

Jenness, R. and Patton. S. 1959. Physical properties of milk. Principles of Dairy Chemistry. 1st Ed. Wiley Eastern Pvt. Ltd. PP: 218.

McCarthy, O.J. 2003. Physical and physicochemical properties of milk. *Encyclopaedia of Dairy Sciences*, Academic Press, PP:1218.

Peeples, J.L. 1962. Forced convection heat transfer characteristics of fluid milk products. A Review, *J. Dairy Sci.* 45: 297.

□□□□

4

Microbiology of Milk

Microorganism is a collective term for all living organisms, which are not visible to the eye, and occupy an intermediate position between the vegetable and animal kingdoms. They are found every where in the atmosphere, in water and in the soil and, as they break down organic materials, they play a very important role in the cycle of the nature.

There are thousands of species which are important to the life and economic structure of the human race. For example, certain species form simple chemical elements during the break down of dead organic material which plants can use again. They increase soil fertility and crop production which results in more food.

Other species are present, and essential, in animal intestines, helping in the digestion of food.

Some microorganisms are used in many food processes, e.g. dahi, yoghurt, cheese, pickles, beer and wine as well as in the acid production to preserve foods. There are microorganisms that produce toxic substances which kill other organisms, e.g. the mould penicillium which produces the substance penicillin.

Many microorganisms cause diseases in animals and plants with a subsequent reduction in the nation's food supply, whereas others cause food deterioration such as mouldy foods, tainted foods, *etc.*

Milk, by its very nature, is a natural growth medium for microorganisms because of its near neutral pH, complex biochemical composition and high water content. Milk when secreted in the healthy udder is almost sterile, however, it is subjected to many sources of microbial contamination. The sources of contamination may be broadly classified as: a) from within the udder, b) from the exterior of the teats and udder, and c) from milk holding and storage equipment.

The microorganisms associated with the teat move up the teat canal and into the interior of the udder. This causes even aseptically drawn milk to contain a small number of microorganisms, mostly bacteria. The surface of the teat may be contaminated with microorganisms from various sources including soil, bedding, manure, and feeds, *etc*. Diverse microflora including spore formers are present in and on materials from these various sources and, depending on the sanitary practices used on a farm, microorganisms from these sources may contaminate the teat and udder and gain entrance into the milk. Bacteria in aseptically drawn milk are usually limited in number and include mostly micrococci, lactococci, and *Corynebacterium bovis*. Freshly drawn milk from healthy cows during routine milking operation may contain from a few to several thousand microorganisms. The number is highly variable among animals and even from quarter to quarter in a given milch animal. Whereas a few microorganisms may enter milk while it is in the udder, most of the microorganisms in raw milk are contaminants from the outside of the udder, milking equipment, and human handlers. The number and types of microorganisms, present in milk are influenced by season, farm hygiene, feed and efficiency of collection, transportation, chilling and storage of milk. The number of bacteria in milk ranges from a few hundred to lacs per milliliter of freshly drawn milk.

Of these some microorganisms are desirable, others are undesirable and still others are harmful and pathogenic. Among the desirable microorganisms (e.g. lactic acid bacteria) there are starter cultures which can be used to produce a variety of fermented dairy products. Undesirable or spoilage microorganisms (e.g. gram-negative psychrotrophs) cause off-flavours and odours and change the texture and appearance of milk and milk products. Pathogenic bacteria (e.g. Salmonella, Listeria) are those capable of causing infection or intoxication. Milk, a highly nutritious food ideally suited for the growth of both spoilage and pathogenic organisms is the basis for an extremely large dairy industry. Milk also plays a protective role for most of the microorganisms.

4.1. Beneficial Microorganisms

Lactic Acid Bacteria: Lactic acid bacteria are found almost everywhere in nature, but they occur particularly in large numbers in places where there is milk. The group includes both bacilli and cocci, which can form chains of varying length but which never form spores. Most of them are killed by heating to 70°C, though the lethal temperature for some is as high as 80°C.

For growth lactic acid bacteria need organic nitrogen compounds. They get them from casein in milk by breaking it down with the help of protein-splitting enzymes. However, the ability to split casein varies greatly from one species to another.

Selected lactic acid bacteria and other microorganisms are used by the Dairy industry to produce fermented products such as dahi, yoghurt and cheese, *etc*. Commercially available starter cultures have been selected for a variety of desirable properties such as: flavour production, lack of associated off-flavours, fast acid production, bacteriophage resistance, salt tolerance, exopolysaccharide production, bacteriocin production and heat sensitivity. These microbial preparations may consist of different species of lactic acid bacteria, propionibacteria, surface ripening bacteria, yeasts and moulds.

Lactic acid bacteria originally found on plants find their way to milk and constitute normal flora. Others are found in the intestine of humans and animals. This group includes facultative anaerobes, non-spore forming (asporogenous), gram positive, catalase negative cocci and rods. These bacteria utilize lactose as a source of carbon and convert it to lactic acid (lactic acid fermentation). Lactic acid fermentation may be homofermentative (exclusive production of lactic acid) or heterofermentative (besides lactic acid, production of other compounds e.g. acetic acid, carbon dioxide, ethanol as end products). The fermentation capacity varies according to the species. Most lactic acid bacteria form between 0.5 to 1.5% lactic acid, but there are species which form up to 3%. Lactic acid bacteria constitute the major group of bacteria involved in dairy fermentation. They are distributed among 11 genera but dairy starter lactic acid bacteria are found only in six of them: Streptococcus, Lactococcus, Leuconostoc, Pediococcus and Enterococcus. Except lactobacillus, which is rod shaped, rest genera are coccus shaped.

All dairy fermentation use lactic acid bacteria for acidification and flavour production. Although lactic acid bacteria are genetically diverse, common characteristics of this group include being gram-positive, non-spore forming, non-pigmented and unable to produce iron-containing porphyrin compounds (catalase and cytochrome), having anaerobic growth but being aero-tolerant and having obligate fermentation of sugar with lactic acid as a major end-product. Lactic acid bacteria tend to be nutritionally fastidious, often requiring specific amino acids, B-vitamins, and other growth factors, while being unable to use complex carbohydrates.

Lactic acid bacteria are generally associated with nutrient-rich habitats containing simple sugars. These include raw milk, meat, fruits, and vegetables. They grow with yeast in wine, beer and bread fermentations. In nature, they are found in the dairy farm environment and in decomposing vegetation, including silage. Some species colonise animal organs including mouth, intestine, and vagina. They are also part of the normal microflora of the streak canal of the mammary gland. Lactic acid bacteria isolated from natural habitats are often physiologically distinct from their starter culture variants. For example, lactococci isolated from plants ferment lactose slowly, if at all.

Lactococci: The genus streptococcus has been divided into four genera, *viz*. Enterococcus, Lactococcus, Streptococcus and Vagococcus. Lactococci also known as lactic streptococci were originally isolated from sour milk and cream. They occur singly, in pairs or in chains and are non- motile, mesophyllic, homofermentative and weakly proteolytic. There are currently five species in this genus but only *Lactococcus lactis* is used as starter culture especially in dahi and cheese. This species has three subsp: *Lactococcus lactis* subsp *lactis, Lactococcus lactis* subsp *cremoris* and *Lactoccus lactis* subsp *diacetylactis. Lactococcus lactis* subsp *diacetylactis* utilizes citrate to produce diacetyl, carbon dioxide and other compounds in cultured milk and cheeses.

Streptococci: Besides lactococci, *Streptococcus thermophillus* is also considered as lactic streptococci which occur in pairs or in long chains. It grows at 45 °C and is homofermentative. It is used to produce acid in dairy products subjected to high temperature during fermentation. It is used as starter in yoghurt, Mozzarella cheese and Swiss cheese in association with *Lactobacillus delbrueckii* subsp *bulgaricus.* It is weakly proteolytic and some strains produce extracellular polysaccharides.

Leuconostoc spp: Leuconostoc species are cocci often ellipsoidal in shape that occur in pairs and chains. They are heterofermentative, gram positive cocci. They produce flavour compounds, diacetyl and acetoin and some strains produce exopolysaccharides. *Leuconostoc mesenteroides* subsp *cremoris* is used in the production of Cottage and cream cheese and cultured milks. *Leuconostoc mesenteroides* subsp. *mesenteroides* and subsp. *dextranicum* often produce slime (glucan, formerly known as dextran) from sucrose. *Leuconostoc paramesenteroides* does not produce glucan and is used in making brined cheese. *Leuconostoc lactis* is also found in milk and dairy products. Leuconostoc sp. reduce an undesirable green flavour in cultured dairy products by converting acetaldehyde to diacetyl, but only grow slowly in milk.

Lactobacilli: *Lactobacillus* species are a genetically and physiologically diverse group of rod-shaped lactic acid bacteria. They are the most acid tolerant of the lactic acid bacteria and produce numerous proteolytic enzymes. There are three groups based on the type of fermentation end products: homofermentative (*Lb. delbrueckii* subsp. *bulgaricus, Lb. delbrueckii* subsp *lactis, Lb. acidophilus, Lb. helveticus* and *Lb. helveticus* subsp. *Jugurti),* facultatively heterofermentative *(Lb. casei, Lb. curvatus* and *Lb. plantarum)* and obligately heterofermentative (*Lb. kefir, Lb. fermentum* and *Lb. bravis).* Some lactobacilli, such as *Lb. acidophilus* are claimed to confer health benefits. Homofermentative lactobacilli are usually thermophillic and are used to produce fermented milk and some cheese varieties that require the use of high temperature during manufacturing. *Lactobacillus casei* and *Lb. plantarum* cannot grow at high temperatures (45° C). They are involved in the ripening of Cheddar and other cheese varieties.

Propionibacterium spp: Propionibacteria are non-spore forming, anaerobic to aero-tolerant, mesophilic, gram-positive rods with optimum temperature of 30° C. They ferment lactate to propionic acid, carbon dioxide and other compounds thus they are responsible for large holes known as eye-formation and flavour production in Swiss cheeses. Propionibacterium *freundenreichii subsp freundenreichii* and *Prop.freudenreichi* subsp *shermanii* are common species used as starter culture in cheese industry.

Coryneform bacteria: Coryneform bacteria are a group of irregular, non-spore forming, gram–positive rods, often found growing on the surface of surface-ripened cheese. This group includes *Bravibacterium, Arthrobacter, Microbacterium, Aureobacterium, Brachybacterium, Rhodococcus* and *Corynebacterium.* These microorganisms are responsible for the viscous, red-orange surface (smear), on surface-ripened cheese varieties. They survive high salt conditions and produce various proteolytic enzymes. Their presence in large numbers causes a slimy rind, discoloured appearance and undesirable flavour in cheese. Currently, the genus *Bravibacterium* is restricted to four species: *Brev. linens, Brev. iodiodinum, Brev. casei,* and *epidermis. Corynebacterium* found in dairy products include *C. ammoniagenes* and *C. variabilis.* The habitats of coryneform bacteria are cheese and human skin. Bravibacteria can grow in presence of high concentration of salt (8-15 %). They do not utilize lactose or citrate, rather they are highly proteolytic, an ability which enables them to produce strong flavour in surface ripened cheese. *Bravibacterium linen* is a common species.

Enterococci: Enterococcus spp are often present in significant numbers in traditional cultures. Enterococci are rapid acid producers, can grow both at 10° and 45° C and in 6.5% salt solution and pH 9.6. Some species are also considered probiotic. Though they possess ideal properties yet their use as starter is disputable due to their faecal origin. Common species are: *Enterococcus faecalis* and *Enterococcus faecium.*

Bifidobacteria: Bifidobacteria are inhabitants of the intestinal tract, which are added to dairy products for probiotic applications. They are non-spore forming, gram-positive, catalase negative, non-motile rods. Though they ferment lactose into lactate and acetate they are not considered as true lactic acid bacteria and rather belong to Actenomycetes group. They grow best at 37-41°C. About two dozen species of Bifidobacteria have been identified. In the manufacture of fermented milks, *Bif. bifidum, Bif. longum* and *Bif. breve* are commonly used in combination with other lactic acid bacteria owing to their slow acid production. Bifidobacteria have been considered as probiotics (organisms that exhibit beneficial effects on health of the host when they are ingested). As a result, a variety of fermented milk products including fermented milks, fermented milk beverages, buttermilk, sour cream, fresh cheese and baby foods have been developed.

Pediococci: Pediococci are the atypical example of only lactic acid bacteria which divide in two planes and form a group of four cells called as tetrads. This genus is homofermenter and comprises 8 species out of which two, *Pediococcus pentosaceus* and *P. acidilactici* are used in association with other lactic acid bacteria as starter organisms. Pediococcus species are salt-tolerant members of the family *Streptococcaceae*, which usually grow as tetrads of cells. Most species can grow at 4-6.5% NaCl. They produce acetic acid and small amounts of lactic acid when growing aerobically and mostly lactic acid when growing anaerobically.

Micrococci: Micrococcus spp are the predominant microorganisms found in raw milk drawn aseptically from the udder. They are constituents of the teat skin and have also been isolated from soil, water and dust. Micrococcus species have proteolytic, lipolytic and esterase activities, which make them important in the ripening of various cheeses especially those that are surface ripened.

Moulds: *Penicillium* species are widely distributed in the environment. The genus includes four subgenera. The surface of soft white cheese can be colonized by *P. camemberti* to produce many different varieties such as Brie and Camembert. This mould produces a white layer of the mycelium on the cheese surface, while spores (candida) are embedded in the curd. The mould metabolises some of lactic acid thereby raising the pH, which allows growth of *Brev. linens* and other ripening microflora. In blue veined cheese varieties, *P. roqueforti* (blue mould) is used in cheese ripening. *Penicillium roqueforti* has a relatively low oxygen requirement for growth (<4.2%) and tolerates 6-10% salt. Both *P. camemberti* and *P. roqueforti* produce lipolytic and proteolytic enzymes. They produce additional compounds that give cheese its distinctive flavour and aroma. *Penicillium casei* is similar to *P. roqueforti* and is found in Swiss cheese. *Penicillium nalgiovense* (Lava), another white mould, tolerates up to 8% salt and is used in some cheese varieties.

Aspergillus niger and *A. awamori* produce lipase and contribute to the flavour of some cheese varieities. *Geotrichum candidum* is often found in raw milk, on milking and dairy processing equipment and on the surface of ripened cheese. It can be used in starter cultures for Brie and Camembert cheese when combined with *Penicillium* species. *Rhizomucor miehei* and *Rm. pusillus* produce chymosin-like enzymes, which are used in cheese manufacture.

Yeasts: *Saccharomyces* species are ascosporogenous yeasts with a capability for vigorous anaerobic or semi-anaerobic fermentation of sugar to produce ethanol and carbon dioxide. None of them utilizes lactose. *Saccharomyces cerevisiae* is the most important species and can be found on the surface of mould-ripened cheeses. *Saccharomyces cerevisiae* metabolises hexoses, lactic acid and other organic acids. Their optimum pH for growth is 4.5-6.5. Oxygen is important to maintain viability but they survive under microaerophilic conditions.

Kluyveromyces marxianus and *K. lactis* can ferment lactose and produce various hydrolytic enzymes. *Kluyveromyces* species are often isolated from Nordic fermented milks. They produce lactase, which can be used to reduce the lactose content of milk and assist digestion of milk by lactose maldigesters.

Debaryomyces species are isolated from soil, water and plants. *Debaryomyces hansenii* is involved in the ripening of mould-ripened soft cheeses. It tolerates high salt concentrations, utilizes lactic acid, produces protease and lipase and grows well at low temperature. *Candida kefyr* is present in the microflora of the fermented milk kefir.

4.2. Spoilage Microorganisms

Spoilage of milk and milk products is manifested as off-flavours and odours and changes in texture and appearance. The most important spoilage microorganisms of milk and milk products are the gram-negative, rod-shaped bacteria (Coliforms and Pseudomonas), gram-positive, spore forming bacteria (Bacillus and Clostridium), lactic acid bacteria, coryneform group, yeasts and moulds.

Coliforms: Coliform bacteria are gram negative, non-spore forming, coccobacilli (short rods), facultative anaerobes with an optimum temperature of 30-37° C. They are found in intestine, soil, manure, contaminated water and on plants. Common species are *Escherechia coli, Enterobacter aerogene, Klebsiella, Proteus, Serratia* and *Citrobacter.* They ferment lactose to lactic acid, other organic acids, carbon dioxide and hydrogen and also bring about proteolysis. Coliforms have been held responsible for excessive gas production in early stage of cheese making (early gas) resulting into development of textural defects and also manifests of flavour defects due to proteolysis. Approximately 10^7 cfu / g of coliform is needed for a gassy defect to be noticed. Klebsiella (*Kl. pneumoniae* and *Kl. oxytoca*) and *Enterobacter aerogenese* are responsible for gas formation in cheese which can lead to swelling of the package. The metabolism of the coli bacteria ceases at pH just below 6.0. This explains their activity at an early stage of fermentation. Other types of spoilage include acid production, slime production in Cottage cheese, bitter flavours and grassy, unclean, medicinal or faecal odours. Cheese varieties in which acid production is delayed are more susceptible to coliform growth. *Serratia marcescens* produces proteolytic enzymes that might cause gelation of the UHT milk. In addition, they produce methanethiol in Cheddar cheese. Coliforms are relatively heat labile and are destroyed by pasteurization. They are used as test organisms for routine bacteriological quality in dairy industry. Their presence indicates post-pasteurization contamination and poor hygienic conditions of dairy plant.

Psychrotrophic bacteria: Most psychrotrophic bacteria present in raw milk belong to the family Pseudomonadaceae, which includes gram-negative, non-spore forming and non-fermentative aerobic rods. *Pseudomonas fluorescens* is the most commonly isolated species in milk with *Ps.fragi* and *Ps. putida* being of less importance. Soil, water, animals and plant materials are natural habitat of psychrotrophic bacteria found in milk. Unable to utilize carbohydrates, they metabolize fat and protein as energy source. Contaminated milk equipment and air provide an additional source of contamination, especially after processing. As little as 1 cfu / ml of raw milk may be enough to spoil milk during cold storage within 5 days. Defects associated with the growth of these organisms in milk include development of bitter and fruity off-flavours. Although psychrophilic, gram-negative bacteria are not heat-resistant, they produce heat-stable extracellular proteolytic and lipolytic enzymes that can spoil heat-treated products. Other spoilage gram-negative rods include *Acinetobacter, Psychrobacter, Flavobacterium, Shevanella putrefaciens* and *Alcaligenes* spp.

Spore-forming Bacteria: Two genera in this group are associated with milk: Bacillus and Clostridium. They are unique spoilage microorganisms because of their ability to form heat- and chemical-resistant spores and their ability to grow over a wide temperature range (0-75° C). Their main habitat is soil, but they can be also found in water, air, fodder and feed.

Bacillus: Bacillus genus includes gram-positive, aerobic, sporogenous, catalase positive rods. They may be psychrophilic, mesophilic but majority of them are thermophilic. They form spores within the cells (endospores) to survive adverse conditions of growth and these spores are not destroyed by ordinary heat treatments but rather are activated and consequently germinate into ordinary vegetative cells. They are actively proteolytic and can spoil the milk by coagulation of milk proteins. Some species are considered pathogenic in nature. Some of the common species are: *Bacillus cereus, B.subtilis, B. stearothermophilus, B.licheniformis, B.circulans and B.polymyxa.*

One potentially pathogenic bacterium in raw milk, *B. cereus,* can be a significant spoilage agent due to the ability of its spores to survive pasteurization and the ability of some strains to proliferate in pasteurized milk at refrigeration temperature. This bacterium can produce enzymes such as proteinase which hydrolyses casein to produce an intensely bitter flavour, and phospholipase, which hydrolyses phospholipids of the milk fat globule membrane and causes instability of the fat emulsion. In unhomogenized milk, this can cause the defect known as bitty cream, but this is not observed in homogenized milk. *B. cereus* in milk seldom causes food poisoning, as the contaminated product develops a strong, unacceptable flavour, and also because toxigenic strains are seldom psychrotrophic. In addition large numbers of this bacterium are required to produce food poisoning. It has been reported that most outbreaks of *B. cereus* poisoning were caused by contamination levels of at least 10^6 cfu/g. *B. cereus* causes defects in high temperature treated milk and cream including sweet curdling (curd formation with no acid production).

B. subtilis survives pasteurization, milk concentration and UHT treatment and produces a variety of enzymes that are capable of hydrolyzing casein and polysaccharides. *B.licheniformis* is a common cause of spoilage in UHT and pasteurized milk. *B. stearothermophilus* is the most heat-resistant Bacillus species, surviving canning and so causing flat, sour spoilage and sweet curdling defects. It is also used to detect antibiotics in milk. *B. coagulans* has also been implicated in UHT and concentrated milk spoilage; it also produces chymosin-like enzymes, which causes sweet curdling. *B. circulans* is a psychrotrophic bacterium, which causes an acid defect in asepically packaged heat-treated milk. *B. marcerans* causes a flat sour defect in canned condensed milk.

Clostridia: Clostridia also known as Butyric Acid Bacteria due to their ability to produce butyric acid, are very common in nature. They are found in soil, on plants and in manure *etc*, and therefore, easily find their way in milk. Poorly stored silage and fodder can be a potent source of contamination of milk with these bacteria at farm, and hence their count is higher in winter when silage feeding is more common. They are anaerobic spore forming bacteria. On the basis of optimum temperature, they can be classified as below:

a) Psychrophile – *Cl. putrefaciens*

b) *Mesophile – Cl. sporogens*

c) *Thermophile – Cl. thermsaccharolyticum*

Many species actively ferment carbohydrates with the production of butyric acid and gases (CO_2 and H_2). Lactose fermenting butyric acid bacteria produce butyric acid during first few weeks of manufacture of cheese. If fermentation occurs later on, it is caused by butyric acid bacteria which ferment lactate. *Cl. butyricum* being lactose and lactate fermenter causes both early and late butyric acid fermentation while *Cl. tyrobutyricm* being lactate fermenter causes late fermentation. Being heat resistant, they can not be destroyed by pasteurization. Their growth can be inhibited by addition of potassium nitrate. However, this practice is prohibited in some countries on account of presumed risk of carcinogens. Alternative methods include bactofugation, microfiltration and use of lysozyme.

Butyric acid bacteria do not grow well in milk, which contains oxygen, but thrive in cheese where more anaerobic condition prevails. *Clostridium* species are important spoilage microorganisms in cheese and canned milk products. Late blowing of some cheese varieties that have a relatively high pH, a high moisture content and a low interior salt content such as Emmental, Gouda and Edam is caused by these microorganisms. *Clostridium tyrobutyricm* and, occasionally, *Cl. sporogenes* and *Cl. butyricum* are involved. These clostridia produce carbon dioxide, hydrogen gas and butyric and acetic acids. The cheese acquires a fermented, ragged texture and a sweetish taste of butyric acid.

Lactic Acid Bacteria and Related Microorganisms: Although lactic acid bacteria are considered beneficial, however, some of the species may cause souring, off-flavour development and texture defects (ropiness, curdling) in milk and milk products. Heterofermentative lactobacilli such as *Lb. brevis* and *Lb. casei* subsp. *pseudoplantarum* cause an open texture in Cheddar and Mozzarella cheese due to gas production. Lactobacilli also convert L (+) - lactate to D (-) - lactate, which reacts with calcium to form calcium lactate, which appears as white insoluble crystal in ripened Cheddar and other cheeses. Salt tolerant lactobacilli produce phenolic and putrid sulphide-like flavours during ripening. *Lb. casei* subsp. *casei* causes a soft body in Mozzarella cheese due to proteolysis. *Lb. delbrueckii* subsp. *bulgaricus* produces a pink discolouration in Italian cheese. *Lb casei* species produce a phenolic flavour in Cheddar cheese.

Lactococcus lactis is commonly used as a starter culture for cheese and for fermented milks. These strains are carefully selected so that they do not produce off-flavours or other defects. Wild strains of lactococci often contaminate raw milk, and if the milk is not kept sufficiently cold they will produce sourness and other off-flavours and odours. One variant, *Lc. lactis* subsp. *lactis* var. *maltigenes,* produces a malty flavour in fluid milk due to the production of 3-methylbutanal. Wild strains of lactococci may also contaminate cheeses and grow during manufacture and ageing. Some of these strains produce fruity flavours due to the production of esters such as ethyl hexanoate and ethyl butyrate.

***Propionibacterium* spp.:** Pigmented strains of *Propionibacterium* cause pink spots in Swiss cheese.

***Enterococcus* spp.:** *Enterococcus faecalis, Ec.faecium* and *Ec. durans* are part of the normal microflora of many cheeses and are sometimes used as starter cultures. Some strains produce undesirable flavours and high levels of amines during cheese ripening.

Micrococcus* spp:* Some strains of *Micrococcus* species are able to survive pasteurization, but spoilage of heat-treated products is also caused by postprocess contamination. *Micrococcus* species can produce swelling in UHT milk packs and have the ability to grow on some cheese varieties. Their growth may be either beneficial or detrimental to cheese flavour, depending on the cheese variety and strains involved.

Putrefaction bacteria: Putrefaction bacteria produce protein-splitting enzymes. They can therefore breakdown proteins all the way to ammonia. This type of break down is known as putrefaction. Some of them are used in dairy processing, but most of them cause trouble.

The category of putrefaction bacteria comprises a very large number of species, both cocci and bacilli, which grow both aerobically and anaerobically. They enter the milk from manure, fodder and water. Many of them also produce the enzyme lipase, which means that they also breakdown fat.

Brevibacterium linens is a putrefaction bacteria which forms a yellowish-red coating on cheese. On the surface of Port Salute cheese it breaks down protein during the ripening period and contributes to the aroma. Unlike many other microorganisms it is highly resistant to salt.

Some unwanted putrefaction bacteria can be found in milk and milk products. One is Pseudomonas fluorescens, normally found in contaminated water and soil. It produces lipase, and therefore is undesirable in butter, which is easily contaminated with this bacterium through rinsing water of poor quality.

Apart from lipase, some unwanted putrefaction bacteria produce a type of rennet-like enzyme. They can therefore coagulate milk without souring (sweet coagulation). In the summer and autumn it sometimes happens that the milk from the odd supplier is heavily infected by these bacteria.

A very typical gas producer is the mobile, spore-forming, anaerobic bacillus Clostridium putrefaciens. It can be found in fermented fodder, water, soil, and also in the intestines. Milk is easily infected by this bacterium or its spores. It can produce a very powerful fermentation in cheese (stinky cheese).

Yeasts: The presence of large numbers of yeasts on a cheese surface may result in a slimy rind, discoloured appearance and undesirable flavours. Nonlactose-fermenting *Saccharomyces* produce gas in fruit yoghurt. Their source is usually a contaminated processing plant environment or unpasterurised fruits. *Saccharomyces cerevisiae* can spoil sweetened and acid dairy products.

Kluyveromyces marxianus var. *lactis, K. marxianus* var. *marxianus, Debaryomyces hansenii* and *Yarrowia lipolytica* spoil acidified refrigerated dairy products such as yoghurt. *Yarrowia lipolytica* does not utilize lactose but metabolises fat, protein and organic acids, allowing it to spoil high-fat products such as butter and cream. It liberates amino and fatty acids and usually causes off-odours and softening of cheese curd. In addition, it produces melanin pigment from tyrosine and causes discolouration of cheese surfaces.

Candida species are potential dairy spoilage organisms because of their ability to digest casein and fat, grow at storage temperatures, and ferment lactose and sucrose. They form surface slime on cream cheese. In yoghurt, they cause yeasty and bitter flavours and gassy texture. The important spoilage species in cheese is *Can. famata* and in yoghurt *Can.famata, Can. versatilis* and *Can. lusitaniae.*

Moulds: *Mucor, Rhizopus, Penicillium* and *Aspergillus* grow at the yoghurt/air interface of undisturbed packages. One mould spore can spoil a carton of yoghurt by producing a visible colony. Moulds also produce off-flavours in contaminated dairy products. *Scopulariopsis brevicaulis* causes odour defects in mould-ripened cheese. *Sporendonema sebi* grows on sweet condensed milk forming discrete colonies (mould buttons). *Geotrichum* grows on most dairy products, especially cheese and butter. Cheese varieties with low salt content are often spoiled by *Mucor* species.

4.3. Pathogenic Microorganisms

Even if produced under highly hygienic conditions, raw milk contains a heterogeneous population of bacteria, some of which are pathogenic and others which can cause spoilage during milk storage. Fortunately, pathogens are generally not determinants of the shelf life of thermally treated milk and dairy products. This is due to their low number in raw milk, their inability to grow at refrigeration temperatures, and their destruction by pasteurization.

The presence of pathogenic bacteria in milk has been a matter of public health concern since the early days of the dairy industry. From the turn of the century to 1940, numerous health hazards were associated with ingesting raw milk and milk products prepared from raw milk. Typhoid fever, the primary milk-borne disease during this period, accounted for 50-80% of all milk related illnesses, with scarlet fever being responsible for an additional 14-27% of the milk –borne infections (Bryan, 1983). Both of these diseases were frequently fatal because suitable treatments such as with antibiotics were unavailable. The high incidence of milk-borne typhoid and scarlet fever, coupled with sporadic dairy-related outbreaks of diphtheria, poliomyelitis, and tuberculosis, soon confirmed the need for increased pasteurization, a process that was used only sporadically during the 1920s and 1930s. After World War II, almost universal adoption of pasteurization, coupled with modernization of milk production practices emphasizing improved farm and dairy factory sanitation, udder health, herd inspection, cooling, handling, and storage of milk have, for all practical purposes eliminated the threat of these diseases, with the last case of milk-borne typhoid fever, scarlet fever, and diphtheria in the United States being reported more than 40 years ago.

Raw milk may contain microorganisms that are pathogenic to humans, and their source may lie either within or out side udder. Historically, the most serious human diseases disseminated by the consumption of contaminated raw milk are tuberculosis and brucellosis. In both diseases, the causative organisms that may be excreted in milk from infected animals are *Mycobacterium bovis* or *M. tuberculosis* and *Brucella abortus, B. melitensis, or B suis*. Often with *Brucella* infections, there is a little change in the milk or udder, but, in the case of tuberculosis mastitis, a pronounced and characteristic change in the milk and udder is observed. In many parts of the world, these diseases have been eradicated from cattle and no longer pose a hazard to human health.

Pathogenic bacteria also may be present in raw milk as a direct consequence of udder disease. Among the organisms commonly producing mastitis, *Streptococcus agalactiae*, *Staphylococcus aureus*, and *Escherichia coli* are pathogens known to humans. *Streptococcus agalactiae* can initiate a variety of clinical conditions, the most serious of which are bacterimia and meningitis of newborns, which are potentially fatal to infected infants.

Pathogenic bacteria are those capable of causing infection or intoxication. The growth of pathogens in milk is inhibited by cooling and the growth of nonpathogenic competing microorganisms. Many pathogens, such as *Mycobacterium tuberculosis* and Brucella species, grow very slowly in milk and others, such as viruses, do not multiply at all. Therefore, the threat associated with their presence in milk will depend on the initial load of milk contamination. Although the potential hazard of pathogens has been minimized by modern milk production and technological practices, disease outbreaks caused by *Listeria monocytogenese, Compylobacter jejuni, Yersinia enterocolitica* and *Escherichia coli* have occurred these days.

The pathogenic organisms may be derived chiefly from: a) dairy animals, b) human handlers, and c) environment. The health of dairy animals is a very important consideration because a number of diseases of cattle including Brucellosis, Q fever, Salmonellosis, Staphylococcal and Streptococcal infections and foot and mouth disease (FMD) virus may be transmitted to the man through the consumption of milk. The organisms of most of these diseases may be transmitted to milk either directly from the udder or indirectly through the infected body discharges that may drop, splash or be blown into milk. The diseased persons may transmit diseases like typhoid fever, scarlet fever, diphtheria, septic soar throat, infantile diarrhoea by contaminated hands, or by coughing, sneezing and talking. Dairy and farm environment may also introduce a variety of pathogens into milk and milk products at different stages of production and processing. Some common air-borne pathogens include: Group A streptococci, Corynebacterium diphtheriae, Mycobacterium tuberculosis, Coxiella burnetii, and some viruses of respiratory origin. Water, fodder and unhygienic conditions at farm and plant level may also contribute pathogens in milk.

Some of the selected groups of pathogens are briefly described as below:

***Staphylococcus* spp**: Staphylococcal spp are nonmotile, nonsporeforming, gram-positive and catalase-positive cocci. They grow well in media containing 10% NaCl and produce protease, lipase and esterases. Staphylococcus aureus is the most important species of this genus associated with milk. It produces heat- stable enterotoxins that are responsible for food poisoning. Its natural habitat includes the skin and mucous membranes of mammals. Most contamination occurs during milking and originates with the cow. Although the presence of St. aureus in milk is difficult to prevent, appropriate cleaning and sanitation of the cow and milking equipment controls initial numbers and cooling the milk prevents growth and toxin production.

***Streptococcus* spp:** Sreptococcus pyogenes is pathogenic to humans and some animals. It resists phagocytosis and produces an erythrogenic toxin and causes scarlet fever. St. agalactiae belongs to group B streptococci and is an important agent of bovine mastitis in some countries and a cause of diseases in humans. The gastrointestinal tract is the main human reservoir. Streptococcus dysgalactiae belongs to Lancefield group C streptococci. It is found mainly in mastitic bovine udders. Streptococcus uberis is found in the lips and skin of cows, udder tissue and milk. It is the main cause of mastitis in some countries, especially during the winter. St. zooepidemicus causes septicaemia and mastitis in cows and food poisoning in humans.

Campylobacter jejuni: *Campylobacter jejuni* is a common cause of human gastroenteritis. It is a gram-negative, spirally curved, slender, motile rod, microaerophilic and is found in food, faeces and water. Although it does not grow in milk, the consumption of fresh raw milk has caused numerous outbreaks of gastroenteritis.

***Yersinia* spp:** The genus *Yersinia* belongs to the family Enterobacteriacae. Members of this genus are gram-negative, motile rods, facultatively anaerobic at 28-29°C but strictly aerobic at 37°C, which can grow at 2-4°C. *Yersinia enterocolitica* is the only species of importance in milk. The most common source of contamination is the rinsing water used at the farm. *Yersinia* species grow well in milk and cause an enteric infection that mimics appendicitis.

***Salmonella* spp**: The genus *Salmonella* (family Enterobacteriacae) consists of small, gram-negative, non-spore forming rods. Most strains are motile. The primary habitat is the intestinal tract. Cows suffering from salmonellosis can excrete large numbers of salmonellae in their faeces and occasionally directly into milk. Milk can be contaminated with *Salmonella* from faeces, humans, water and dust. Many outbreaks of salmonellosis have been attributed to milk and milk products. Unlike staphylococcal food poisoning, the ingestion of viable cells of *Salmonella* is necessary for salmonellosis. Growth of *Salmonella* in milk is not necessary as ingestion of only a few cells can cause the disease.

Escherichia coli: Escherichia coli is a member of the family Enterobacteriacae. It is a gram-negative rod, facultatively anaerobic and ferments lactose. Four categories of pathogenic *E.coli* are recognized: enteropathogenic, enterotoxigenic, enteroinvasive and enterohaemorrhagic. Enterotoxigenic *E. coli* produces enterotoxins that cause diarrhoea.Humans are the main reservoir. To cause diarrhoea, sufficient numbers of toxigenic *E coli* must be ingested and adhere to the small intestine. In recent years, enterohaemorrhagic *E coli,* mainly *E. coli* O157:H7, have caused milk- borne illness. These pathogens cause haemorrhagic colitis (bloody diarrhoea), an illness that can lead to renal failure in children. The dairy cow gut is a reservoir for *E coli* O157: H7. Haemorrhagic strains of *E. coli* do not ferment sorbitol and the incubation temperature used to detect faecal coliforms (44-45°C) will not allow *E. coli* O157:H7 to grow. The strain of E.coliO157:H_7, a food-borne pathogen of international importance, is unable to grow in pasteurized milk at temperatures below 10° C. In addition, it is really destroyed by pasteurization, and hence consumption of pasteurized milk does not pose a significant risk for this pathogen.

***Listeria* spp:** Within the genus *Listeria*, only *Li. monocytogenes* and *Li. ivanovii* are considered virulent with *Li. monocytogenes* being the only species of public health concern. *Listeria innocua* is the most frequently encountered nonpathogenic *Listeria* species. *Listeria monocytogenes* is a gram-positive, short rod with rounded ends that occurs singly, in parallel or in V- shapes. It grows slowly in milk at refrigeration temperature. *Listeria monocytogenes* causes mastitis and abortion in animals. In humans, it causes miscarriages and meningitis in its severe form and flu-like symptoms in its mild form. Raw milk can be contaminated from faeces, cows suffering from mastitis, poor quality silage and milking equipments. It produces hemolysin (hemolysis) and an endotoxin that causes meningoencephalitis. Although *L. monocytogenes* is more heat tolerant than most other non-spore-forming pathogens, pasteurization should result in its total destruction; however, some evidence exists of it being linked to a serious food poisoning incident involving pasteurized milk in the U.S. during 1983 (Ryser, 1998).

***Mycobacterium* spp:** *Mycobacterium tuberculosis* is a slender, straight or slightly rod shaped, nonmotile, nonspore-forming, aerobic and acid fast bacterium. It is one of the most heat–resistant pathogenic microorganisms likely to be present in milk. *Mycobacterium tuberculosis* may gain access to milk from infected animals through milk secretion and faecal contamination or from milkers and other environmental sources. The organism does not multiply in milk but survives in unpasteurized milk and milk products.

Mycobacterium paratuberculosis causes the infection commonly known as Johne's disease. Detectable numbers of this organism have been reported In the milk of both clinically affected and asymptomatic cattle. Pasteurization inactivates *Mycobacterium paratuberculosis* when present at levels associated with milk from asymptomatic cattle. It is unknown whether this microorganism is pathogenic for man.

Mycobacterium bovis causes infection in animals and humans. Compared with *Mb. tuberculosis,* growth of *M. bovis* is less luxuriant and it adapts to aerobic growth after repeated subculturing. Contaminated milk, faeces, soil and water are the main sources of infection.

***Brucella* spp:** *Brucella* species are Gram-negative, aerobic, short rods that do not ferment carbohydrates. They survive well in milk and dairy products and are pathogenic to humans and animals. The most important causes of brucellosis in milk are *Br. abortus* and *Br. Melitensis.*)

***Coxiella burnetii*:** *Coxiella burnetii* is a rickettsia (family Rickettsiaceae), which causes Q fever in humans. Ricketssiae are obligate intracellular parasites. *Coxiella burnetti* is a small pleomorphic, sometimes filamentous, non- motile rod that produces a capsule like structure. It is highly resistant to chemical and physical disinfectants and is the most heat resistant pathogen found in milk.

***Clostridium* spp:** Clostridia are Gram-positive, sporeforming rods, which are usually found in sediments, the intestinal tract of humans and animals, soil, dust, faeces and silage. They are anerobic and often poisoned by atmospheric oxygen unless in the spore form.

Clostridium perfringes causes food poisoning and gas gangrene in man and a variety of disease in animals. Milk and milk products provide a ready medium for transmission of *Cl. Perfringes.* Vegetative cells sporulate in the gut and release exterotoxin, which is responsible for symptoms such as profuse diarrhoea, sudden acute inflammation of the abdomen and severe abdominal pain. Large numbers of cells must be consumed for illness to occur.

Botulism is an intoxication attacking the nervous system caused by ingestion of toxins produced by *Cl. Botulinum.* Very low levels (<1 spore ml^{-1}) of these organisms are common in milk. They do not germinate or grow in raw or pasteurized milk, but cheese and cheese products can support growth if they are not sufficiently acidic.

***Klebsiella pneumoniae*:** *Klebsiella pneumoniae* belongs to the family Enterobacteriaceae and is an agent for pneumonia, urinary tract infection and gastroenteritis and mastitis. It is present in animal bedding and water.

***Serratia* spp:** *Serratia* species are Gram-negative, facultative, anaerobic rods of the family Enterobacteriaceae. They are distributed in soil, air, water and plants. Some strains produce haemolysins and infected animals produce contaminated milk. Their presence in pasteurized dairy products indicates poor sanitation practices since they are heat sensitive. *Serratia marcescens* is the most important species and causes mastitis.

***Proteus* spp:** *Proteus* species are Gram-negative, non-sporeforming rods belonging to the family Enterobacteriaceae. They are commonly found in the faeces of humans and animals, soil and plants. They frequently cause a variety of infections in humans, especially urinary tract infections. *Proteus mirabilis* is the most common species followed by *Pr. vulgaris* and *Pr. penneri.*

Moulds and Yeasts: Many different genera of moulds such as *Aspergillus, Pennicilium* and *Fusarium* produce mycotoxins in milk and dairy products. Mycotoxins are secondary metabolites that are acutely toxic, carcinogenic, emetic, oestrogenic, hallucinogenic, mutagenic of teratogenic. *Aspergillus flavus* and some other *Aspergillus* species produce aflatoxins when growing on cheeses. Some strains of *Geotrichum* might cause infection in humans. *Candida albicans* is pathogenic to humans and animals.

Viruses: Viruses are genetic elements that replicate inside cells and also have an extracellular nonreplicating state. Replication of the virus often destroys the host cell causing illness. The extracellular form of the virus is a submicroscopic particle and can be transmitted between hosts. Viruses do not multiply in milk but some may survive for long periods. Viruses can be infective at very low doses and most that are found in milk produce gastroenteritis and originate with the cow. Viruses in milk are inactivated by pasteurization.

Rotaviruses can produce severe diarrhoeal illnesses. Milk may be a vector for this virus but detection in raw milk is prevented by the presence of antiviral antibodies (immunoglobulins; IgG). The antibody / virus complex is dissociated in the highly acidic conditions of the stomach.

Hepatitis A virus enters milk through faecal contamination or polluted water. This virus causes symptoms of fever, vomiting, nausea and abdominal discomfort. The virus eventually affects the liver, causing enlargement and jaundice.

Poliovirus causes the acute infections disease poliomyelitis, which is characterized by fever, vomiting and headache. The poliovirus might infect the central nervous system and cause paralysis. It can be transmitted to milk through faecal contamination.

Protozoa: *Toxoplasma gondii* is a parasite of humans and many warm-blooded animals, especially dairy goats. Infection occurs as a result of ingestion of foods or water contaminated with oocysts. Contaminated milk is considered a potential source of human toxoplasmosis.

Cryptosporidiosis is an infection caused by *Cryptosporidium muris* and *Cr. parvum*. Diarrhoea is the primary symptom of infection. Cows can shed *Cr. muris* oocysts in their faeces, which may lead to milk contamination. Drinking water is the most common vehicle for transmission of this disease.

Entamoeba histolytica is a protozoan that causes amoebiasis, the third most common cause of death by parasites in the world. Transmission occurs via ingestion of cysts in contaminated foods or water or through poor personal hygiene.

Giardia intestinalis is a flagellated protozoan that inhabits tracts of humans and animals. Cysts survive well in the environment and are transmitted via contaminated hands, drinking water and food contaminated with faeces.

4.4. Microbial Population Dynamics in Milk

Microbial population in milk are continually changing and interacting with the milk components and with each other. The initial microbial population of raw milk is affected by factors such as equipment and animal cleanliness, season, feed and cow health. The initial microflora of good quality milk consists mainly of organisms found within the udder and of the normal teat skin flora. These microorganisms include nonthermoduric micrococci and streptococci, which do not grow well at low temperatures. Pathogens will predominate in milk from mastitic cows. Seasonal factors include feed source and housing, both of which influence the level of bacterial spores in milk. Psychrotrophic bacteria (those that grow at refrigeration temperatures) are at low or even undetectable levels in the best quality fresh raw milk. They originate from the water and milking equipment. After collection, milk is cooled, which initiates a change in microbial population from Gram-positive rods and cocci, which do not grow, to Gram-negative rods, which can grow slowly at low temperatures. These Gram-negative rods are primarily Pseudomonas sp and are capable of causing various off-flavours when population exceeds 10^6 cells/ml.

When raw milk is not kept cold, lactic acid bacteria will grow. The resulting increase in acidity will inhibit growth of many other microorganisms including sporeforming Bacillus and Clostridium sp, and Gram-negative Pseudomonas species and coliforms. Growth of lactic acid bacteria is rapid at 20° C, slows as the temperature decreases. Many strains of lactic acid bacteria produce bacteriocins, which inhibit other lactic acid bacteria as well as some pathogens such as *Listeria* and *E. coli.*

Both the lactic acid bacteria and the psychrotrophic bacteria that grow in raw milk are heat sensitive, so when milk is pasteurized, microorganisms that have previously grown in the product are greatly reduced in number. The surviving microflora consists mainly of sporeforming bacteria, micrococci and lactobacilli. Pasteurized milk that is not recontaminated with the microorganisms will often keep at refrigeration temperature for 3 weeks or longer, because the surviving microorganisms grow slowly or not at all in the cold milk. Spoilage may occur more rapidly if significant amounts psychrotrophic *B. cereus* are present in the raw milk. Most pasteurized milk is recontaminated with low numbers of psychrotrophic bacteria resulting in shorter shelf life.

Developments of closed milking systems, use of bulk tanks to store and transport raw milk and improvement in refrigeration systems have caused the microflora naturally present in raw milk to change from predominantly gram-positive, acid producing bacteria to gram-negative, psychrotrophic microorganisms chiefly species of genus pseudomonas.

Types of Microflora: Microorganisms found in milk can also be described according to their optimum temperature for growth and heat resistance. This is a very practical consideration since milk is preserved by employing low temperatures to prevent changes due to microbial activity and by high temperatures to reduce microbial population and destroy pathogens. All the four types of microorganisms i.e. mesophilic, thermoduric, thermophilic and psychrophilic are found in milk.

1. **Mesophilic:** The microorganisms growing optimally at 30- 32°C are called as mesophilic. The most important mesophilic bacteria are streptococci, lactobacilli and coliforms, which produce acid and gas and off flavours. Other microorganisms in this group are Micrococci, Corynebacterium spp, Mycobacterium spp, yeasts and moulds, *etc.* They are killed in the pasteurization.

2. **Thermoduric**: Thermoduric microorganisms are those which survive pasteurization conditions but do not grow at pasteurization temperature. Most of them do not multiply well at ambient temperatures. The most common thermoduric bacteria are found in the genera Microbacterium, Corynebacterium, Micrococcus, Streptococcus and Bacillus. Excessive numbers of thermoduric bacteria in milk make it difficult to meet the grading standard.

3. **Thermophilic**: Thermophilic bacteria grow well at the temperature used in pasteurization, specially when the low temperature holding method is followed. These bacteria can grow at 55°C and most of them have an upper limit of growth at about 70° C. Although some facultative thermophiles may grow at 37°C or lower in standard plate count (SPC) analysis, the standard method of enumerating this group of organisms is to incubate agar plates at 55°C. Most thermophilic forms are found in two genera, Bacillus and Clostridium.

4. **Psychrophilic:** Psychrophilic bacteria are those which are able to grow at refrigeration temperatures (2-7°C) regardless of their optimum growth temperature. Usually the term 'psychrophilic' is used for organisms that have an optimum temperature below 20° C. In the psychrophilic microflora of milk and milk products, very few are classical psychrophiles and majority of them are mesophilic (optimum temperature: 20-32°C) in nature. They produce a wide variety of spoilage defects. The defects may result in the production of

many "off" flavours and odours. The most commonly encountered psychrophilic bacteria are members of the genera Pseudomonas, Achromobacter, Vibrio, Flavobacterium and Alcaligenes, They arc killed in the pasteurization process, but are sometimes found in pasteurized milk. The contamination takes place after pasteurization from equipment, cans, bottles, and water.

The psychrotrophic bacteria detected (5-7°C in 7 to 10 days) in raw milk belong to two broad categories, viz, gram-negative rods and gram-positive rods or cocci. The psychrotrophic gram-negative bacteria belong to different genera, namely *Pseudomonas, Acinetobacter ,Flavobacterium, Alcaligenes and Enterobacter (coliforms).* Among these, Pseudomanas constitute about half of the total gram-negative rods. The gram-negative rods or cocci consist of the following bacteria: *Bacillus* spp (spores), e.g., *B. coagulans, B. circulans* and *B. subtilis, Arthrobacter* spp and *Streptococcus* spp (Yadav, *et al.*, 1993)

4.5. Effect of Processing on the Microbiology of Milk

The principal milk processing operations include separation and clarification, homogenization, pasteurization, sterilization, chilling and packaging. Contamination with microorganisms is minimal to many thousands, depending upon whether the equipment is properly cleaned and sanitized. Vigorous agitation, such as with the use of pumps, may increase the number of microorganisms in milk by disrupting bacterial clumps into individual cells, each of which can give rise to a colony in plate count procedure. Generally, water supplies do not contain sufficient chlorine to destroy the gram-negative bacteria. Therefore, equipment washed with such water must be sanitized before use to control these bacteria.

During separation, many microorganisms are physically removed from milk and deposited along with somatic cells and other particulate matter in the slime that contains large number of microorganisms.

The heat treatment of milk is the key unit operation to control the microbial quality of milk. The scientific basis for the specific conditions used for heat treating milk and milk products is derived from the concepts of microbial thermal death times in which the destruction of the organisms is assumed to be dependent on a linear, semilogarithmic relationship of temperature to time. The overall objectives of the heat treatments applied to market milks are to a) eliminate or reduce the risk of disease associated with pathogens common to raw milk and b) extend the shelf life of milk by inactivation of potential spoilage organisms and degradative enzymes. The specific objectives are to ensure that all particles of milk are heated to the desired temperature for the desired time and to avoid significantly damaging the flavour or other quality characteristics of milk. Rapid cooling after heat process is also essential to minimize product heat damage and to control the growth of microorganisms that may survive the heat process. In general, the higher the heat treatment, the greater the efficiency of microbial destruction, but also the greater the chance that the quality of milk will be affected. The specific heat treatments and their effect on microorganisms is given in Chapter-5.

4.6. Clean Milk Production

Although India has emerged as the largest producer of milk, its contribution to the world dairy trade is negligible. One of the major factors for low export of our dairy products has been the quality and safety aspects of milk and milk products. Consumers all over the world have become quality conscious and prefer high quality products. Due to liberlization and globalization of world economy, abundant opportunities are emerging for India to take its due place in the world dairy market. Since the international market has become demanding in terms of quality, safety and delivery of dairy products, one has to start with raw milk received at the dairy plant. The adoption of clean milk production practices at the producer level coupled with Good Manufacturing Practices (GMP) and Hazard Analysis of Critical Control Point (HACCP) at plant level would provide competitive edge to milk and milk supplies in the international market.

Quality of Raw Milk: At present the quality of raw milk is of major concern. It has been observed that while the raw milk at the cow / buffalo udder level in India compares well with that of any developed countries (Table 4.6.1), it is the manner in which milk is handled subsequent to milking which affects the quality of raw milk reaching the dairy dock or at chilling centre.

Table 4.6.1: Comparison of the status of milk quality in India vs developed countries

Category	Indian condition (SPC cfu/ml)	Developed Countries (SPC cfu/ml)
Raw Milk Quality,Producer Level	1,000-10,000	2,000-10,000
Collection Centres (Dairy Co-op. Society)	20.000-5,00,000	Not applicable
Dairy Dock through bulk coolers & road tankers	1,00,000- 10,00,000	10,000-1,00,000
Pasteurized milk quality at Dispatch Dock	50,000/ml (shelf life - 3 days under refrigeration ≤ 4°C	5,000/ml (shelf life–14 days under refrigeration at ≤ 4°C)
Consumer level	50,000-1,00,000 due to lack of cold chain with MBRT, 2.30h or so	5,000-10,000 due to cold chain distribution & MBRT, 8h or so

Source: Chauhan (2000)

The microbial counts in raw milk may usually vary from less than one thousand to more than one million (10^6) per ml. The total microbial load may be estimated by standard plate count (SPC) or by conducting methylene blue reduction (MBRT) test. Based on the results of these tests, raw milk can be graded for its microbiological quality. The Bureau of Indian Standards (BIS) has laid down such standards for grading raw milk (Table 4.6.2). In general, the microbial quality of milk in our country is quite poor. The higher microbial load in the milk also creates other implications such as higher acidity, higher pasteurization temperature, protein denaturation and presence of toxins in the milk.

Table 4.6.2: Bacteriological standard for raw milk (BIS)

Grade	Standard Plate Count (per ml)	MBRT (Hr)	One hour Resazurindisc number	Presumptive coliform test
Very good	Not over 200,000	5 and above	4 or higher	Absent in 0.01 ml.
Good	200,000 to 1million	3 and 4	4 or higher	Absent in 0.01 ml.
Fair	1 million to 5 million	1 and 2	3.5 to 1.0	Absent in 0.01 ml.
Poor	> 5 million	0.5 0	0.5 to 0	Present in 0.01 ml.

Regarding clean milk production various findings have been reported which are diverse. In a study sponsored by Indian Council of Agricultural Research ICAR) during 1986-87, the Kaira Cooperative Milk Union reported that quality of milk as delivered by most farmers was quite satisfactory in that over 93% of the samples showed an average MBR (methylene blue reduction) time of more than two hours. The study covering 11 milk routes in different directions and different distances, further revealed that the deterioration of quality had set in at the village society level as only 73% of samples there had an MBR time of more than two hours. Thus, the study attributed that the main cause of concern was improper cleaning of milk cans and other milk collection equipment. The situation aggravated further due to undue long exposure of milk to high ambient temperature leading to rapid spoilage; consequently, only 4% samples had an MBR time of more than two hours. Findings from the other places also revealed the necessity of chilling the milk at village society level to control the microbiological, chemical and physical reactions from taking place.

The performance reported in this study by the Kaira Union cannot be generalized since the things are comparatively well organized there due to extensive work done in the last 50 years. On all India basis, the things are different to look at. It is reported that it is not uncommon for dairy plants to receive raw milk with a plate count of five to ten million per ml or a spore count of 500 to 2,000 per ml whereas in North America, milk from the producer can be rejected if it has a count for more than 75,000 per ml If we compare this then we see a long road ahead to achieve the target of clean milk production.

Siva *et al.* (1993) studied the bacteriological quality of raw milk from cow and buffalo collected from individual producers, collection centers and dairy plants. The total plate count of cow and buffalo milk samples from individual producers averaged 1± 4.15x 1 million (range, 0.7-17 x I million) and 32 ± 23 x 1 million (range, <0.1-100 x 1 million) cfu per ml, respectively. The average total plate count of cow and buffalo milk collected from collection centers was found to be 9.1 ± 1.6 x 1 million (range, 4.6-12 x 1 million) and 5.1± 1.65 x 1 million (range, 0.46-8 x 1 million) cfu per ml, respectively. The average total plate count of cow and buffalo milk collected from dairy plants was found to be 17 ± 0.43 x 1 million (range, 0.1-85 x 1 million) and 23 ± 5.7 x 1 million (range, 0.3-120 x 1 million) cfu per ml, respectively. It is apparent that the bacteriological quality of milk collected from individual producers, collection centers and dairy plants were not satisfactory.

They also studied the coliform counts of cow and buffalo milk collected from individual producers, collection centers and dairy plants. The average coliform count of cow and buffalo milk collected from individual producers was $0.63 \pm 031 \times 10^4$ (range, $< 0.1\text{-}082 \times 10^4$) cfu per ml, respectively. The average coliform count from cow and buffalo milk from collection centers were $66 \pm 38 \times 10^4$(range, $1.7\text{-}150 \times 10^4$) and $22 \pm 21.5 \times 10^4$ (range,$0.18\text{-}86 \times 10^4$) cfu per ml, respectively. Similarly the average coliform counts in cow and buffalo milk collected from dairy plants were $150 \pm 0.82 \times 10^4$ (range, $0.1\text{-} 2000 \times 10^4$) and $140 \pm 0.82 \times 10^4$(range, $0.5\text{-}1100 \times 10^4$) cfu per ml, respectively. It is apparent that the number of coliforms were too high indicating unhygienic production of milk. The study showed that there was no significant difference in bacteriological quality of cow and buffalo milk. The authors also reported that the chilling of raw milk at the collection center helped in arresting the growth of bacteria during transportation. The bacteriological quality of pasteurized milk was satisfactory meeting the BSI standard of <50,000 cfu per ml.

Overall, this study showed that bacteriological quality of raw milk at various stages of collection was far from satisfactory. The high counts in raw milk samples indicated unhygienic production and handling at farm and during transportation under Indian conditions.

It has also been reported that the volume of borderline souring in India is estimated to be up to 10 per cent of milk collected by dairies in summer months (Chakraborty, *et al*, 1986).

Hence the need for massive movement for Clean Milk Production has been felt and a multi-pronged approach has been adopted by the dairies. This includes awareness campaign, training, focus on clean hands, teat dip after milking, use of clean SS vessels for milk handling, istallation of insectocutors at the collection centers, SS 304 cans in place of aluminium cans, bulk cooling of milk at Society (collection center) level and transport by SS-304 road milk tankers, *etc.*

Concept of Clean Milk Production: In view of the immense dietary importance of milk, the need to produce safe, clean and wholesome milk is of profound significance. Clean milk does not mean milk in which all visible dirt is absent or milk from which it has been removed, rather it denotes 'raw milk from healthy animal, that has been produced and handled under hygienic conditions, that contains only small number of harmless bacteria and that possesses a good keeping quality without being heat treated'. There is a strong correlation between the quality of raw milk and finished products.

Considering the bacteriological quality of raw milk reaching the dairy plants presently there exists scope for improvement. The two principles that universally guide the quality of raw milk are:

a) avoiding or minimizing contamination at various stages of handling raw milk, and

b) reducing the growth and activity of microorganisms in raw milk

Knowledge of the possible unhygienic practices that lead to the gross contamination of milk will be useful in realizing the gravity of the situation and in evolving improved strategies. The possible undesirable practices that are prevalent may broadly be classified into following categories:

a) Practices related to milch animals: unhealthy animal, unclean body and udder,

b) Practices related to milking process: unhealthy milker, unclean hands and cloths, unhygienic personal habits, incomplete milking, wrong milking procedures, unclean vessels for milk collection,

c) Practices related to environment: poor housing and feeding of the animal, unhygienic surroundings.

d) Post-milking practices: chilling and prompt transport of milk.

e) Contaminants in milk.

a) Practices Related to Milch Animals

Healthy Animals: The milch animal is the starting point in the production of clean, low count milk. The udder is not an important source of bacteria in milk unless pathological condition exists. Normally milk contains few bacteria at the time it is drawn. The milch animals should be kept in good health. This calls for prevention through vaccination and timely treatment against sporadic diseases. The animals should be screened for TB and mastitis at frequent intervals since these diseases are harmful to public health. Any animal with physical disability such as inflamed or defective udders or teats or enlarged glands should be isolated and her milk not mixed with regular produce.

Clean Animals: Clean milk can not be produced from dirty animals. If the flanks, belly, udder, teats and tail of the animal are soiled with manure, earth, bedding or loose hair, considerable extraneous materials may fall into the pail. Before each milking, the cows should be groomed to remove the loose hairs, dandruff, dust, manure, soil or other accumulations from their bodies. The grooming should be completed at least half-an – hour before milking in order that an excessive quantity of dust will not be in the stable air. In addition, udders and teats should be washed with a wet cloth and dried with another cloth that has been rinsed in and wrung from clean water. If udder and teats are not dried, dirty water may fall from them into the milk pail and the moisture may cause the teats to become chapped and cracked during winter. The clipping of the flanks, udder, belly and tail facilitates washing and grooming.

b) Practices Related to Milking

Milker: The milker should be healthy with clean habits. Unhealthy milker may directly transmit disease-producing microbes to the milk through sneezing, coughing, *etc*. Unclean hands and cloths of the milker may also be a potential source of contamination. Unhygienic personal habits, sneezing, coughing, etc by milker are also undesirable. The milker has to follow hygienic practices from beginning to the end. He should be in good health not suffering from any disease like TB or flu. He should wear clean clothes and cover his head at the time of milking. His fingernails should be trimmed so as not to cause any injury to the teats. He should ensure that his sweat drops do not enter the milk. Similarly, he should wash his hands before commencing his work. The milker should not smoke during milking.

Milking Process: The milker should practice dry milking. The usual tendency is to dip the fingertips in milk or apply oil which is really not necessary and allows dirt to enter milk. The animal should be milked completely. At the end of milking the teats should be dipped in disinfectant solution (iodophor) which also helps in closure of teat sphincters thereby reducing the entry of mastitis germs. It should be ensured that the animals having any disease are milked last, and most importantly their milk should be disposed of separately. Similarly, the milk from the animals receiving antibiotic treatment should be handled separately for a period of 72 hours after stoppage of treatment.

Machine milking is very common in Western countries. It has been found that milk drawn with the help of machines may be as low in bacterial content as that produced with the most scrupulous care in hand milking provided that proper methods of cleaning, sterilization and operation are carried out. However, if the parts of milking machines are not properly washed and sterilized, it may increase the bacterial content.

One common objection to milking machines has been the belief that the udders of the animals were injured and that milk production decreased. In recent years numerous workers have reported that the modern types of milking machines, properly operated, have no such ill effects.

Special precaution should be taken in cleaning of the milking machines. Immediately after milking, the surfaces of the rubber parts of the machine should be rinsed before the milk solids get dried onto them and become difficult to remove.

Milk Vessels: Most of the dirt or sediment that enters milk drops from the body of the animals during the milking process. The use of small-topped milk pail will keep out at least 50% of such dirt. The vessels used for drawing milk should be properly cleaned and sanitized. The use of properly sanitized utensils is the most important single factor in producing milk with a low bacterial content. The delayed washing of utensils results in a larger bacterial count than the utensils washed immediately. The milk utensils should be made of a non-rusting and non-absorbent material such as aluminium or galvanized iron. Stainless steel would be ideal, but for the cost considerations. The utensils should be free from dents, cracks and crevices.

The utensils should be rinsed with tap or lukewarm water immediately after milking and then brushed thoroughly on all surfaces with washing solution heated to a temperature between 40-50° C. Finally, they should be rinsed with clean water and then sterilized. The "sterilization" of dairy equipment usually refers to the destruction, either by heat or by chemicals, of bacteria in vegetative or spore forms remaining on the equipment after washing.

c) Practices Related to Environment

Hygienic Milking Environment: The place where housing, feeding and milking of the animals are done need special care in order to minimize contamination of milk. The sanitary construction, location and arrangement of dairy-farm buildings are necessary for low count milk production. The animal shed should be at a well-elevated place with good drainage. It should be properly ventilated with windows admitting daylight. The shed should be fitted with fly-proof wire mesh wherever possible. Floors and gutters should have adequate slope for easy drainage and removal of dung. The animal shed should be properly illuminated. It is equally important to clean the shed from time to time. It is recommended to clean (sweep) the animal shed at least 30 minutes ahead of actual milking so that the flying dust is allowed to settle on the ground which prevents its entry in milk pail. Brooming the cattle shed and removal of dung from time to time will control the flies which are a major menace and source of infection. Similarly, the feed materials having off-flavours should be kept away from the milking area since these flavours are known to enter milk.

Feed: The feed given to the animal should be of good quality and free from mould or decomposed materials. Mouldy hay or grains, decomposed silage or feeds badly fermented are undesirable in market milk production. Feeds that are old, stale, infested and vegetables like cabbage, turnip, onions, garlic are bound to cause off-flavours. Therefore, these should be stored away and not be given to milch animals within a couple of hours of milking.

One major cause of concern emerged recently pertains to entry of insecticides and pesticides into milk via mainly feed materials. This is happening through injudicious use of these poisonous formulations as crop protection measures. Often, these chemicals are used beyond their recommended dosages. The farmers have to be careful while spraying chemicals like malathion and it should be noted that there is a complete ban on the manufacture and use of DDT and BHC. Since these chemicals find their way in oils and fats in the crops, it is better to use deoiled ingredients in animal feed which will eliminate the risk of pesticide contamination of milk.

d) Post-milking Operations

Straining Milk at the Farm: Ordinarily, noticeable quantities of foreign materials, such as particles of dust, dirt, feeds, bedding, manure, hair, flies, and many other undesirable substances may find their way into milk because of careless handling of milk at the dairy farm. Many of these foreign substances carry large number of bacteria, yeasts and moulds. To remove these foreign matters straining is practiced. This straining is accomplished at the dairy farm by means of miscellaneous pieces of cloth, cotton batting, wire gauge, cellulose pads or specially prepared strainer pads. These materials are able to remove principally the large particles.

In order to carry the clinsing of milk a step further, various devices have been suggested for filtering milk through filters possessing pores much smaller than the ordinary strainers, cloth or metal. Milk filtering devices which are provided with closely woven cotton cloths or cellulose pads are available. The mesh of these filters is very fine and provides a much more efficient filtering capacity. It is intended that these filter pads should be used but once and then discarded, since their efficiency is impaired or destroyed by washing. They are effective in removing visible sediments from milk but do not filter out leucocytes, epithelial cells, cell fragments or microorganisms unless these are trapped on the larger particles which make up the visible sediment.

The most effective method of removing foreign matters from the milk is clarification. It works on the principle of cream separator.

Chilling of Milk: Healthy and clean animals, clean and sanitized utensils, hygienic milking environment are necessary to produce milk of low bacterial content. The bacteriological quality of raw milk in India at the time of milking is comparable with that in leading milk exporting countries (including EU, Australia and New Zealand). However, there is significant deterioration in milk quality from farm to factory. The deterioration takes place on two accounts.

- Infrastructure issues: lack of all-weather roads, electrical supply for chilling centers, potable water supply and sewage disposal, *etc.*
- Contamination through equipment, loss of time and lack of temperature controlled storage / transportation.

The time lag coupled with transportation at ambient temperature results in deterioration of quality in terms of sensory properties (odour, taste, colour), composition (fat, SNF, protein, etc), hygiene (bacteriological-pathogenic, spoilage, somatic cells) and also leads to adulteration (water, foreign substances).

An increase in temperature prior to pasteurization can lead to an exponential increase in bacterial count in milk, which is highlighted in Table 4.6.3 (EU standards allow a maximum of 1,00,000 / ml). Hence transportation and storage in controlled temperature conditions is critical to preserve the quality of milk. However, cooling does not replace the need for hygienic milking conditions. An example of the impact of milking conditions on quality is shown in Table 4.6.4.

The solution to these issues lies in identifying and addressing handling, storage and transportation practices from the producer to the dairy plant and onward to the consumer, and facilitating improvement of hygiene, sanitation and food safety and operating efficiency in dairy plants. The action plan includes:

a) Increasing awareness about the importance of good quality milk among farmers.

b) Training of farmers on hygienic habits at farm level and collection centers.

b) Giving incentive to farmers through higher remuneration for quality milk.

c) Setting up quality testing infrastructure at the collection center. This involves testing of bacterial count, acidity, smell / taste, somatic cell count, *etc.*

Installation of bulk coolers for efficient collection is critical to preserving and improving the quality of milk. Benefits of bulk cooling include:

- Longer collecting intervals (milk can be collected once a day instead of the current practice of twice a day) which reduces the cost of transportation.
- Flexibility in milk delivery and pick up time.
- Handling of cans are eliminated.
- Increased potential for collection from producers in remote locations.
- Maintenance of good hygienic conditions.

The Government should give incentives to dairies to invest in clean milk production and bulk cooling. The incentives could be in the form of reimbursing a part of the cost of equipment for collection and testing. The Government can develop a quality mark for milk on the lines of Agmark, which should include every important trait of milk quality, like:

- Hygienic quality: bacteriological and cytological traits, absence of pathogens and other contaminants.
- Sensory quality.
- Nutritional quality.
- Technological quality.

This quality mark can be used by processors to differentiate their products vis-à-vis competition in local and export markets.

Table 4.6.3: Bacterial count in milk at various temperatures and time intervals (cfu x 10^3/ml)

Temperature (°C)	Fresh	24 Hr	48 Hr	72 Hr
4.4	4	4	5	8
10	4	15	125	6,000
15	4	16	33,000	326,000

Source: Mathur, H. 2007

Table 4.6.4: Bacterial count in different milking conditions (cfu × 10^3/ml)

Milking Conditions	Fresh	24 Hr	48 Hr	72 Hr
Clean cows, environment, utensils	4	4	5	8
Dirty cows, environment, utensils	136	281	538	749

Source: Mathur, H. 2007

Thus prompt chilling of milk is necessary in controlling the growth of organisms present in milk at the time it is drawn from the udder. The milk then should be stored in protected environment until it is delivered to the milk plant or receiving station. Even low count milk must be held below 10°C, if it is to be stored for a day or two. At 5°C, practically no growth occurs, until after 48 hours, thereafter, the reproduction of bacteria is very slow.

In places where milk is stored in cans before transportation, bulk can coolers are the best options. Some of the other cooling options practiced may be air cooling, water cooling, ice cooling and mechanical cooling. The cooling aids usually used are household refrigeration, direct expansion surface cooler, expansion bulk tank, ice bank and chilled water.

Speedy Transportation: The basic system of milk transport in India comprises the transport of milk from the form to the collection center (in small vessels or cans), from the collection center to the chilling center (in cans or small tankers) and from the chilling center to the processing plant (in insulated road tankers). The quality of milk will deteriorate during transit if it is not properly chilled. The milk should be held for a minimum time at ambient temperature. In general, the transport of uncooled milk can be justified only if great care has been taken in its production (number of cfu <100,000/ml) and if the milk is processed or chilled to a low temperature not more than 3 hour after its production.

It is essential to reduce the time gap between milking and its reception at the dairy dock. Therefore, the first step may be to organize easy transportation of milk from village societies and collection centres, closer to dairy plants. The conventional milk routes need to be split into two groups: one, those which can bring in the best quality milk, and the other for the balance milk. The smaller (3-5 tonnes) energy efficient trucks can greatly help in using milk routes effectively and in optimization of transportation costs.

4.7. Contaminants in Milk

When we talk about quality, it does not restrict ourselves to the bacteriological but also physical and chemical quality of raw milk before it reaches even the first chilling station. As per the definition of adulteration the presence of residues of pesticides, heavy metals, antibiotics, aflatoxins, drugs, hormones, etc in excess quantities indicates adulteration. As these residues are not inherent to milk, so directed measures should be employed so that these residues can be eliminated and even if they are present, their level does not exceed the established standards.

Insecticides/Pesticides: Insecticides/pesticides are the chemicals which are used to kill insects / pests to save the crops. When these chemicals are used irrationally could prove injurious to the health of the consumers. Dairies should have infrastructure like gas liquid chromatographs having electron capture detector (ECD) to detect organo-chlorine pesticides like DDT, aldrin, dialdrin, HCN, lindane, BHC, *etc.* The standard laid down by the PFA for pesticide residues in milk and milk products should be adhered to. This is only possible if we have the commitment and infrastructure to check the residue levels. Dairies are not adding or removing pesticides, the message has to flow to the farmers about the uses and their harmful effects if used in excess.

The use of certain pesticides have been prohibited because the residues of the chemicals may pass into the milk. Likewise, certain sprays for crops which will later be eaten by milch animals have been prohibited or their use permitted only at certain periods of development because they may be recovered in the milk supply. During 1960s it was reported that milk frequently contained pesticides, however, their levels were well below the safety limits. However, some reports in India have indicated that the residues of the pesticides do sometimes exceed the permissible limit prescribed by PFA.

Antibiotics: In recent years, the dairy industry has come to use considerable quantities of antibiotics in the treatment of animal diseases, notably mastitis. When such treatments are made, the milk from the treated animal is not supposed to be used for human consumption for at least 72 hours following the treatment. If such milk is added to milk from untreated animals before the 72 hours period is completed, residual antibiotics may be detected in the entire supply. These antibiotics may enter the milk directly, as in inter-mammary treatments for mastitis, or indirectly through the blood stream of an animal which has been intravenously injected with antibiotic preparations for some pathological conditions. There are also reports that large amounts of antibiotic supplements in grain may result in the detection of residues in the milk. The presence of antibiotics in milk or other dairy products has serious health implications and hence they must be used only as specified. Penicillin apparently has greater influence on public health than other antibiotics in common use and thus has held the main interest in developing test procedures for residual antibiotics.

Industrial Chemicals: Toxic industrial chemicals are a source of environmental contamination and also a source of serious exposure to certain workplaces. Heavy metals, for example, lead, mercury, cadmium, arsenic, *etc* have been reported in milk and milk products. These environmental contaminants are harmful / toxic if they are ingested in higher concentration than what is prescribed by PFA act. Lead and mercury are most frequently studied because they have been the cause of infant poisoning through milk. Lead is the single most common heavy metal pollutant of environment. In general, urban dwellers are at greater risk than rural residents. Higher values of lead in milk of urban populations compared to rural ones, and higher values in colostrum compared to mature milk, have been reported. At world level, concerns are being expressed for their harmful effects and their prescribed limits are being lowered frequently in order to ensure that the food available to the consumers is safe.

Aflatoxins: Aflatoxins are fungal metabolites found as toxic contaminants of foods. Aflatoxins are produced by the common moulds,*Aspergillus flavus* and *A. parasiticus by* virtue of their ability to produce aflatoxin. These can be secreted in milk by the milch animal which has been fed with aflatoxin containing feeds. Upon ingestion, the Aspergillus toxins are metabolized by the milch animals and are secreted into milk in the form of M_1 and M_2 which are also toxic to the milk consumers.

Physical Contaminants: physical contamination / hazards found in milk and milk products could be metal fragments, glass, wood splinters, stones, dirt, plastics, insects, etc. The presence of these can cut the mouth, break teeth, cause choking or perforation in the alimentary tract. If proper care is taken during production, transportation, processing and handling these physical contamination can be avoided.

References

Bryan, F.L. 1983. Epidemiology of milk- borne diseases. *J. Food Prot*. 46:637.

Burton, H. 1984. *J. Dairy Res.*, 51:341.

Burton, H. 1988. Ultra-high Temperature Processing of Milk and Milk Products. Elsevier Applied Science, New York.

Chakraborty, B.K., Chaudhary, S.S., Alex, K.A., Jacob, G. and Soni, G.J. 1986. *Milchwissenchaft,* 41:16.

Chauhan, R.S. 2000. Quality challenges for sustenance of Indian dairy industry. *Indian Dairyman,* 52(12):113.

Douglas, S.A., Gray, M.J., Crandall, A.D. and Boor, K.J. 2000. *J. Food Prot.*, 63:516.

Frank, J.F. and Hassan, A.N. 2003. Microorganisms associated with milk, *Encyclopaedia of Dairy Science,* Academic Press, pp: 1786.

Hinrichs, J. and Kessler, H.G. 1995. In Heat-induced Changes in Milk, 2nd Ed., International Dairy Federation, Brussels, Belgium, pp: 9.

Jay, J., 1996. Modern Food Microbiology, 5th Ed. Chapman and Hall, New York.

Mathur,H. 2007.Dairy India. 6th Ed. pp:43.

Mottar, J.F. 1989. Enzymes of Psychrotrophs in Raw Food. R.C. Mckellar, ed. CRC Press, Boca Raton, Fl. pp: 227.

Muir, D.D. 1996. *J. Soc. Dairy Technol.*, 49(1): 24.

Patel, G.B. and Blankenagel, G. 1972. *J. Milk Food Technol*, 35: 203.

Ralyea, R.D., Wiedman, B. M.,and Boor, K.G. 1998. *J. Food Prot.*, 61:1203.

Ryser,E.T. 1998. Public health concerns. In: Applied Dairy Microbiology, by Marth, E.H.and Steele, J. L. New York: Marcel Dekker, pp 263.

Siva, C.V., Patel, D.A. and Sannabhadti, S.S. 1993. Microbiological status of raw and pasteurized milk. *Indian J. Dairy Sci.*, 46:2.

Yadav, J.S., Grover, S. and Batish, V.K. 1993. Hygienic milk production. A Comprehensive Dairy Microbiology, 1st. Ed. PP: 124.

PART II
Processing and Preservation of Milk

5

Processing and Preservation of Milk

Milk is a highly perishable commodity. The shelf life of raw milk is in hours. In order to harness its full potential for the well being of the humanity, it is essential to extend its shelf life not only in days but also in months and years. This can be achieved by judicious application of processing and preservation technologies.

Preservation is any purposeful treatment or processing of a food which prevents spoilage and extends the shelf life of raw material to a longer than its natural keeping quality.

During storage and distribution foods are exposed to a wide range of environmental conditions. Environmental factors such as temperature, humidity, oxygen and light can trigger several reactions that may lead to food deterioration. As a result foods may be altered to such an extent that they are either rejected by the consumer or are harmful to the person consuming them. It is, therefore, essential that the good knowledge of different reactions that cause food deterioration is gained prior to understanding the principles of food preservation.

The deterioration in foods may be caused either due to internal or external chemical or microbial reactions occurring in milk. The changes may be either latent to senses of consumer, or they may be discernible by the human senses. The consumer cannot perceive latent changes visually, olfactorily or otherwise, and laboratory measurements are the only method to detect them. Still the nutritional value of such materials may be seriously impaired. Such changes include fermentation, oxidation of lipids, loss of vitamins and changes in the contents and composition of nitrogenous substances.

Non-microbial changes in foods, perceptible to human senses, may often lead to serious deterioration noticeable to the average consumer. These include discolouration and changes in odor, taste and consistency. Microbial changes may result in alteration of original properties of milk making it unfit for further processing, deterioration in flavour quality, loss of nutrients and toxin production.

Preservation methods: The preservation methods are based on the principle of reduction of microbial contamination and creation of unfavourable conditions for the occurrence of undesirable chemical and microbial reactions. This can be achieved as follows:

1. Reduction of microbial contamination of milk- clean milk production,
2. Removal of microorganisms from milk- clarification, bactofugation, microfiltration.
3. Direct inactivation of microorganisms - pasteurization, sterilization, thermization
4. Indirect inactivation of microorganisms:

a) Removal of moisture – concentration using an evaporator, drying, sweetening, salting,

b) Reducing temperature - chilling, freezing,

c) Removal of oxygen and storage at modified atmosphere.

These concepts and methods are elaborated in subsequent chapters.

5.1. Market Milk

Historically, market milk has been defined as fluid milk products sold for direct human consumption. Although the collection and use of milk for human consumption can be traced back to some of the earliest recorded history, the concept of market milk has developed in more recent times. In general, the market milk industry has grown in coincidence with the establishment of major metropolitan areas, which typically are not amenable to individual ownership of milch animals for personal milk collection. Until the end of nineteenth century, market milk was primarily raw milk collected from the farms, distributed fresh to consumers and consumed fresh. Currently, these practices would be considered unacceptable because of public health concern as well as perishability of raw milk. The development of pasteurization and other heat processes for dairy products has transformed the market milk industry and dramatically expanded product distribution capabilities all over the world.

Dairy products are traditionally classified into two broad categories: a) fluid or market milk products and b) manufactured milk products. Processing facilities are designed to produce either fluid milk products or one of the manufactured products. The dairy products sold to the consumers in the fluid form are commonly known as fluid or market milk products, the terms fluid and market are used interchangeably. Some of the more common foods which are normally considered fluid milk products include whole milk, skim milk, double toned milk, toned milk, standardized milk, full cream milk, mixed milk, recombined milk, special milks, butter milk and lassi, *etc.* Several of the products have modifications. The product may be modified with vitamins or minerals. Solids may be added. Fat content may be adjusted to suit the consumers' use and legal requirements. Process conditions may be varied to produce pasteurized, homogenized or other types of special products. Recently new products like calcium-enriched milk, low-lactose milk, iron-fortified milk, chilled coffee, sports drinks, etc have been introduced in market milk. UHT milk is finding wide application in our country as well as abroad.

Despite the profound historical heritage, ethnic and modern traditions that have lead to establishing milk as an integral part of dietary regimen in many cultures of the world, dairy industry has faced adverse campaigns from the competing food industry that have raised several concerns in the minds of the consumers. Milk fat has been projected as the villain in coronary heart diseases. Elevated levels of LDL cholesterol have been linked to hypertension and increased risk of myocardial infarction. Concerns have also been raised about the involvement of milk in allergies, lactose intolerance, mucus formation, cancers, diabetes, cataract and Crohn's disease. The general validity of each of these contentions can be effectively countered on scientific grounds. Although it is clear that some individuals may have specific intolerance to milk constituents under certain conditions of physiological stress.

However, the dairy industry has remained unwittingly passive towards such unfavourable onslaught of reprehensions. Recent nutritional and biochemical research has reinforced newer confidence in the healthful and extranutritional attributes of milk. Fluid milk is a unique source of calcium with high bioassimilability which counters osteoporosis and contributes very effectively towards counterbalancing the loss of calcium from bones in post-menopause women. Milk has shot into prominence in certain ethnic cultures such as the Japanese where inadequate calcium intake has become a national concern. Optimum intake of calcium is also regarded essential for maintaining normalcy of cardiovascular function in the body. Several other extranutritional and bioprotective factors present in the milk such as lactoferrin, lactoperoxidase, immunoglobulins, lysozyme and vitamin binding proteins have been known to provide protection against enteropathogenic microorganisms and rotavirus. Intake of milk also promotes establishment of healthy microflora in the microecological system of the gut. The R&D managers in the proactive dairy industry are now engaged in developing a range of health promoting, nutritional, refreshing beverages from milk through the application of biotechnology to further enhance the health attributes of milk. A glance at the dairy counter of any large supermarket is sufficient to show us the vast array of forms in which milk is presented. Very prominent among these are milk beverages in a multitude of fat levels, enriched or flavoured in varying ways, and aimed at various section of the market-pregnant women, breast feeding mothers, toddlers, children, adolescents, slimmer's, active adults, pensioners, *etc.*

Biotechnology has also been employed for the enzymatic degradation of lactose as well as production of galacto-oligosaccharides. Such product variations of the market milk are intended for alleviating the symptoms of lactose intolerance through ingestion of milk. These products are marketed commercially in South-European countries and have been introduced by certain multinational companies in South Asia also. Processed milk containing live microorganisms, such as *Lactobacillus acidophilus* and *Bifidobacterium bifidum* are being marketed commercially in various parts of North America and Europe.

Manufactured milk products include most of the non-beverage products, such as khoa, chhana, paneer, butter, butter oil, ghee, condensed milk, dry milks, cheese, frozen desserts, an assortment of sweets, *etc.*

The production of high-quality dairy products require high quality raw materials. Market milk and its associated products require a raw milk supply of higher quality than any other segment of the dairy industry in respect to healthfulness, sanitary quality, flavour, keeping quality and aesthetic background.

Volume of Market Milk: The market milk industry is one of the tremendously large size considered either from the amount of the product concerned, the number of people involved or the capital represented. India has a unique pattern of production, processing and marketing / consumption of milk which is not comparable with any large milk producing country. Approximately 70 million rural households (primarily small and marginal farmers and landless labourers) in the country are engaged in milk production. Over 11 million farmers are organized into about 0.1 million village Dairy Cooperative Societies (DCSs) (about 110 farmers per DCS). The cumulative milk handled by DCSs across the country is about 18 million kg per day. These cooperatives form part of the national milk grid (NMG) which links the milk producers throughout India with consumers in more than 700 towns and cities bridging the gaps on account of seasonal and regional variations in availability of milk. The Anand model which involves setting up institutional infrastructure at the village, district and state levels (owned and operated by the farmers) has progressively and largely eliminated the middlemen, enabling direct interface of producers with processors (Mathur, 2007).

In India, milk is mostly produced in small quantities of two-four litres by small and marginal farmers spread over 5,00,000 villages. The country has a long tradition of keeping milch animals as part of the farming household. Buffalo and cow and to a limited extent, goat are the main milch animals in the Indian sub-continent. Buffalo contributes some 55 per cent, cow 41 per cent and goat 4 per cent to India's total milk production. Presently, the milk production in India serves three main user groups:

- The household sector, mainly for the purpose of drinking and secondly, for conversion into milk products, such as dahi, makhan, buttermilk, lassi and ghee for family use.
- The non-organized sector (dudhwala and halwais) for urban liquid milk marketing and production of mithais and other traditional products, and
- The organized sector that processes milk into pasteurized liquid milk and largely western products.

The first two user segments account for over 82% of milk produced in India. The remaining 18% is handled by the organized sector. A few of the dairy plants process over one million litres of milk per day. About 45% of India's milk production is utilized for making indigenous milk products such as khoa, chhana, paneer, makhan, ghee and dahi. These products provide a profitable outlet to the organized sector. The product-wise milk utilization pattern is presented in Table 5.1.1. Interestingly, the household sector coverts milk mainly into products for immediate consumption, while the traditional sector makes products of short shelf life. On the other hand, the modern dairy sector manufactures western dairy products such as cheese, butter, milk powders and ice cream as well as ghee which have longer shelf life.

Table 5.1.1: Milk utilization pattern in India

Products	Year			
	1943*	1956	2001	2005
Milk Production (Million tonnes)	23.5	17.8	84.6	94.5
Milk Utilization (Per cent)	100	100	100	100
A. Liquid Milk (%)	28.0	39.2	46.0	50
B. Traditional Dairy Products (%)	72.0	60.8	50.0	45.0
Ghee / Makhan (%)	58.7	46.0	33	
Dahi (curd / Chakka) (%)	5.2	8.8	7.0	
Khoa (Partially desiccated milk) (%)	5.0	4.4	7.0	
Chhana & Paeer (%)	3.1	1.6	3.0	
Western Products (%)	Neg**	Neg**	4.0	5.6

*Includes Pakistan & Bangladesh, ** Negligible

Sources: (1) Report on ' Marketing of milk in India and Burma.' Manager of Publications, Govt. of India, Delhi, 1943. (2) Report on 'Marketing of Ghee and Other Milk Products', Manager of Publication, Govt. of India, Delhi, 1957. (3) Dairy India, 1997, Delhi. (4) Technology of Indian Milk Products, 2002.

5.2. Pattern of Consumption

As the consumer expenditure on milk and milk products increases, the consumption preference shifts from liquid milk to products like dahi, butter, ghee, paneer, cheese, ice cream and sweets, etc. It is estimated that of the total production, 46% is consumed as fluid milk. Ghee and butter together account for about 34 per cent. The three additional milk products, *viz*, dahi, including 'lassi' and 'chhachh, paneer and khoa add another 15%. The balance 5% is accounted for by milk powder, ice cream and other specialized western dairy products. The increasing disposable income among the middle- and low- income groups in the urban and rural areas is bringing to the surface the hitherto suppressed demand for sweets and milk products.

Per Capita Availability: India's per capita availability of market milk is not commensurate with its ranking as world's top milk producer. However, the present per capita availability of 240 g / day (88 kg/year) is much higher than the average for the developing countries in the Asia / Pacific region, but lower than the world average. It is noteworthy that during the last ten years, the per capita availability in India has gone up significantly despite the booming population. By 2011, it is expected to reach 280 g/day when the population would be 1,178 million.

The minimum consumption recommended by the Nutritional Advisory Committee of the ICMR is 220 g/day (80.3 kg/year). This was equaled in 2000-01 but is considered low as compared to the nutritional recommendation of 283 g per day by the WHO. Various studies indicate that the top 10% of the India's population consumes 30% of the milk produced, while the bottom 30% manages only with 10% of the milk. The rich class in India consumes milk largely as liquid or in the form of products, while the lower income groups use it as whitener in tea/coffee.

Fluid Milk: The fluid milk market has emerged as the most dynamic segment of the dairy industry growing at a compound annual growth rate (CAGR) of 10 per cent. The urban dairy market, dominated by fluid milk, has many exciting opportunities for the entrepreneurs. It cannot be regarded as homogeneous, but layered, with each layer offering its own rewards. In the organized sectors, the share of 3% fat toned milk exceeds 50%, 4.5% fat standardized milk stood at 33%, and 6% fat full-cream milk was 9%.

The cooperative and public sector dairies meet 40% of the demand of fluid milk in Class-I cities. The balance is shared by the private organized and traditional non-organized sectors. Presently, only some 1,000 out of 5000 cities and towns in India are served by its milk distribution network, dispensing hygienically packaged wholesome, quality pasteurized milk. Rising awareness about hygienic standards and adulteration of loose milk has led consumers in the urban areas to switch to pasteurized packaged milk.

The organized sector is beginning to tap the demand for low-fat milk in 200 ml sachets and is selling milk in small towns with an average demand of 10,000 litres per day. The traditional 'dudhwala' scores over the organized sector by selling small quantities (100–250 ml) of milk, ensuring home delivery and giving milk on credit for one month. It wins the consumer's confidence with the concepts of 'malai' and 'fresh' milk. To compete with him, some cooperatives have initiated home delivery free of cost.

Market Potential: India's dairy market is multi-layered, shaped like pyramid with the base made up of vast market of low-cost milk. The narrow tip at the top is a small but affluent market for western type milk products. The bulk of the demand for milk, however, is among the poor in urban areas (bottom of the pyramid) whose individual requirement is small. Nevertheless, it adds up to a sizable volume millions of litres per day in major urban centers where lies the immense growth potential. Presently, barely 1,000 out of 5,000 cities and towns are served by the milk distribution network of the organized sector.

The effective milk market is largely confined to urban areas, inhabited by over 25% of the country's population having a household income of Rs. 5,000. this is a large target group for branded milk and milk products. An estimated 50% of the total milk produced is consumed here. In the next 5 years (by 2011), the urban population is expected to touch 360 million – a growth of about 2.5%. The projected age distribution of Indian consumers shows a steadily rising percentage in the 20-34 age group which is most receptive to experiment new products. The age group, which was about 25 per cent of the total population, is growing steadily. As demographic changes take place, there would be increasing number of nuclear families and working women in urban India. The emergence of organized food retail chains / super markets will also lead to growth in the sale of packaged dairy and food products. The expected phenomenal rise in urban population would be a boon to Indian dairying.

5.3. Types of Market Milk

The fluid milk industry has become increasingly diversified in recent years, distributing a wide variety of fluid milks and technologically compatible products. In India, different types of milk, as given under PFA rules 1955 (as amended December, 1985) are defined as follows:

Pasteurized Milk: The term pasteurization, when used in association with milk and milk products means heating milk of different classes by a heat treatment as indicated below and cooling to a suitable temperature before distribution. Pasteurized milk of different classes shall show a negative phosphatase test. The terms 'pasteurization,' 'pasteurized' and similar terms shall be taken to refer to the process of heating every particle of milk of different classes to at least 63°C and holding at such temperature continuously for at least 30 minutes or heating it to at least 71.5° C, and holding at such temperature continuously for at least 15 seconds or an approved temperature –time combination that will serve to give negative phosphatase test. The pasteurized milk of different classes shall be cooled immediately to a temperature of 10° C or less. Pasteurized milk shall contain not more than 50,000 cfu per ml. Coliforms shall be absent in 0.01 ml

Sterilized Milk: The term sterilization, when used in association with milk, means heating continuously to a temperature of 115° C for 15 minutes or 145° C for 3 seconds or equivalent approved temperature-time combination to ensure preservation at room temperature for a period of not less than 15 days from the date of manufacture. Sterilized milk shall show absence of albumin by a negative turbidity test. Sterilized milk shall be sold only in the container in which it was sterilized.

Standardized milk, mixed milk, toned milk, double toned milk, recombined milk and flavoured milk have already been defined in Chapter 1.

When milk is offered for sale without any designation, the standards prescribed for buffalo milk (which vary for different regions, viz. milk fat, 5 or 6% and SNF, 9%) shall apply.

Special Milks: When natural constituents of whole milk have been altered by addition, removal, exchange and/ or treatment, the resultant milk is designated as special milk. Recent years have witnessed a large increase in the market penetration of special milks into the total fluid milk market. In many countries, now a large portion of fluid milk is consumed in the form of special milks. Manufacturers of special milks offer numerous advantages that are broadly related to dietary, cost and scarcity aspects.

Though milk is considered as nature's almost perfect food, however, sometimes it is not considered suitable for some people on health ground or they do not like its flavour. Under such circumstances manufacture of special milks such as dietetic, low-fat and flavoured milks, *etc* can solve the problems.

Fat is one of the most expensive constituents of milk. The price of milk is determined by and large by its fat content. High-fat milk is priced at higher level which can not be afforded by poor segment of the society. Therefore, low-fat milk like toned and double toned were introduced in India to overcome this problem. Replacement of milk fat with vegetable fat could also help in reducing the cost of milk.

Due to seasonal fluctuation in milk production, there is acute shortage of milk during the lean period in our country. In certain parts of the world fresh milk is not produced at all. Manufacture of reconstituted and recombined milk from anhydrous milk solids can overcome such milk shortages. These anhydrous milk solids could either be prepared from the domestic surpluses or marketed from those countries that have surplus milk production.

5.4. Collection and Transportation of Milk

The production of high quality products requires high quality raw milk. Characteristics of raw milk supply are influenced markedly by milk producing and handling systems, which in turn are associated with the practices followed by plants, interstate shipment of milk and roles played by dairy plants and producers in obtaining and maintaining a good raw milk supply.

The dairy industry in India is unique in several ways. Nowhere else in the world have we dairy industry of such a magnitude based on the efforts of individual producers who produce milk from anywhere near one litre to a few litres per day. Most often, in all countries production of milk is confined to rural areas, while its demand is mostly from urban areas. Availability of inputs required for production of milk is cheaply and conveniently available in rural areas, whereas densely populated potential consumers are in urban areas. In addition, rural people, in general, face lot of marketing problems due to scanty and scattered nature of milk production, habitants and unavailability of proper infrastructure. Hence milk has to be collected, transported and marketed from villages to towns/cities for better return.

The milk collection system, chosen must reflect the local conditions in terms of technical competency, cost, infrastructure and climate. Milk collection from producers through collection points is done mostly in rural areas with a large number of small suppliers and thus, eliminates the need for their own chilling and storage facilities. Collection points must comply with the same hygienic requirements as the dairies, in addition to infra-structural facilities of quick transportation. In no case, milk after milking should take more than 4 hours, particularly in temperate countries, to reach to a point where it is chilled promptly to less than 4° C.

Planning Milk Collection: Well-adapted handling techniques for milk and dairy products of milk collection of some other countries, found economically sound are being practiced in most of the countries since long. Thus under similar environmental conditions, a successfully adapted model of milk collection of some other countries, found economically sound and technically reliable, can be taken up cautiously, of course, if required, with certain modifications in light of local existing conditions and developing features. The ultimate aim of any collection system is to provide regularly 'safe' milk for the processing units and / or customers to meet their demand at economical cost. The important considerations are as follows:

1. Climatic conditions: Climatic considerations like temperature and humidity with sharp seasonal variations play an important role in planning a suitable milk collection system. High climatic temperatures and humidity are very conducive for the growth of microorganisms. Therefore, provision should be made to introduce chilling facilities at the collection point to bring down the temperature of milk to below the 4°C within 4 hours of milking.

2. Developmental features: Planning of a collection system must be done in view of the actual stage of development which is subject to change with the development of the locality. The developmental features include: communication network, availability of technical know-how for maintenance and replacement of equipment, education and skill level, purchasing power of the people of the locality and basic amenities and infrastructure particularly transport.

3. Inherent characteristics of milk: Due to perishability of milk a collection system needs to: provide suitable containers, viz. utensils, cans, tanks or tankers to affect transport, storage and processing; to give fair measure (volume or weight) for payment; facilities for platform and laboratory tests.
4. Size of dairy plant: Depending upon the potentiality of milk production suitable capacity and size of reception and chilling facilities should be planned.
5. Density of milk supply: If milk is supplied to large dairy plants over a long distance from the production site, the milk collection centers are established to collect sufficient milk to justify a call for lorry or tanker. Intermediate collection points are more likely to be required when milk is to be collected from a low- density production area at a long distance. Large collection center will supply milk directly to the factory.

Organizing Milk Collection: After planning milk collection, steps are taken to organize collection system. The first step is to undertake extensive survey in the milk-shed area. Availability of milk at various collection points is ascertained based on the number of milch animals, future potential for development and the presence of competitors. This is followed by route planning and finalization of location for collection and chilling centre. Since organization involves interests of producer, processor and consumer, the collection system must be well organized and operated under tight and well controlled manner.

5.5. Types of Milk Collection Systems

A number of milk collection systems have been developed and are being used throughout the world to provide market to the milk producers and obtain sufficiency of milk for processing plant.

Direct from Producers: The milk produced near the city is generally transported by the individual farmers in small containers. This practice suits also to the large producers located near the city / processing plant. There is no obligation of any kind on either side.

The processor is in daily contact with the milk producers. Quality control can be performed in the presence of the producer. Adulteration can be dealt with in the presence of suppliers. The relative nearness and personal contact between producers and processors is excellent. Additional job opportunities among rural people can be created.

Dairy has the right to fix the price of milk. Generally low price is offered to producers. Milk producers are normally exploited. Dairy may deny taking the milk on various grounds. There is no assured market for milk throughout the year. The dairy because of seasonal variation may not accept all the milk supplied by producers. Producers do not get incentive for increasing milk production. Neither facilities to increase milk production are provided by dairy nor social and economic needs are taken care of. The profits earned by the dairy are not shared by milk producers.

Through Contractors: The traditional middleman (contractor) acts as a interface between the dairy plant and small milk producers. He collects milk from the farmers and transports it in large cans on cycle, rikshaw, tanga or tankers depending on the volume of milk handled. Apparently it seems to be simple and flexible system. It saves time of small milk producers / suppliers. All such milk is transported without chilling. In this procurement system, the milk processor has little control on the quality of milk procured by the contractor from milk producers. Price for the milk received by the producers is generally low. Producers do not get any incentive or help for milk production.

Through Agent: Some dairies enter into an agreement with the authorized agents for the supply of certain quantity of milk for specific period. Normally, the prices for the milk, its quality and quantity in different seasons are mutually agreed upon. Other details such as mode of payment, timings, transportation of milk, settlement of disputes, if any, and penalties for failures, etc are decided at the time of making agreement. The agents have their own arrangements to collect, chill and transport the milk in cans, tankers and bulk tanks etc by their own vehicles. Dairy is in no way concerned with milk production and management of milk collection, transportation and incurring expenses on it. Dairy has not to deal with large number of producers but only with few contractors.

Milk producers are, invariably, exploited by the agents and the dairy as well. Quality of milk, in general, is poor, adulterated and fabricated. Once becoming dependent on the supply of milk by agents, dairy yields to their dictate. Producers get very low price for their milk and profits are taken by the agents. Often milk producers remain debtor to the agent and they do not have freedom to sell their produce elsewhere. No facilities for increasing milk production nor for their social upliftment are provided. This system of milk procurement encourages red tapeism / corruption.

Through Cooperatives: At the village level, farmers organize themselves in a cooperative society, which establishes milk collection centres. The society members deliver milk twice a day to the milk collection centres where milk is weighed, tested and price is paid to the farmers according to its quantity and quality. The payment is based on the percentage of fat, SNF or total solids in milk. The village society supplies/sells milk to its own district cooperative dairy plant. It transports milk in cans by truck or insulated road milk tanker, if there is a chilling centre. Besides milk collection, the dairy society also provides technical input services such as artificial insemination, veterinary aid, concentrated cattle feed and fodder seeds and counseling to the society members to enhance milk production.

Unlike the other systems of procurement, the milk producer is the owner of the dairy. He has right to decide the price of milk and also to get the share of profit made by the dairy. This system gives self-reliance to the producers for solving their problems in a collective manner. This is a foolproof system to eliminate all the demerits of other types of milk collection.

Through Chilling Centres: If the dairy plant is far away from the collection center, then the collected milk is first brought to a centralized chilling centre. The milk is chilled to 4° C and is stored in insulated storage tanks of 5,000 to 20,000-litre capacity. Subsequently, the chilled milk is transported in the insulated road milk tanker to the dairy plant. The transportation of milk from the chilling center to the dairy plant usually takes place once a day. The distance between chilling centers and plants varies from 20-170 kms. On an average, area covered by a chilling centre is about 40 sq. kms with the range of 25-125 kms.

This has made possible shipment of milk from places hundreds of miles away from the metropolitan cities such as Bombay, Calcutta, Delhi and Madras. In some cases chilled milk is transported by train such as from Anand to Bombay. Sometimes frozen milk is transported in refrigerated tankers from such far away places as Mehsana to Delhi, about 1000 miles away.

5.6. Transportation of Raw Milk

The dairy plants organize the collection and transportation of milk in its collection area. Route plans need to be established and continuously optimized for an effective utilization of the transport facilities and keeping transport cost low. Some sorts of transport are also required to carry the milk from points of production to the points of collection, pick up, chilling or processing.

Milk being perishable commodity, it becomes necessary to transport the fresh raw milk to the consumer or chilling/processing plant within 4 hours of its production. Thus transportation becomes an integral part of milk collection system. An efficient and suitable facility is selected on the basis of the raw milk collection as well as regional requirements.

The different modes of transport of milk used in India have been summarized in Table 5.6.1

Table 5.6.1. Different modes of transport of milk

Mode	Optimum Load (kg)	Optimum Distance (km)	Remarks
Head load	15-25	3-8	Generally employed for small load and distance, important in hilly areas
Shoulder sling	20-40	5-10	Meant for heavier load and shorter distances, hilly areas
Pack animal	40-80	5-10	Ponies, horses, donkeys, bullocks
Bullock cart	300-400	10-12	In villages where no road exists, Rather slow
Tonga (Horse cart)	250-300	12-15	Faster than above modes, needs road
Bicycle	40 or more	10-15	Quick and handy, easily accessible to milk producer's consumer's home
Motor cycle	100 or more	15 or more	Heavier duty than bicycle
Cycle rickshaw	150-250	10 or more	More carrying capacity than cycle
Boat	40-200	2-8	When required through rivers
Auto rickshaw	250-500	15 or more	More capacity & faster than cycle rickshaw
Motor truck	0.5 to 3.5 tonnes	100 or more	Carry milk in cans, bulk tanks; most efficient
Railway wagon	10-12 tonnes or more	100 or more	Most dependable & economical for long distance but less popular
Road tankers	3-12 tonnes	100-1000	Insulated stainless steel tanks mounted on road truck chasis
Rail tanker	10-50 tonnes	500-3,000	Insulated and refrigerated stainless steel tanks mounted on rail truck/chasis

Transport Vessels

- Milk cans: 40-50 litre cans up to 3,000 litres per truck.
- Farm containers: Made of stainless steel, mobile and insulated (partially with chilling), 200 to 500 litre capacity.

- Tanks installed on trucks: Insulated and/or refrigerated, capacity 600 to 3,000 litre tanks mounted on truck to receive milk on the route.
- Milk tankers: Separated into several chambers with and without an integrated reception device and data recording, capacity 3,000 to 5,000 litre milk.
- Transport pipes: Subterranean pipelines made of stainless steel in developed countries for transporting milk between the dairy and collecting point. Milk is pushed or flowing by gravity at suitable location.

Types of Transport: Roadways, railways, waterways and airways are the possible types of transport. Sometimes combination of two or more can also be used for transporting milk. In selecting suitability of a type of transport, volume of milk, geographical location of the area, availability of facilities and ultimately the cost of transportation are taken into account. The comparative advantages of different types of transport is given in Table 5.6.2.

Table 5.6.2: Comparative advantages of different types of transport

Type of Transport		Advantages
Milk can	i)	Handling small quantities of milk possible
	ii)	Hygienic, if cleaned and sanitized properly
Tanker	i)	Quicker mode of transport
	ii)	Lower cost for large quantity of milk
	iii)	Better temperature control
	iv)	Less risk of contamination from dust, etc.
	v)	Time and labour saving in loading and unloading
	vi)	Overall saving of detergent, etc.
Railways	i)	Cheaper than roadways over long distances.
	ii)	Larger quantity of milk can be handled at a time.
Roadways	i)	most economic to transport milk in containers by using bicycle, tricycle, motor cycle, carts,; trucks, lorries and tankers.
	ii)	Loading and unloading possible directly at godowns of seller and buyer.
	iii)	Cheaper than rails over short distances.
	iv)	Most convenient and less time consuming

5.7. Cooling of Raw Milk

When milk is freshly drawn its temperature is about 38° C which is very conducive for the growth of microorganisms. If milk is not chilled immediately, bacterial deterioration may set in. Therefore, freshly drawn milk should be promptly chilled and held at 4° C till processing to preserve it against bacterial deterioration. Chilled milk can easily and safely be transported without having appreciable deteriorative changes due to microbial growth. Thus, raw milk is chilled to (a) limit the growth of bacteria, (b) minimize micro-induced changes and (c) maximize its shelf life. However, chilling milk involves additional expenses which increase the cost of processing. Importantly, chilling process does not destroy microorganisms nor it renders milk safe for human consumption. It is only a means of checking the growth of microorganisms for a certain period.

Effect on Microbial Growth: Generally milk is chilled immediately after milking to below 10° C, within 4 hours to prevent/retard the multiplication of mesophilic and thermophilic bacteria including disease producing and food poisoning microorganisms until the milk reaches the dairy. The extent of control of the growth of microorganisms is dependent on type of organisms. Staphylococci do not grow below 10° C. Growth stops for most types of *B. coli, B. proteus* and *Micrococci* between 0 and 5° C. If milk is stored cold for too long time, there can be an undesirable increase in psychrotrophic organisms which produce extremely heat resistant lipases and proteases.

The time factor is critical in arresting bacterial growth in fresh milk. As the milk from the udder of healthy animal has low bacterial count, there is a lag phase immediately after milking, for about 4 hours, before bacterial multiplication begins to take place. The quicker the milk is cooled, the better the quality and in the ideal condition, milk is cooled immediately after milking to 4°C or below and held at that temperature till it is processed.

Effect on Keeping Quality: Fresh raw milk is chilled to 4° C to extend its shelf life (freshness). At this temperature, the activity of enzymes, the growth of microorganisms and metabolic processes are all slowed down. As a result, prolonged holding of chilled milk is bound to cause significant deteriorative alterations in keeping quality of milk. In addition, cooling causes a considerable dissociation of β-casein, calcium and phosphate ions and proteases from the casein micelles. The milk loses its suitability for cheese making, has longer coagulation time and lower curd tension of coagulum.

Chemical and biochemical processes are considerably slowed down by cooling. However, milk which has been stored for long time, sometimes has a bitter off-flavour. Enzymes and microorganisms can cause chemical changes which are accompanied by a lower pH value and change in nitrogen containing compounds. Psychrophilic microorganisms cause proteolysis of casein and, together with enzymes, also that of albumin. Protein breakdown products (polypeptides) are formed. Certain bacteria are responsible for the hydrolysis of fats causing rancid flavour development. Several enzymes such as oxidase, catalase and reductase are active for a long time, even at 0° C. Hence, if the time between milk reception and processing is 2-3 days, the storage temperature should be kept between 2-3° C for minimum effect on keeping quality of milk.

Equipment and Methods of Chilling

Can Immersion: The fresh milk immediately after milking, is placed in a container (preferably metal) which is gently lowered into a tank / trough of cooling water. Cooling of milk will slowly take place and if the water is cold enough, the milk temperature will be reduced low enough to allow milk to be marketed / processed. The milk inside the cans may be stirred with the help of plunger for uniform quick cooling.

In-can cooling: Portable refrigeration units may be employed for in-can cooling of milk by direct immersion of cooling coil. The cooling coil is kept immersed in the can till the desired cooling temperature is attained. Such a unit is fitted on a trolley and is suitable for cooling 5-7 cans (200-280 litres of milk) at the farm.

Rotor Freeze: Rotor freeze provides spray of chilled water outside the cans obtained by mechanical refrigeration system and passing through the perforated tubes around the neck of the can. With this system, milk temperature is brought down to 10°C from 35°C within 15 minutes.

Surface Cooler: An improvement of water cooling is a metal surface cooler, where water flows through the inner side and the milk flows over the outer surface in thin film. A well designed water cooler will reduce milk temperature almost instantaneously. The cooled milk is received below in a receiving trough, from which it is discharged by gravity or a pump.

Bulk milk cooler: This consists of a double jacketed vat fitted with a mechanical agitator. It also has a provision for circulation of chilled water which comes from the chilled water tank. Normally, milk is chilled and subsequently stored at low temperature until transported to the processing units. Bulk milk coolers are generally installed at chilling centers.

This method is more suitable for handling 500-2,500 litres milk/day. It is being increasingly used by village level milk collection centres in India. From the bulk coolers, milk is pumped into insulated milk tankers for transportation to the dairy plant. Bulk milk coolers are usually horizontal, semi-circular, or vertical cylindrical tanks with an inner jacket and an outer insulated body. To effect cooling, the inner shell of the tank has provision for either chilled water around its external periphery or a direct expansion cooling coil from a mechanical refrigeration system. Milk is either directly poured into the tank or pumped through a balance tank. Milk coming in contact with the inner shell of the tank is cooled to around 4° C. The agitator inside the tank helps to maintain uniform cooling of milk.

Plate Chiller: This is the most widely used very effective equipment for chilling of milk by the commercial dairy plants. It is widely used for large scale cooling of milk (5,000-50,000 litres/day) at the chilling centers. They are highly efficient, compact and easily cleanable. In a chiller, a number of gasketed plates are tightly held between the frames. These plates are so arranged that a flow passage for milk exists on one side of the plate and the cooling medium (usually chilled water) on the other side. There is a counter-current flow between the milk and the chilled water through alternate plates. It helps in efficient transfer of heat from milk to the cooling medium-chilled water which results in quick chilling of milk. The chilled milk flows from the plate cooler to the insulated or chilled water-jacketed milk storage tank for storing milk at 4° C. A mechanical refrigeration system with ice bank tank ensures supply of chilled water to the plate cooler.

Tubular Cooler: This consists of two concentric tubes, inner tube usually carries the milk to be chilled while cold water is passing through the hollow space in between the pipes. The length and diameter of both the tubes are determined according to the capacity of the plant. The flow of milk and chilled water is in opposite direction, i.e., counter-current. The tubular cooler is efficient and milk is not exposed to the atmosphere.

Brine Cooling: The direct expansion coil is used to cool brine which is then circulated by a pump around the product to be cooled. Brine system of cooling may be of a) brine circulating type, b) brine storage type, and c) congealing tank type. This system has the advantages of being safe with ammonia and of causing less damage in case of leakage and the temperature can be easily controlled. It also allows the storing up of refrigeration in the cold brine and, therefore, allows heavy refrigeration load of short duration to be carried with a system having a much smaller compressor than direct expansion system used. The overall thermal efficiency of a brine system is usually less than the direct expansion system on account of the one extra heat transfer and added radiation losses.

Ice Cooling: Ice, produced by commercial ice plants, is used in some countries to cool milk. The use of ice for cooling is generally fairly expensive and not particularly effective due to the problems in getting an optimum and rapid heat transfer from the liquid milk to the solid ice. Different methods of cooling milk by ice are:

- **Putting ice around metal cans of milk:** It is the simplest form of cooling milk in which ice slabs are stacked around the metal cans of milk on the delivery vehicle and the system relies on heat transfer by contact.
- **In-can cooling:** In this method, ice is placed in metal container, known as ice gum or ice cone, which is inserted into the can of milk. This permits the more effective heat exchange rate by giving off latent heat of ice and sensible heat of melted water but reduces the volume of milk that can be carried in the milk can. When ice is completely melted in the ice cone and there is no more heat transfer, the water is thrown and the fresh ice pieces are put in. the process of cooling milk by this method continues even during transportation from collection centres to processing unit.

5.8. Grading of Milk

Testing of quality of milk at the receiving dock is usually done based on a set of quick tests. These tests can be classified in two major groups: A) Platform Tests and B) Laboratory Tests. The platform tests refer to all those tests, which are performed to check the quality of incoming milk on the receiving platform so as to make a quick decision regarding its acceptance or rejection. They are performed on each can or tanker of milk with the object of detecting milk of inferior or doubtful quality from being mixed with the high-grade milk. The main purpose of the examination of raw milk at the reception dock is to assess i) freshness, ii) hygienic quality and iii) composition.

A) The platform tests

1. Organoleptic tests
2. Temperature
3. Sedimentation test
4. Clot-on-Boiling test (COB)
5. Alcohol test
6. Alcohol-Alizerin test
7. Neutralizer test

B) Laboratory tests

1. Acidity test
2. Fat test
3. SNF test (solids-not-fat)
4. Methylene Blue Reduction (MBR) test
5. 1-Hour Resazurin Reduction test
6. Direct Microscopic Count (DMC) test
7. Standard Plate Count (SPC) test
8. Presumptive Coliform test

A) Platform tests

Organoleptic Tests: Organoleptic or sensory tests are performed with the help of five sense organs, viz eye, nose, tongue, ear and skin. Organoleptic tests are quick, cheap and with growing experience of the assessor, very reliable. Since practically no equipment is needed, the sensory tests can be carried out anywhere and any time. However, sensory tests are subjective and would depend on the assessor's faculty of perception.

This includes testing for odour, appearance, colour, presence of foreign particles and partially churned fat globules at the surface of milk. All these observations are made immediately but simultaneously after opening the lid of can, rail or road tanker. Odour of the milk is most simple and valuable test to decide fitness of milk for processing. The lid of each can is removed, inverted and raised to the nose to receive the odour. The odour will be representative of the milk in the can. Then the milk is vigorously shaken using a plunger and odour is tested again. With practice, one can differentiate among odours produced by feed, rancidity, products of bacterial growth and absorption after the milk is produced. Sourness due to bacterial contamination can be identified by the smell and can be further confirmed, if required, by the taste as well. If the odours are pronounced and unpleasant, the milk should be rejected.

Appearance of milk should be inspected for any floating extraneous matter, colour change and partial churning of fat. Normal milk should be free from these. Presence of visible dirt, straw or manure indicates that the milk has been handled in an unhygienic way. If extraneous matters are present, the producers should be instructed to adopt hygienic method during milking and transportation. Normally cow milk should be yellowish whereas buffalo milk, white. If there is any significant deviation from the normal colour, the reason should be traced out. Sometimes due to destabilization of fat globules, churning of fat takes place and clumps of fat start floating on the surface of milk. This may arise due to agitation of milk during transportation, particularly if the temperature is high. This may create problem in sampling, analysis and processing of milk.

Temperature: The temperature of incoming milk should be checked. The temperature at which milk is transported and delivered at the processing plant is often an indication of its quality. In the tropical countries, like ours, where temperature is very favourable for the bacterial growth, cooling of milk before transportation is desirable. If the temperature of milk is kept below 10°C during transportation, the shelf life of milk can be enhanced and factors like delay in processing of milk or breakdown during journey will not cause serious concern for spoilage of milk. Temperature of milk coming from chilling centers should be checked. Temperature of more than 5°C indicates bacterial action and reflects quality. However, milk in small quantities from the individual producers, and from very short distances can be accepted even if it is not cooled.

Sedimentation test: The sediment test presents a simple, rapid and a quantitative measure indicating the cleanliness of milk with respect to visible dirt. The hygienic conditions adopted during production, transportation and handling of milk at different stages can be indicated with the help of this test. But this test could have its fullest usefulness only if there were assurance that the milk has not been strained. Only with this limitation, this test is used as a supplement to other intake tests for the acceptance or rejection of milk. However, the test can be very useful in teaching the producers or suppliers of milk to maintain proper sanitary conditions.

This test is carried out by allowing a measured quantity of milk (usually 500 ml) to pass through a fixed area of a filter disc and comparing the sediment left with the prepared standards.

Clot-on-Boiling test (COB): This is a quick test to determine the suitability of milk for heat processing. This is an index of developed acidity. If the acidity of milk exceeds 0.17%, it may lead to the appearance of clots on boiling.

A 5 ml sample of milk is transferred in a test tube. The test tube is placed in a boiling water bath for 5 min. Observe formation of clots or flakes on the test tube wall. Formation of clots or flakes indicates positive test showing that milk has high developed acidity and is not fit for heat processing.

Alcohol test: The alcohol test is used for rapid assessment of stability of milk during heat processing, particularly for condensing, sterilization and drying. It is an indication of mineral balance of milk and not so much as an index of developed acidity. The test aids in detecting abnormal milk such as colostrum, milk from animals at late lactation or suffering from mastitis and milk in which mineral balance has been disturbed.

This test is performed by mixing equal parts (5 ml) of milk and ethyl alcohol (75% for cow milk and 68% for buffalo milk). Appearance of any flakes on the wall of the test tube is an indication of positive test. This shows that milk is not fit to be subjected to high heat treatment.

Alcohol-Alizarin test: This is similar to the above tests, but it helps to indicate the approximate percentage of titratable acidity. Thus it is used to determine the suitability of milk for high heat treatment.

Procedure of doing the test is also similar as that for alcohol, but in this the contents of the test tubes after proper mixing are observed for the colour besides the presence of size of flakes. The test is performed by mixing equal parts (5 ml) milk and alcohol-alizarin solution (0.2%). The formation of flakes and colour are observed. The interpretation of the results is shown in Table 5.8.1.

Table 5.8.1. Interpretation of alcohol-alizarin test

Colour	Size of Flakes	Approx. Acidity (%)	Heat Stability
Lilac or pale red	No flakes	Up to 0.14	Good (low acidity)
Lilac or pale red	Small flakes	0.14 to 0.17	Poor (sweet curdling)
Violet or purple (alkaline)	Small flakes	0.17	Poor (late lactation or mastitis
Reddish brown (acidic)	Small flakes	0.17 to 0.20	Very poor
Brownish yellow to yellow (highly acidic)	Large flakes	0.20	Very poor

Neutralizer test: Neutralizer test is conducted to detect the presence of added neutralizers, *viz.* caustic soda and carbonated salts. The test is performed by mixing equal parts (5 ml) milk and ethyl alcohol (75%) with few drops of 1% aqueous solution of rosalic acid. Presence of rose-red colour indicates addition of carbonate neutralizer in milk.

B) Laboratory tests

Acidity test: The titratable acidity of milk is used to ascertain whether the milk is fit for giving heat treatment. Natural or apparent acidity does not make the milk sour, but developed acidity due to excess lactic acid adversely affects the quality of milk and alters its behaviour upon heat treatment.

The titratable acidity is determined by titrating a known amount of milk sample (10 ml) by a standard alkali solution (N/10 or N/9) using phenolphthalein as the indicator. Appearance of light pink colour indicates the completion of reaction. Note the titre value. The percent acidity is calculated as lactic acid.

Fat tests

a) Gerber Method: Gerber method is used to determine fat content in milk. The fat percentage in milk is commonly used as the basis for payment of milk. When a definite quantity of sulphuric acid and amyl alcohol are added to a definite volume of milk, the proteins get dissolved and the fat globules are set free which remains in liquid state due to heat produced by the acid. Upon centrifugation, fat being lighter separates on the top of the solution.

The procedure involves transferring 10 ml of sulphuric acid (Gerber acid) into milk butyrometer (range, 0-10%) using automatic measure. An aliquot of 10.75 ml of well mixed milk is transferred slowly by the side of butyrometer wall taking care not to wet the neck of the butyrometer. Add 1.0 ml of amyl alcohol using automatic measure to the mixture of milk and acid. Stopper the butyrometer with a lock stopper, using the key, and shake the contents well. Butyrometer is kept in a water bath at 65° C for 5 min followed by centrifugation at 1100-1200 rpm for 5 min. Again the butyrometer is kept in the water bath at 65° C for 5 min before taking the reading directly on the butyrometer stem.

b) Gravimetric Method: For quantitative separation of fat it is necessary to break the protective film surrounding the fat globule by suitable agent (ammonia). The passage of fat globules from aqueous phase to solvent is facilitated by alcohol. The mixed solvent system brings about extraction of fat from non-fatty solids in the solution. This principle is used in Rose-Gottleib/ Mojonnier Method of fat determination.

The procedure involves transferring 10 g of well mixed sample of milk into Rose-Gottleib tube / Mojonnier flask. Add 1 ml of concentrated ammonia and mix well by gentle swirling motion. Add I ml of alcohol and again mix well. Add 25 ml of diethyl ether, stopper the tube with cork and shake vigorously for 1 min. Remove the cork and add 25 ml petroleum ether, stopper and shake well for 30 seconds. Allow the tube to stand until the ethereal layer is separated clearly from the aqueous layer (for Rose-Gottleib method). In case of Mojonnier method – centrifuge the Mojonnier flask for 10 min. Decant the clear ethereal layer into a previously weighed aluminium fat dish. Repeat extraction with 15 ml portions each of diethyl ether and petroleum ether twice to completely extract fat from the sample. Transfer the ethereal layers from each extraction into the fat dish. Place the dish on a hot plate (60-65°C) and allow the ether layer to evaporate slowly. Dry the residual fat at 98° C in an oven and then allow the fat dish to cool by placing in a desiccator. Weigh the fat dish and note the weight. Repeat heating, cooling and weighing until successive weighing do not differ by more than 1 mg. Calculate amount of fat by difference of weight in fat dish before and after extraction (reading 'A'). Divide reading 'A' by weight of the sample and multiply by 100 to get percent fat in sample.

Now, Milko-tester minor or semiautomatic butterfat analyzer is used for determining the fat content in milk. This is based on the principle of scattering of light by milk fat globules. Light transmission through the milk-mix is measured photometrically and red directly as the fat percentage in milk samples on digital display. Accuracy of the result is approximately the same as for the Gerber fat test.

Total Solids (TS) and Solids-Not-Fat (SNF) Content: Lactometers are used for rapid determination of specific gravity of milk. Based on the lactometer reading of milk taken under standard conditions and knowing the fat percentage, it is possible to calculate TS and SNF by using the well known Richmond's formula which differs for the type of lactometer.

The method is based on the principle of floatation, which states that when a solid is immersed in a liquid it is subjected to upward thrust equal to the weight of liquid displaced by it and acting vertically upwards. Lactometers are variable immersion type hydrometers and calibrated before hand with liquid of known specific gravity.

The SNF content of milk is calculated on the basis of its specific gravity. The specific gravity of milk is determined by using lactometer reading. Milk drawn from the udder contains a large volume of air bubbles and the milk fat undergoes a gradual solidification. Due to these factors a gradual contraction in the volume of milk takes place with a slow increase in specific gravity to a maximum (Racknagal phenomenon). The specific gravity of milk will, therefore, vary with the duration and temperature of storage. This variation may be overcome by ensuring that the fat is completely in the liquid state before the specific gravity reading is taken. This is achieved by pre-warming the milk.

The sample of milk is warmed to a temperature of 40-45°C and maintained within this range for 5 minutes during which time the contents of the bottle are adequately mixed. Care shall be taken to avoid the formation of air bubbles or froth when mixing the sample. The sample is then water cooled to 27 ±2°C and held within this range until the specific gravity reading is taken. The sample shall not be held for more than one hour. The reading is then taken according to the following procedure:

The sample bottle is gently inverted two or thee times. The milk is then poured down the side of the lactometer jar so as to avoid the formation of air bubbles. Sufficient milk will be poured into the jar to ensure that some of it overflows when the lactometer is inserted. The lactometer, held by the stem, is inserted in the sample and released when it is approximately in its position of equilibrium thus avoiding wetting more than a very short length of the stem above the milk surface. As soon as the lactometer is at rest, the scale reading corresponding to the top of the meniscus of the milk is noted. The lactometer jar shall be vertical and the bulb of the lactometer shall not touch the side.

It is advisable to repeat the reading after depressing the lactometer about 3 mm and allowing it to come to rest. Note the temperature of the milk with the help of the thermometer. Get the corrected value (CLR) from the standard Table for corresponding temperature. Calculate SNF content using the following formula:

Specific gravity = CLR/1000 + 1

Percent SNF =C LR/4 + 0.25x fat % + 44

Per cent TS = CLR/4 + 1.25 x fat %+ 44

Dye Reduction tests

Dye reduction test involves testing the time required for reducing dyes such as methylene blue or resazurine. Colour of these dyes are altered by change in oxidation-reduction potential of milk. Hence the rate at which discharge of colour takes place is an indication of metabolic rate and thus bacterial activity of milk. Rate of colour change varies depending upon the types of organisms present and their activity at a particular temperature. Greater the number of bacteria, shorter will be the time required for dye reduction and thus the rate of dye reduction indicates quality of milk.

Methylene Blue Reduction test (MBR): The methylene blue test is the simplest method for grading raw milk. It does not determine the number of bacteria, but measures one type of bacterial activity, i.e., the rate at which microorganisms utilize oxygen. If all bacteria utilize oxygen at the same rate, the test could be used to indicate the number of bacteria present. Since microorganisms vary in this respect, the test has definite limitations.

Methylene blue gives blue colour to milk which disappears upon reduction. If the disappearance of blue colour occurs within 30 minutes, such milk cannot be accepted.

The procedure involves transferring 10 ml of milk in a test tube, adding 1 ml of working solution of methylene blue. Stopper the tube and shake well. Place the tube in a water bath at 37°C. Observe discolouration of the contents against control sample. Note the time of discolouration. Make control sample by mixing 10 ml of milk + 1 ml of water and 10 ml of milk + 1 ml of methylene blue dye. Keep them in boiling water bath for 3 minutes. Based on this test milk can be graded as shown in Table 4.6.2.

One-Hour Resazurin Test: The resazurin test has the same advantages and limitations as the methylene blue test. Resazurin undergoes a series of colour changes in comparison to only one for methylene blue.

In resazurin reduction test instead of methylene blue resazurin is used, which is more sensitive dye, hence requires less time. Usually for resazurin reduction, tubes are incubated for only 10 minutes and the colour is compared with the resazurin disc in comparator. However, one-hour resazurin test gives a better indication of the quality of milk than 10-minute resazurin test. Reading of 4 or more is considered satisfactory.

Resazurin reduction occurs in two stages, the first an irreversible change from the blue resazurin to the pink resorufin and the second, a reversible change from the pink resorufin to the colourless dihydroresorufin. The first stage of reduction or colour change from blue to pink is fairly easily brought about so that the quality of milk is assessed in much shorter time. Taking advantage of the two-stage reduction, several procedures have been proposed for reading the end point of resazurin test.

The procedure involves transferring 10 ml of milk in a sterile test tube aseptically and adding 1 ml of resazurin test solution. Stopper the tube and shake well. Place the tube in water bath at 37°C for 1 hour. Compare the colour developed in a Lovibond comparator using resazurin disc. Grade the milk as per BIS standard as given in Table 4.6.7.

Direct Microscopic Count: The direct microscopic method consists of examining, under a compound microscope, stained films of a measured volume of milk spread on glass slides over specified area. It enables the rapid estimation of the total bacterial population of a sample of milk and also reveals useful information for tracing the sources of contamination of milk. The microscope is first calibrated so that the exact area of the microscopic field is known. Then the measured quantity of milk (0.01 ml) spread over a measured area (1 sq.cm.) on a clean glass slide so that each microscopic field examined represents a quantitative aliquot of the sample. The milk is allowed to dry, and the film is defatted, fixed and stained with a suitable dye. The average number of bacteria per microscopic field is determined after examining between 5 and 60 fields, depending on the microscopic factor and the number of bacteria per field. Either the total cells or clumps can be counted, but the clump count agrees more closely with results obtained by the agar plate method than does the total cell count.

This method offers the most rapid technique for determining the extent of bacterial contamination in milk and requires 10 to 15 minutes for examining one sample. The additional advantages of this method are: general morphology of microorganisms can be determined, mastitic milk can be detected and a permanent record is made available. It has been used for the classification of raw milk samples into different grades on the basis of clump counts, for screening milk samples for 'acceptable' quality, and for obtaining information regarding likely sources of contamination. The microscopic appearance (types and arrangement of cells) of the milk film will give indication of any udder infections as well as the cause of high counts due to utensil contamination or inadequate cooling.

Estimates of bacterial counts by this method may be expected to be relatively more accurate in the case of poor quality milk having high bacterial counts. In the case of low count samples, examination of a large number of fields is necessary to obtain some accuracy in the estimates. Other sources of error in this method are those caused by (a) variable distribution of bacteria in films, especially those prepared from samples of high sanitary quality; (b) inaccurate measurement of 0.01 ml quantities and faulty preparation and staining of slides, (c) failure of this method to distinguish between the dead and living organisms; and (d) mistakes in observation and calculation.

As per BIS standard the bacteriological quality of milk is assessed on the basis of direct microscopic count as follows:

Bacterial Count Grade (per ml)

Less than 5, 00,000 → Good

5, 00,001 to 40, 00,000 → Fair

40, 00,001 to 2, 00, 00, 000 → Poor

Over 2, 00, 00, 000 → Very poor

Standard Plate Count: The standard plate count is the most satisfactory method for enumerating bacteria in raw and pasteurized milk. It is most expensive of the methods discussed, but is also the most accurate. The necessary equipment for the standard plate count can be utilized for many other purposes such as coliform counts, laboratory pasteurized counts, thermophilic counts, *etc.* The standard plate count method is used for determining the total number of viable bacteria in milk and consists of mixing appropriate quantity of milk with a suitable nutrient agar medium in a petri dish and counting the bacterial colonies developed after incubation at a specified temperature for a definite period of time. The grading of raw milk on the basis of standard plate count is shown in Table 4.6.2.

Presumptive Coliform Test: This group of bacteria is important in quality control of milk as it is indicative of possible faecal contamination and due to its ability to produce acid and taints in milk. The presence of this group in milk considered to be an indicator of the degree of unhygienic practices during production, processing or storage and is intended to measure general care taken in handling this product. The members of this group are generally destroyed during pasteurization and, therefore, any positive coliform test in the case of pasteurized milk is considered to indicate post-pasteurization contamination.

The procedure involves inoculation of a series of brilliant green bile or MacConkey broth fermentation tubes with appropriate volumes (such as 10 ml, 1 ml, 0.1ml and 0.01ml) of the sample dilution in triplicate. The tubes are incubated at 37 ± 0.5° C for 48 h or 30 ± 0.5° C for 72 h. Acid and gas formation in at least two tubes out of three constitute a positive presumptive test.

5.9. Processing of Milk

Various unit operations performed for processing of milk are:

1. Reception and storage
2. Centrifugal operations (clarification, separation, standardization, clarifixation)
3. Heat processing (pasteurization, sterilization, thermization)
4. Homogenization
5. Packaging
6. Storage
7. Distribution

The sequence of processing treatment may vary from plant to plant and certain operations may be combined in a single integrated system. For example, pasteurization and homogenization can be accomplished as one continuous process. The processing of raw milk received at the dairy plant is essential for the following reasons:

- To meet the quality standards to conform to the law of the country. In India it is the Prevention of Food Adulteration (PFA) Act, 1954 & rules 1955,
- To comply with certification requirements of agencies like Agmark and Bureau of Indian Standards (BIS), International Standards Organization (ISO), Codex Alimentarius Commission (CAC) prior to marketing products
- To enhance the shelf life of products, and
- To satisfy consumer taste.

5.9.1. Reception and storage of milk

Milk may be delivered to the dairy plant either in cans or in tankers (road/rail). The place in the dairy plant, where milk first arrives and is received after grading for acceptance, is known as milk reception dock or platform. Dairy reception dock is especially designed and equipped to facilitate rapid reception of milk and cleaning and sterilization of used containers.

Since further processing of milk mainly depends upon its quality, the decision of accepting the milk, must be done quickly immediately after arrival and thorough investigation. The milk reception should be so planned and the equipment so chosen that the intake operations are expedited, particularly where large volumes of milk is received. Delay may lead to deterioration of milk awaiting dumping and may increase in labour and operating costs of the can washer. Therefore, the deliveries of milk should follow a schedule and reception be completed within stipulated period of 2-3 hours to facilitate the following plant operations uninterrupted, especially in tropical countries.

Upon arrival of milk at chilling center or dairy plant it is subjected to certain preliminary examination in order to assess its general quality and decide whether to accept or reject. At the point of reception, the milk should be clean, sweet with pleasant odour, taste and free from extraneous matters. Sanitary quality of milk on receiving platform depends on its production situation at the farm and situations of handling and transportation. Milk may be arriving in cans or tankers and before emptying, the milk is inspected for gross changes in organoleptic quality and is done to find whether a particular lot of milk is fit for processing or not.

Milk cans are unloaded from the vehicle and are taken to the emptying point, where the lids are removed and milk is inspected. If there is no gross abnormality of quality, milk is poured into a weighing tank and the weight is recorded. Simultaneously a sample of milk is collected for detail testing of quality. Emptied cans and lids are taken to can washer. From the weighing tank milk is transferred to a dump tank and from which pumping of milk is done through cooling coil into a raw milk storage tank kept at higher level to permit gravity flow to the pasteurizer. With this method the storage tanks should be sufficiently insulated to maintain a low temperature until the milk is further processed. Each storage tank should be equipped with an agitator with which the milk is mixed before being drawn from the tanks for pasteurization

Milk coming in tankers is also thoroughly inspected for quality. For unloading outlets of the tanker is connected to sanitary pipes and milk is then pumped into the storage tank. The tanker is then subjected to thorough washing and sanitization. Milk coming from chilling center might be graded, weighed, sampled and chilled already. However, milk is usually weighed and sampled again at the dairy plant in order to rule out any variation in the quantity and quality. In order to minimize deterioration of quality due to delay in processing, milk reception should be completed within 3 to 4 hours.

The purpose of storage tank is to hold milk at low temperature so as to maintain continuity in milk processing operations and prevent any deterioration in quality during holding and processing period. Storage tanks also facilitate standardization of milk in bulk, which ensures uniform composition.

The insulated storage tanks are either horizontal or vertical in design. Selection of the type of storage tank depends on the layout and requirements of the floor space availability in the dairy plant. For handling small volumes, horizontal tank (5,000 to 15,000 litre capacity) may be used, while for large handling silo tanks with 25,000 to 1, 00, 000 litre capacity are preferred. This will reduce the cost of building, capital cost of tanks as well as operation, cleaning and maintenance costs, since the number of units required for any desired capacity is considerably few. The total capacity of raw milk storage tanks would be, under normal circumstances, equal to daily intake at the plant. With a coordinated programme of rate and time of receiving at the plant and the rate of processing, some raw milk storage capacity could be reduced. These silo tanks are fitted with an agitation system (mechanical/pneumatic) to gently stir the stored milk to prevent cream separation by gravity. In some plants, storage tanks are located on the upper floor as it saves space on the ground floor and help unload milk by gravity.

5.9.2. Centrifugal operations

Processes based on application of centrifugal separation of material of varying densities, are increasing in number and significance in modern fluid milk operations. Present centrifugal processes involve:

1. Clarification: Centrifugal removal of dense foreign matter, dirt, cellular debris, *etc.*
2. Separation: Centrifugal separation of fat and skim milk.
3. Standardization: Centrifugal removal of fat to adjust fat content to a desirable level by either batch or continuous processes.
4. Bactofugation: Centrifugal removal of bacterial cells in milk by a single pass through a centrifugal machine.
5. Clarifixation: Centrifugal homogenization or emulsion stabilization.
6. Solid concentration: Centrifugal separation of milk solids during shrikhand and quarg cheese manufacture, recovery of whey protein solids or coagulated milk proteins, *etc.*
7. Centrifugal evaporation: Use of force to improve drying efficiency- limited dairy applications but used in orange juice concentration.

Clarification, separation and standardization are operations utilized in almost all fluid milk plants, with many plants utilizing a single centrifugal machine to perform all three operations.

5.9.2.1. Filtration and clarification

During handling of milk at the farm and its transportation, certain visible particles and dirt may find access to milk. These may be removed either by straining, filtration or centrifugal clarification. Straining and filtration are simple and comparatively inexpensive but inefficient in comparison with clarification. The filtration has been discussed briefly in Chapter-4, clean milk production. Relatively large pieces of extraneous materials are usually removed by 'straining' (passing the milk through a fine metal-guage strainer or metallic sieve on the farm, at the collection center or at the processing plant). Tubular sieves located in the milk inlet pipe to the processing unit (pasteurizer) are also used.

However, finer foreign matters to be removed require clarification using a special filter or a clarifier. These steps of aesthetic improvement of product are particularly useful for overcoming the problem of sediment in fluid milk and liquid milk products in general, and homogenized milk in particular.

Filtration: Filtration (or, clarification using a filter bag) refers to making the milk pass through a filter cloth or filter pad. The filtering medium has a pore size (25-100 μm) that permits most of the foreign matters to be retained on it. The milk filter consists of a nylon filter-bag or a filter-pad supported on a perforated stainless steel (SS) support held in an SS enclosure with a tight fitting lid, milk distributor, and inlet- and out-let connections. Milk usually passes from top to bottom. In case of twin filters, three-way volves in the inlet and outlet lines enable switching from one filter to the other when first is to be cleaned. Sometimes, filters may be provided in the form of cylindrical bags or 'stockings' fitted over perforated SS tubes as in the modern continuous pasteurizing plants (high-temperature short-time, or HTST pasteurizers).

Filtration can be carried out either on cold milk (~10° C) or warm milk (40-45° C). since warm milk filtration is more rapid due to lower viscosity of warm milk, it is universally used. For cold filtration, the filter is located in the line connecting the milk receiving tank or holding tank and the pasteurizer. Since warm filtration requires preheating, the filter of this type is placed between the regeneration and the final heating section of the HTST pasteurizer.

The filter-bag must periodically be cleaned. Accordingly, the operation run may vary from 2-10 h depending on the level of foreign matter and the filter pore size. Generally, twin filters located in parallel are employed to permit cleaning of one filter while other is in use. This enables continuous process run. Filtration removes only gross impurities, and does not remove bacteria from milk. Accordingly, it does not improve the keeping quality of milk. In fact, bacteria may grow in the filters if they are used for unusually long time without cleaning.

Clarification: Application of centrifugal force to remove dirt and other particles heavier than milk is called clarification. The clarifier is very similar to the separator in construction and in operation except there is no cream spout. The principle of clarification involves introduction of milk between two adjacent rotating conical discs (in a stack of several discs) of a centrifugal bowl and subjecting it to centrifugal force. This force causes the heavier dirt particles to be thrown out into the sludge space surrounding the discs where it is collected during the run, while the comparatively lighter milk continuously flows inward and upward to the outlet. While filtration removes the suspended foreign particles by the straining process, clarification removes, by centrifugal sedimentation, dirt and debris which has gained entry to the milk incidental to its production as well as leucocytes, epithelial cells from the udder, coagulated milk protein particles including calcium phosphate and other mineral, fat-bacterial clusters, occasional red blood corpuscles and to some extent bacteria in the form of clarifier sludge. There is no separation of fat globules (cream) and skim milk in the clarifier.

Operation of Clarifier: The normal operating speeds of clarifiers, 4,000-8,000 rpm, are presumed to be without significant effect on the fat globules of milk. This is prevented further by the construction of the discs in certain types of centrifugal clarifiers, which compels all of the milk to be subjected to the same degree of centrifugal force by passing near the periphery of the bowl. Depending upon the temperature conditions, there may be some release of membrane material into the skim milk phase as a result of centrifugal force. Since viscosity of milk decreases with increasing temperature, warming of the milk to at least 31-35° C increases the efficiency of operation.

In a centrifugal clarifier, the milk is introduced into the separation channels at the outer edge of the disc stack, flows radially inwards through the channels towards the axis of rotation and leaves through the outer at the top. On the way through the disc stack the solid impurities are separated and thrown back along the undersides of the discs to the periphery of the clarifier bowl. There they are collected in the sediment space. As the milk passes along the full radial width of the discs, the time of passage also allows very small particles to be separated.

The accumulated sludge is removed from the bowl by dismantling the clarifier at regular intervals. The interval may range from 1 to 8 hours depending on the size of clarifier and the amount of impurities in milk. However, most large-size modern clarifiers are 'self-desludging' or 'partial desludging' type in which periodical sludge removal takes place during the clarification process without interruption of the clarifier operation. Such desludging results in about 0.05-0.10% of milk being lost and the sludge being liquid rather than solid as in the non-self-desludging machines.

The clarifier may be located in the raw milk line between the raw milk tank and pasteurizer. Alternatively, milk may be clarified warm by placing the clarifier at a suitable point in the regeneration section of the HTST unit or between the regeneration and final heating section.

Clarification can be accomplished successfully at almost any stage of processing but when applied to warm milk in which the fat is liquid, it may initiate rancidity unless the milk is pasteurized quickly thereafter to destroy the activity of the lipase activity.

The clarifier sludge or clarifier slime consists primarily of foreign matters, dust and dirt particles, milk proteins, fat, calcium phosphate and other minerals, leucocytes and microorganisms. The amount of slime varies with the amount of foreign matter, stage of lactation, acidity of milk clarifying temperature, bowl velocity and length of running time. Its composition will depend on whether it is liquid (82-86% water, 6-8% protein), or solid (65-69% water, 24-28% protein). On an average a clarifier slime may contain about 73% moisture, 3% lipids, 18% proteins, 2.6% organic solids and 3% ash.

Some clarifier designs permit continuous removal of sludge during operation. This eliminates the need to shut down the machine to open the bowl to remove sludge. A clarifier may be operated, depending on the size for periods ranging from 2 to 8 h on cold milk (5-10° C) and from 1 to 4 h on warm milk (57° C) without cleaning.

There are certain advantages and disadvantages for cold and warm clarification. The warm clarification has the following features:

- The efficiency is greater because of higher temperature, viscosity of the milk decreases, resulting in efficient removal of suspended particles
- Running time is reduced because of rapid sludge build-up.
- Operation of the entire system is more critical with a high-pressure drop through the clarifier on one side of the pump and suction on the other side.

Cold clarifier has the following features:

- Efficiency is quite low because of high viscosity of milk at low temperature.
- Operating time is more because smaller amounts of heavier particles are thrown out as sludge.
- Quality of processed milk is better because the soluble dirt has been removed from the milk before heat is applied.

When the clarifier itself is clean and well sterilized before use, the actual number of microorganisms in clarified milk would be considerably reduced since a large number of organisms would be thrown out into the clarifier slime. If the plate count is higher after clarification, it means that the clarifier has not been properly cleaned.

5.9.2.2. Cream separation

The process of fractionation of whole milk into skim milk and cream is known as separation. This process utilizes the differential in the relative densities of fat and milk serum for effecting separation of two components. Fat globules are lighter, less dense with lower specific gravity of 0.93, than the surrounding liquid phase or serum (specific gravity, 1.036) and rise to the surface when milk is left undisturbed. The fat-rich layer thus formed is called ' cream' and the fat-poor layer called 'skim milk'. This process is called 'creaming'. It is possible to separate two layers mechanically.

Because of the ease with which fat can be separated from milk, the process of cream separation is very commonly employed in the dairy industry. Cream separation enables the processor to manufacture a variety of fat-rich products such as cream of various types, butter, butter-oil, ghee, *etc.* Cream separation also makes it possible to adjust the composition of milk with respect to its fat and SNF contents. Such compositional modification may be desired for product manufacture as also for meeting the legal requirements of different types of market milk.

Methods of Separation: Two methods of separation of cream from milk are commonly used: (a) gravity separation and (b) centrifugal separation. Both these methods rely on the basic principle of separation of two immiscible liquids having different densities, under the influence of gravitational or centrifugal force.

(a) Gravity Separation: As mentioned above, when milk is allowed to stand undisturbed for some time, a layer of cream (*malai*) forms on the top due to rising of fat globules which are initially dispersed throughout the bulk of milk. The upward movement of the lighter fat globules (density, 0.93 at 20° C) in the heavier serum (density, 1.036) takes place owing to gravity. Creaming may become evident in as short time as half-an-hour.

The presence of cream layer on milk may be important from consumer's standpoint, but beyond this, the phenomenon involves properties of fat globules, such as clustering, that are broadly significant in the behaviour of milk and its various products.

Principle of Creaming: The rate of rise of a spherical particle in a liquid medium is represented by the following equation, which in essence is Stokes' law:

$$V = \frac{2gr^2(d_1-d_2)}{9\eta}$$

Where V = velocity of rise in centimeters per second,

r = radius of the sphere in centimeters,

d_1 = density of dispersion medium,

d_2 = density of the sphere,

g = gravitational force (981 dynes), and

η = viscosity of the liquid in poises.

The rate of cream separation is directly proportional to the difference between the densities of fat and serum and to the square of fat globule diameter, and inversely proportional to the viscosity of serum. Thus, for a given sample of milk, the creaming rate will be maximum when the density difference is maximum and viscosity is minimum. Both these factors are, in turn, affected by temperature of milk. As the temperature rises, the ratio of the density difference and the serum viscosity increases favouring the separation process. This increase is particularly prominent between 10 and 30°C and much less above 50° C.

It has been reported that the fat globules of milk rise in close accord with Stokes' law. However, average fat globules of approximately 4μ in diameter would take several hours to rise 1 inch according to the Stokes' equation. It is clear that other factors must enter into the phenomenon for a cream layer to appear on milk in as little as 30 minutes. The principal factor that aids the creaming process is clustering of the individual fat globules. As the milk is drawn from the udder the globules exist largely as separate entities. In the quiescent state, globules in milk begin to rise. As shown in the equation, the velocity of rise is directly proportion to the square of the radius of the globule. Therefore the larger globules overtake the smaller ones rather quickly. At this point the factor of clustering comes into play. When a larger globule comes in contact with the smaller globule, it is held there, and the two joined globules rise together at an even more rapid rate primarily because of their greater effective radius. Incidental to their rise they come in contact with other globules until clusters of substantial size are formed, which rise much more rapidly than any of the individual globules. It is true that any of these clusters do not rise strictly in accord with Stokes' law since they are irregular in shape and contain considerable occluded serum.

It then is logical to ask: What causes clustering? What makes the fat globules stick together? These questions have never been answered in a completely satisfactory manner. It has been reported that a protein classified as a euglobulin (also known as fat agglutinin) in the milk is essential to the clustering of fat globules and the formation of cream layer. The protein that facilitates creaming appears to act in much the same manner as bacterial agglutinins and alters the surface properties of the fat globules in some way to make them adhere to one another. When the milk fat is in solid state, separation of the milk yields skim milk that is euglobulin-poor whereas separation at 50° C yields a skim milk that is euglobulin-rich. It seems that euglobulin helps in clustering by lowering interfacial tension on the surface of fat globules. That surface tension activity is associated with the euglobulin is suggested also by the tendency toward excessive foaming in euglobulin-rich skim milk.

Factors Affecting Creaming: Maximum cream layer volume is secured with milks of high fat content and relatively large fat globules. Such milk will contain more clusters of larger size with greater amounts of occluded serum. Since buffalo milk contains higher fat content with relatively larger fat globules, the cream layer formed in buffalo milk is considerably thicker than that of cow milk. In addition, heat treatment and extent of agitation of milk also affect creaming process.

In the case of raw milk, the deepest cream layer volume is secured when the milk is chilled promptly and quickly to 10°C and stored at 4°C or lower. Cream layer volume in pasteurized milk, equivalent to that obtainable with raw milk, can be secured if the milk is (a) processed without unduly rigorous agitation, (b) pasteurized at minimal conditions (63° C for 30 min or 72° C for 15 sec) and (c) promptly chilled to 3 to 4°C. Excessive heat treatment can irreversibly denature the euglobulin of milk. Thus, as the heat treatments of milk are intensified beyond that for conventional pasteurization, progressive loss of cream layer volume occurs. Adsorption of euglobulin on the surface of the fat globules after pasteurization is favoured by rapid chilling to low temperatures. Apparently the adsorption process is favoured by having the fat in a solid or semisolid state. Where the cooling process is slow the adsorption of euglobulin does not go to completion, and as a consequence the clusters are small, rise slowly in the milk, and form a shallow, indistinct cream layer. The normal pasteurization process is somewhat like "wiping the slate clean" so far the creaming process is concerned. Exclusive of agitation so rigorous during processing as to disrupt the normal emulsion of the fat, pasteurization can be considered as a treatment to regain the normal creaming potential of the milk. In the heating process all of the euglobulin is desorbed from the fat globule surface, and on cooling conditions can be made optimum for the re-adsorption process.

In general, the two principal factors involved in agitation and its effect on cream layer volume are intensity and temperature. As a rule excessive agitation should be avoided because of its disrupting effect on normal cluster formation and the possibility of its denaturing euglobulin. Excessive agitation is to be avoided particularly after the milk has been pasteurized. Normal agitation during the pasteurization process is without effect on creaming potential for the globules are dispersed rather completely at that time. The creaming process in cold milk may actually be facilitated by the mild agitation since such treatment would favour larger clusters which would be more loosely packed.

Cream separation by gravity is, however, a very slow and inefficient process. It is of little practical value for commercial purposes. Therefore, mechanized cream separation employing a centrifugal machine is most commonly used in the dairy industry. Such machines develop force equal to 5 to 10 thousand times that of gravity. Even for a small scale separation involving, say 10-20 litres of milk, a centrifugal separator is used, be it hand-driven or motor-driven.

Centrifugal Separation

Historical: Cream has been considered very valuable component of milk. For centuries, housewives knew just one way of extracting cream from milk: They boiled the milk, cooled it, then spooned of the surface cream. The method was unhygienic and inefficient. So began the search for a cream separator. A number of inventors took up the challenge.

The first continuous centrifugal milk separator was patented by Gustaf de Laval in Stockholm, Sweden in 1878. Hand-power separators were sold on the market in 1886. The first Alfa-Laval separator made its appearance, incorporating von Bechtolsheim's Alpha disks in 1890. The world saw the first hermetic (solid bowl) milk separator made by Alfa-Laval in 1933. In 1962, the first self -cleaning milk separator arrived. In 1974 Alfa-Laval made the first hermetic self-cleaning separator.

The dairy industry introduced centrifugal separation in the late nineteenth century. Starting from hand-driven machines, the development of electrical drives and the overall efficiency and capacity was the main focus for decades. At the end of 1970s automatic discharging separators were introduced into the dairy industry with the capability of operating much longer, without stopping for cleaning. Today, skimming centrifuges can handle throughputs of up to 60,000 l per hour on a single machine. The applications for the skimming centrifuges in the dairy industry are the separation of: warm milk, cold milk, whey, buttermilk, butter oil and retentates.

The separation of fat and water phases can be accelerated by the use of centrifugal force which makes the separation complete and almost instantaneous. As explained in the preceding section on creaming, the fat globules of milk have a normal disposition to separate by rising from the skim milk phase. This is a relatively slow and inefficient means of recovering cream and the cream separator has proven extremely useful in both hastening the process and increasing its efficiency.

The rate of rise of fat globules in milk through the force of gravity is accurately expressed by the Stokes equation and the force constant (g) for gravity in this equation is 981 dynes. To determine this constant in terms of the acceleration produced in a centrifugal machine, such as a separator, the following equation is used:

$$g = \frac{(2\pi S)^2 R}{(60)^2}$$

in which S is bowl speed in r.p.m. and R is distance of a given globule from the axis of rotation. By using the expression of g in the Stokes equation and reducing the resulting equation to simplest terms, the rate of separation (V) is given as:

$$V = \frac{0.00244(d_1 - d_2)r^2 S^2 R}{\eta}$$

It becomes evident from this equation that the rate of separation of fat globules will increase with increase in r, the radius of the fat globules; S, the speed of the separator; R, the distance from the bowl axis; and with decrease in η, the viscosity of the milk. Temperature is a factor of related importance since it influences r, η and $(d_1 - d_2)$, as discussed subsequently.

Construction of Centrifugal Separator: The modern cream separator consists of a bowl which can be rotated at high speed by means of suitable gears and arrangements for supplying milk to the bowl and removing the cream and skim milk. The chief parts of the bowls are: (1) the shell, (2) the inside fixtures, and the spindle which supports the weight and by means of which the rotation is accomplished. The construction of the separator may be depicted. Inside the bowl there are number of discs provided in which the milk is stratified. The remainder of the machine is essentially a set of gears so arranged as to make possible the turning of the spindle on which the bowl is carried at a high rate of speed. The gears are generally housed in a tight case in which they dip in the oil while operating.

If the separator has been in operation for some time, a thin layer of a sticky substance, possibly showing some evidence of solid impurities will be found adhering to the wall of the bowl. This is separator slime. Next in order comes a layer of skim milk, while at the inner edge of the upright wall of fluid the fat globules are packed closely together forming cream. This gathering of the cream near the center of the bowl is the first and most important step in centrifugal separation.

All that remains is to lead the two layers out of the bowl without mixing. The separate removal of these two layers is accomplished by establishing two outlets at proper distances from the axis of the bowl, one of which connects with the cream layer in the bowl, the other with the outer edge of the bowl where the skim milk is found.

The skim milk from near the outer edge of the bowl cavity moves between the dividing discs and the inside shell of the bowl. At the top of the disc the space between it and the shell of the bowl connects with a slot in the neck of the bowl. This slot is the skim milk outlet. The skim milk which comes from the outlet with some force is gathered in the so called 'skim-milk pan' from which it flows through the spout provided for that purpose. A second outlet, located on the neck of the bowl above the skim milk outlet, connects with the inner side of the dividing disc and serves to conduct the cream from the bowl into the cream pan.

Mechanism of Cream Separation: As the milk enters a rapidly revolving bowl, it is acted upon both by gravity and by the centrifugal force generated by rotation. The centrifugal force is so much stronger than that of gravity that the effect of latter becomes negligible. Consequently milk entering the bowl is thrown to the outer wall of the bowl rather than the bottom. This means that the bowl fills from the outside toward the centre rather than from the bottom toward the top.

The milk entering the rapidly revolving bowl is subjected at once to a very powerful centrifugal force. The milk serum has higher specific gravity than the fat, and for this reason is brought to the outer part of the bowl while cream is forced towards the centre of the bowl.

Operation of Centrifugal Separator: The centrifugal separator is similar to the clarifier, but milk entering through the bottom of the separator bowl holding a stack of conical discs rises up through holes located somewhere in the middle of the inner and outer edges of the discs. The milk between discs is subjected to a centrifugal force in the rotating bowl and thereby tends to fly out from the centre. The skim milk fraction, being heavier, moves away and forms a layer on the outer edge of the discs, whereas the fat globules gather on the inside edge. The incoming un-separated milk forces the separating layers further and upward out at the top of the bowl. Thus, there are two outlets in a cream separator, one for skim milk and the other for cream, the cream outlet being nearer to the centre.

Factors Affecting Efficiency of Separation: Since fat removal from milk is the principal function of a cream separator, the efficiency of process, also called skimming efficiency, is determined by the effectiveness with which the fat content of the out-coming skim milk is reduced. The residual fat content of skim milk is usually in the range of 0.01-0.05% in the modern machines. A fat content higher than 0.06% represents poor separation efficiency. The skim milk fat content is inversely related to fat recovery in cream. Hence, the skimming efficiency is often defined as the percentage of total fat in whole milk recovered in the cream separated from it. For a given fat content of whole milk, the higher the fat content in skim milk, the lower the skimming efficiency.

There are number of factors that influence efficiency of separation or, more particularly, the fat content of skim milk and cream. These factors fall into three general groups:

i) The design and state of repair of the separator

ii) Certain characteristics of milk to be separated, and

iii) The manner in which the separation is carried out.

For any given separator in good working order, the relative efficiency in performance is more or less fixed, so that the separator itself does not serve as a variable. With respect to the milk, the principal factors are size of fat globules and fat content. Actually these two factors are related, since higher fat test is closely correlated with larger average globule sizes. Fat globules of diameter 2μ and lower are very incompletely recovered by the cream separator. Thus the distribution pattern of globule sizes may have some bearing on the efficiency of separation. The total amount of fat in a given milk will determine the fat content of the cream using a given setting of cream or skim milk screw in the separator. This results from the fact that adjustment of these screws (there being either one or the other on a separator) determines a ratio of discharge for the cream and skim milk fractions. If the machine is so adjusted as to yield 5 volumes of skim milk for one volume of cream, this ratio will be constant irrespective of the fat content of milk going into the separator. Consequently, variations in the fat test of the milk will reflect themselves in the fat test of cream. The thumb rule is that for every 0.1% change in fat test of milk, there is 1% change in the fat test of cream.

The principal variable of importance in the separating process is temperature of the milk. Temperature bears on the following factors: (a) the difference in density between fat globules and the skim milk phase, (b) the viscosity of the milk, and (c) the radii of fat globules. Referring to the equation (p.31) dealing with velocity of separation (V), increase in temperature tends to increase the difference (d_1-d_2), decrease viscosity of milk (ç) and increase the radii of the globules (r). Thus, temperature of milk has significant effect on skimming efficiency. It has been reported that by increasing the separating temperature of milk from 5° to 40° C the effective force tending to separate the cream increases by 380% but in going from 40° to 80° C, the increase is only 95%.

As the density and dynamic viscosity are functions of the temperature, warm milk separation is always more efficient than cold milk separation. The optimum temperature for the separation of milk is about 55° C. At temperatures above 60° C, there is some precipitation of proteins, which have a negative effect on separation efficiency. These proteins form a thin film on the surface of the discs and with disc interspaces of only 0.3-0.6 mm, these deposits have a detrimental effect on the conditions of flow.

A reduction in temperature from the optimum reduces the separation efficiency due to the increase in viscosity until, at about 20-25° C, a blockage of the cream flow occurs. Therefore, cold milk separators differ from warm milk separators in two main respects, they are:

- A large disc interspace
- An open or hermetic cream discharge.

Currently there is a trend towards lower separating temperatures, which, in general, have been made possible through improvements in the design and efficiency of separators. Cold milk separators usually operate at a temperature between 4 and 12° C, and yield a skim milk testing 0.01% fat. As a general rule, any long-term mechanical treatment of milk should be avoided at a temperature between 15 and 50° C because increased lipase activity will result as an increased level of free fatty acids.

Long cooling periods of, e.g. over 2-3 days change the chemical properties of the fat globules because of the absorption of more water, which increases their density. This influences the skimming ability.

Skimming efficiency is considered to be optimum when the skim milk tests no more than 0.01% fat by Gerber method. Such efficiency is possible with most of the available separators provided that they are in good working condition and the milk is separated within recommended temperatures. Fat test of the skim milk is an obvious means of evaluating separator performance.

The rate at which the milk is fed to a separator influences separating efficiency simply because the longer the milk is in the separator the longer it is exposed to the action of the centrifugal force. It can be seen also in this connection that the speed of the separator bowl is involved in a similar manner. The lower the bowl speed, the lower the centrifugal force is, the slower and less complete the separation, and higher the loss of fat in the skim milk. A higher bowl speed gives higher skimming efficiency but, since increased speed requires greater energy input, normal range of 4,000 to7, 000 rpm (sometimes as low as about 2,000 rpm) giving efficient separation is normally not exceeded in the separator design.

There are certain other factors which may also affect skimming efficiency. Intense agitation of milk prior to separation, air incorporation (foaming) and high acidity of milk adversely affect the separation efficiency. Poor disc condition (mis-shaped, dirty or scratched one), vibrations of the separators and defective gaskets in the cream section could cause unacceptable efficiency. Excessive slime getting collected in the sludge space of the bowl would also have an adverse effect on the separator performance.

The poor efficiency of separation could be due to faulty operations such as low temperature, over capacity cream seal or check valve leaks, inclusion of homogenized milk, too long a run or mechanical failures such as bowl under speed, damaged outlet parts, worn seals and bowl out of balance.

Factors Affecting Yield and Fat Content of Cream: The yield of cream and skim milk can be given by the following formulae:

i) Yield of cream (% feed of milk) $= \dfrac{f_m - f_s}{f_c - f_s} \times 100$ .... (Eq. 1)

ii) Yield of skim milk (%of feed milk) $= \dfrac{f_c - f_m}{f_c - f_s} \times 100$ .... (Eq. 2)

where,

t_{m} = fat in milk, percent

t_{s} = fat in skim milk, percent

t_{c} = fat in cream, percent.

All those factors which affect the skimming efficiency can be expected to influence the cream yield too. Conditions leading to a higher skimming efficiency would give a better yield. However, the fat content of cream is obviously the major factor influencing the yield of cream. Accordingly, the adjustment of the cream screw or skim milk screw is critical with regard to cream yield.

The position of the cream screw, i.e. a valve provided in the cream outlet controls the flow rate of the cream being discharged. Turning the 'inward' reduces the cream discharge rate thereby increasing the fat content of cream. Adjusting the valve by 'outward' movement has the opposite effect. Similarly, manipulation of the skim milk screw so as to decrease the flow rate of the existing skim milk will decrease the fat concentration of cream and vice-versa. Thus, changing the position of the cream screw or skim milk screw alters the ratio of cream to skim milk; an increased ratio decreases the fat content of cream and a decreased one raises it.

Further, a lower temperature and a higher fat content of milk lead to an increased fat content of cream, whereas an increased feed rate causes a decreased richness of cream, and vice-versa.

Basic Design of the Centrifugal Separator: A section through a self-cleaning separator shows that a bowl consists of two major parts, the body and the hood. They are held together by a threaded lock ring. The disc stack is clamped between the hood and distributor at the centre of the bowl.

Modern separators are of two types, semi-open and hermetic.

Semi-open design: Centrifugal separators with paring discs at the outlet are known as semi-open types (as opposed to the older open models with overflow discharge).

In the semi-open separator the milk is supplied to the separator bowl from an inlet, normally in the top through a stationary axial inlet tube. When the milk enters the ribbed distributor, it is accelerated to the speed of rotation of the bowl before it continues into the separation channels in the disc stack. The centrifugal force throws the milk outwards to form a ring with a cylindrical inner surface. This is in contact with air at atmospheric pressure which means that the pressure of the milk at the surface is also atmospheric. The pressure increases progressively with increasing distance from the axis of rotation to a maximum at the periphery of the bowl.

The heavier solid particles settle outwards and are deposited in the sediment space. Cream moves inwards towards the axis of rotation and passes through channels to the cream paring chamber. The skim milk leaves the disc stack at the outer edge and passes between the top disc and the bowl hood to the skim milk paring chamber.

Paring disc: In the semi-open separator the cream and skim milk outlets have special outlet devices-paring discs. Because of the outlet design the semi-open separators are usually called paring- disc separators.

The rims of the stationary paring discs dip into the rotating columns of liquid continuously paring out a certain amount. The kinetic energy of the rotating liquid is converted into pressure in the paring disc and the pressure is always equal to the pressure drop in the downstream line.

An increase in downstream pressure means that the liquid level in the bowl moves inwards. In this way the effect of throttling at the outlets are automatically counteracted. In order to prevent aeration of the product it is important that the paring discs are sufficiently covered with liquids.

Hermetic design: Before the 1930s, centrifugal separators were of the open type. Milk entered at the top in a free jet, and skimmilk and cream emerged from separate outlets. As air mixed freely with milk, foam were produced. The foam created various problems.

The hermetically-sealed separator solved this problem. In this machine milk entered from the bottom under pressure and completely filled the bowl. Inlet and outlet seals prevented contact with air. As air was absent, the separation was foamless.

Milk is fed from below and enters the bowl through the hollow, rotating spindle. It completely fills the system and is prevented from escaping by seals at the inlet and the outlets. The pressure drop in the bowl is overcome by a built in centrifugal pump, which creates sufficient excess pressure to overcome the back pressure of a subsequent plate heat exchanger as well. The actual separation takes place in the bow, and the cream and skim milk are discharged under pressure. The required cream concentration can be obtained through regulation of the cream outlet, and the quantity is measured on a cream flow meter.

With the help of supplementary equipment such as a remixing or standardizing device, the operator can clarify the milk by merely turning a three-way cock which remixes the cream and milk. The concentration of the cream can be adjusted during operation over a wide range. Standardizing is simplified and accurate – by turning the cock, adjusting an additional valve and reading a second flow-meter installed for the purpose.

Benefits of Hermetic Separation

- **Gentle treatment of milk:** There is no turbulence. So fat globules are prevented from breaking up and more cream is obtained.
- **Hygienic separation:** There is no contact with air. This means no bacterial contamination of milk, no oxidation of fat and no rancidity.
- **No foaming:** With air absent, there is no foaming which causes reduced capacity utilization of subsequent equipment on the production line.
- **Processing versatility:** The capacity can be adjusted to suit individual requirement.

Limitation: The hermetic separators (solid bowl) swiftly became indispensable in leading dairies. However, they still presented one problem: cleaning. At intervals each machine had to be opened and milk sludge cleaned out – a wet, messy, back-breaking job which ate up production time. Frequent dismantling also increased wear and tear. Moreover, cleaning by hand inevitably put a limit on machine size. And as world milk volume shot up, larger separators were needed.

Self-cleaning Hermetic Separator: The answer to these problems came in the form of an amazing new development in dairy engineering. In 1974, Alfa-Laval developed the world's first self-cleaning separator which could perform the almost unimaginable feat of cleaning itself without stopping. The arrival of this machine carried dairymen into an exciting new phase in cream separation. This revolutionary machine has speeded up milk processing and boosted cream output. It discharges sludge automatically, saves time and labour. It does away with frequent dismantling and reassembly which makes for longer machine life. The self-cleaning hermetic cream separator can run almost indefinitely with sustained skimming efficiency. It need to be stopped only every other month or so for inspection.

Discharge Process: solid particles accumulated in the angled sediment space of the bowl are automatically ejected at pre-set intervals. A hydraulic impulse is delivered to the spring-loaded valve at the bowl bottom. These open very briefly (< 0.5 sec.) to drain the operating water space. The sliding bowl bottom drops and exposes the ejection ports. In 'partial discharge' , the slots open for only 0.5 sec. As milk escaping with the discharge is negligible, feed to the separator need not to be interrupted. In 'total discharge' the slots open long enough to empty the entire contents of the bowl. This is required in the rinsing stage of the CIP programme.

Clean-in-Place (CIP) Programme: In this programme, the centrifuge is flushed clean by detergents circulating in a closed system. Cleaning includes all parts in contact with milk, inside and outside the bowl, inside the frame hood, and the sludge outlet.

The cleaning cycle is controlled by a programme timer and normally comprises the stages given in the following Table: The total time of the program is about 65 minutes.

Stage	Operation	Approx time (min)	ApproxTemp(°C)
1.	Pre - rinse with water.	4	-
2.	Acid wash (0.5 – 0.8% nitric acid solution). . Returned to tank after use	15	65
3.	Intermediate rinse. Water displaces acid, and goes to drain after regenerative cooling.	6	65
4.	Lye wash (1% caustic soda solution with wetting agent and phosphate additives). Returned to tank after use.	25	65
5.	Hot-water sterilization. Water displaces lye and	10	90-95
6.	Cooling.	5	-

Control of Fat Content in Cream

Paring disc separator: The volume of cream discharged from the paring disc separator is controlled by the throttling valve in the cream outlet. Progressively larger amounts of cream, with progressively diminishing fat content, will be discharged from the cream outlet if the valve is gradually opened.

A given rate of discharge consequently corresponds to a given fat content in the cream. If the fat content of whole milk is 4% and cream with 40% is required, the discharge from the cream outlet must be adjusted to 2,000 l / h. The pressure on the skim milk outlet is set by means of a regulating valve at a certain value according to the separator and the throughput. Then the throttling valve in the cream outlet is adjusted to give the flow volume corresponding to the required fat content.

Any change in the cream discharge will be matched by an equal and opposite alteration in the skim milk discharge. An automatic constant pressure unit is fitted in the skim milk outlet to keep the back pressure at the outlet constant regardless of changes in the rate of cream flow.

Cream flow meter: In paring disc separators the volume of the cream discharged is controlled by a cream valve with a built-in flow meter. The size of the valve aperture is adjusted with a screw and the throttled flow passes through a graduated glass tube. The tube contains a spool-shaped float which is lifted by the cream flow to a position on the graduated scale which varies according to the flow rate and viscosity of cream.

By analyzing the fat content of the incoming whole milk and calculating the volume of cream flow at the required fat content, it is possible to arrive at a coarse setting of the flow rate and to adjust the throttling screw accordingly. Fine adjustment can be made when the fat content of the cream has been analyzed. The operator then knows the float reading when the fat content of the cream is correct.

The fat content of cream is affected by the flow variations in the line. Other type of instruments are used, for example, automatic in-line systems to measure the fat content of cream in combination with control systems which keep the fat content at a constant value.

Hermetic Separator: An automatic constant pressure unit for a hermetic separator. The valve shown is a diaphragm valve and the required product pressure is adjusted by means of compressed air above the diaphragm.

During the separation the diaphragm is affected by the constant air pressure above and the product (skim milk) pressure below. The preset air pressure will force the diaphragm down if the pressure in the skim milk drops. The valve plug fixed to the diaphragm then moves downwards and reduces the passage. This throttling increases the skim milk outlet pressure to the preset value. The opposite reaction takes place when there is an increase in the skim milk pressure, and the preset pressure is again restored.

Difference in outlet performance of hermetic and paring-disc separators: There is a difference between the cream outlets on a paring-disc and hermetic separators. In the paring-disc separator the outer diameter of the paring-disc must penetrate into the rotating liquid column. The distance is determined by the fat content of cream. The fat content is highest at the inner, free cream level in the separator. From there the fat content is gradually reduced as the diameter increases.

An increased fat content in the cream from the separator increases the distance from the inner, free liquid level of the cream to the outer periphery of the paring disc by the cream level being forced inwards. The fat content at the inner, free cream level must consequently be considerably higher if for instance 40% cream is to be discharged. The cream must be over-concentrated to a higher fat content, compared with the cream leaving the separator. This could result in destruction of fat globules in the inner most zone facing the air column, as a result of increased friction. The result would be destruction of fat globules which will cause sticking problems and increased sensitivity to oxidation and hydrolysis.

Cream from the hermetic separator is removed from the center where the fat content is highest. Over-concentration is, therefore, not necessary.

When removing cream that has a high fat content, the difference in outlet performance is even more important. At 72% the fat is concentrated to such an extent that the fat globules are actually touching each other. It would be impossible to obtain cream with this fat content from a paring-disc separator, as the cream would have to be considerably over-concentrated. The required pressure cannot be created in a paring-disc separator. High pressures can be created in the hermetic separator, which makes it possible to separate cream with a fat content exceeding 72% globular fat.

Operational Precautions: To ensure proper operation the following steps should be followed in operating the separator:

1. correctly assemble and securely close the bowl,
2. adjust the cream screw to proper setting based on past performance,
3. start machine and before any milk is run, be sure that it is revolving at rated speed. In some machines it is necessary to fill the bowl with water before starting in order to avoid severe vibrations,
4. it is advisable to flush the bowl with warm milk before introducing milk (warm milk separators),
5. warm milk to the desired temperature just before it goes to the separator. For warm milk separation it is recommended to use temperatures of 32-35°C although separation at 55-60°C is fairly a common practice today.,
6. run milk at rated capacity and run at a uniform rate,
7. cool cream to about 10° C as soon as it comes out of separator. Minimize agitation between 10-27°C
8. remove separator slime as needed. Generally every four hours with warm milk separators.

5.9.2.3. Standardization

Standardization is a process of adjusting the fat/SNF content of milk to certain predetermined level. Adjustment could be either raising or lowering the fat / SNF content and is done by adding skim milk or cream as required. For example, for raising SNF, skim milk has to be added into the milk or fat has to be removed to the required level, while for enhancing fat content, cream has to be added into the milk.

The process of standardization can be carried out in two different ways: batch standardization and direct in-line standardization. The first stage in both methods is to separate whole milk into cream and skimmilk.

Various methods exist for calculating the quantities of products with different fat contents that must be mixed to obtain a given final fat content. These cover mixtures of whole milk with skim milk, cream with whole milk, cream with skim milk and skim milk with anhydrous milk fat (butter oil).

The calculation of the quantity of cream or skim milk to be added to milk, or cream or skim milk to be separated from it can be made by a simple method known as the Pearson's square method (Fig 5.9.1). It consists in drawing an arbitrary squire, placing at the left corners of the squire, the desired fat percentage. Then, subtractions are made diagonally across the squire, the smaller value being deducted from the larger one, and the differences are entered at the correspondingly opposite corners on the right-hand side. These two new values at the right corners are summed to obtain a third value. All the three values placed at the right represent the proportions or relative amounts of the given products to be mixed (top right figure for the amount of the product to the top left, bottom right figure for the product to the bottom left, and the sum for the final product). The following is an example of such a calculation:

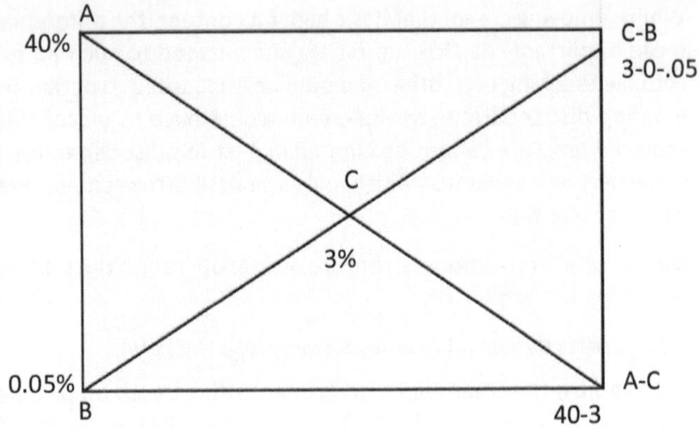

Fig. 5.9.1. Pearson's square method

How many kg of cream of A% fat must be mixed with skim milk of B% fat to make a mixture containing C% fat? The answer is obtained from a square Fig 5.9.9 where the given figures for fat content are placed.

A Cream fat content 40%

B Skim milk fat content 0.05%

C Fat content of the end product 3%

Subtract the fat content values on the diagonals to give C-B = 2.95 and A-C =37.

The mixture is then 2.95 kg of 40% cream and 37 kg of 0.05% skim milk to obtain 39.95 kg of a standardized product containing 3% fat.

From the equations below it is then possible to calculate the amounts of A and B needed to obtain the desired quantity (x) of C.

Two methods, prestandardization and poststandardization, are used in batch processing. Prestandardization means that the milk is standardized before pasteurization. When standardizing to a fat content higher than the raw milk fat content, cream is mixed with the milk in the tanks in the proportions which give the required fat content. In order to standardize to a lower fat content, the raw whole milk is diluted with separated skimmilk. The standardized milk is pasteurized after analysis and adjustment.

Poststandardization means that pasteurized whole milk is mixed in tanks with cream or skimmilk, according to whether the fat content is to be adjusted upwards or downwards, in the same way as for prestandardization. Some risk of reinfection is involved as poststandardization involves mixing already pasteurized products. Both methods require large tanks and the analysis and adjustment are labour-intensive.

The second method, direct standardization, has therefore been an attractive alternative for many years. In this method the fat content is adjusted to the required level by remixing of a calculated proportion of the cream from the separator to the skimmilk line. The difficulty of obtaining separated cream with a precisely controlled fat content has often made it necessary to analyze the standardized milk afterwards and carry out a final adjustment in tanks.

Direct in-line standardization

Principle: In modern milk processing plants with a diversified product range, direct in-line standardization is usually combined with separation. Previously the standardization was done manually, along with increased volumes to process the need for fast, constant and correct standardization methods, independent of seasonal fluctuations of the raw milk fat content, has increased. Control valves, flow and density meters and a computerized control loop are used to adjust the fat content of milk and cream to desired values.

The pressure in the skim milk outlet must be kept constant in order to enable accurate standardization. This pressure must be maintained regardless of variations in flow or pressure drop caused by the equipment after separation, and this is done with constant-pressure valve located close to the skim milk outlet.

For precision in the process it is necessary to measure variable parameters such as:

- fluctuations in the fat content of incoming milk,
- fluctuations in throughput,
- fluctuations in preheating temperature.

Most of the variables are interdependent; any deviation in one stage of the process often results in deviation in all stages. The cream fat content can be regulated to any value within the performance range of the separator, with a standard deviation based on repeatability between 0.2-0.3% fat. For standardized milk the standard deviation based on repeatability should be less than 0.3%.

Most commonly the whole milk is heated to 55-65°C in the pasteurizer before being separated. Following separation the cream is standardized at preset fat content and subsequently, the calculated amount of cream intended for standardization of milk (market milk, cheese milk, etc.) is routed and remixed with an adequate amount of skim milk. The surplus cream is directed to the cream pasteurizer.

Under certain circumstances it is also possible to apply an inline standardization system to cold milk centrifugal separator. However, it is then very important that all fat fractions of the milk fat are given enough time at low temperature (10-12 h) for complete crystallization. The reason is that the density will vary with the degree of crystallization and will thus jeopardize the measuring accuracy of the density transmitter, which is always calibrated at prevailing conditions after having been installed.

Operation: The direct automatic standardization systems are designed for on-line standardization of the fat content for standardized milk and cream. These systems usually have two control loops: one for the cream fat content and one for the standardized fat content. The fat content of the cream is obtained by adjusting its throughput via signals from the mass flow meter installed in the cream line. The fat content of the standardized milk is obtained by dosing part of the cream to the skim milk.

Two flow transmitters and one mass flow meter are available for measuring the throughputs of:

- cream from the centrifuge.
- cream to be incorporated.
- raw milk.

With the information, the computer can calculate the throughputs of other systems, namely:

- standardized milk from the centrifuge.
- skim milk from the centrifuge.
- surplus standardized cream.

The mass flow meter measures the cream density and quantity. The computer transforms this density into fat content. Combining the information for fat content and throughput data, the computer regulates the system control valves for:

- achieving the fat content required for the standardized cream.
- reincorporating the necessary amount of standardized cream into the skim milk, in order to obtain the required fat content of the standardized milk.

5.9.2.4. Bactofugation

Bactofugation is a process in which a specially designed centrifuge called a bactofuge is used to separate microorganisms from milk. Originally the bactofuge was developed to improve the keeping quality of market milk. At the present time bactofugation is also used to improve the bacteriological quality of milk intended for other products like cheese, milk powders, UHT- milk, whey for baby food.

Bacteria, especially heat resistant spores, have a significantly higher density than the milk. A bactofuge is, therefore, a particularly efficient means of ridding milk of bacterial spores. Since these spores are also resistant to heat treatment, the bactofuge makes a useful complement to thermization, pasteurization and sterilization.

The bactofuge is a high-speed clarifier (up to 20,000 rpm) provided with discharge nozzles in the bowl wall. The centrifugal force generated is up to 10,000 g (g = gravitational acceleration). The bacteria in milk being bactofuged are collected in the form of 'bactofugate' in the sludge space. The bactofugate is approximately 3% of the feed volume and contains primarily bacterial spores and milk proteins. Anaerobic spores are removed to an extent of 98-99%. A double bactofuge treatment at 73°C yields more than 99.9% reduction in bacterial spores of milk.

The original bactofuge was a solid bowl centrifuge with nozzles in the periphery of the bowl. It was long considered necessary to have a continuous flow of the heavy phase, either through a peripheral nozzle or over the heavy phase outlet of the bactofuge, to achieve efficient separation. This was possibly true of the old solid-bowl centrifuges with vertical cylindrical walls, but in modern self-cleaning separators with a sludge space outside the disc stack, bacteria and spores can be collected over a period of time and intermittently discharged at preset intervals.

There are two types of modern centrifuge:

- The two-phase bactofuge has two outlets at the top: one for continuous discharge of bacteria concentrate (bactofugate) via a special top disc, and one for the bacteria-reduced phase.
- The one-phase bactofuge has only one outlet at the top of the bowl for the bacteria-reduced milk. The bactofugate is collected in the sludge space of the bowl and discharged at the preset intervals.

The amount of bactofugate from the two-phase bactofuge is about 3% of the feed, while the corresponding amount from the one-phase bactofuge can be as low as 0.15% of the feed.

Bactofugate always has a higher dry matter content than the milk from which it originates. This is because some of the larger casein micelles are separated out together with the bacteria and spores. Higher bactofugation temperature increases the amount of protein in the bactofugate. The optimum bactofugation temperature is 55-60° C.

The reduction effect on bacteria is expressed in percent. Bacteria belonging to the genus Clostridium, an anaerobic spore-forming bacteria, are among the most feared by cheese makers, as they can cause late blowing of cheese even if present in small numbers. That is why cheese milk is mostly bactofugated.

Bactofugation of milk is always a part of milk pretreatment. In applications where quality of milk for cheese and powder production is the objective, the bactofuge is installed in series with centrifugal separator, either downstream or upstream of it.

In order to destroy the bacteria contained in bactofugate and improve the economy of the process by utilizing the milk protein in it, a process called 'Bactotherm' has been evolved. Clarified and standardized milk is bactofuged at 60-75°C followed by pasteurization employing HTST process. The bactofugate is deaerated in a vacuum chamber and sterilized at 130-140° C for 3-4 seconds using steam injection, and finally mixed with chilled bactofugated milk for further processing.

5.9.2.5. Clarifixation

Another special application of centrifugal force has been a partial homogenization with an apparatus called a 'clarifixator'. A clarifixator is a centrifuge which, besides clarifying also homogenizes the milk to a certain extent. To meet these requirements the bowl of the clarifixator is of a special design but works in principle as an ordinary separator bowl.

The milk is led from the regeneration section of the pasteurizer at a temperature of 55-60°C to the clarifixator and is distributed in the bowl in the ordinary way. The separated cream passes over the clarifixator disc. The clarifixator disc has a number of teeth (Fig 5.9.2) as if for kneading purposes. These teeth are grounded. The break down of fat globules is brought about by the spikes or protrusions on the paring disc provided in the cream passage at the top of the centrifuge. A paring disc is a fixed circular structure as a stationary centripetal pump. The cream separated from milk strikes the protruding obstacles before entering the paring disc. The fat globules, thus experiencing an intense turbulence or shearing action, are broken down to a smaller size (less than 2μ). As the cream passes over the disc, there will be a partial vacuum due to the rotation of the disc. The disc is rotated at a high speed. Due to the partial vacuum, there will be instantaneous evaporation of water and as the cream passes towards the higher pressure side, there will be condensation of the water vapour. The evaporation and condensation is instantaneous. As it condenses on the fat globules, this will release lot of energy which causes mechanical shear on the fat globules and causes them to crack down to smaller size. The homogenization depends upon the speed and number of teeth of the disc. But the speed can not be continuously increased because it causes increasing turbulence (Re. Number). The cream is then mixed with the incoming milk to be recycled through the bowl. The fat globules of sufficiently reduced size will not get re-separated when the cream passes through the bowl discs again and will, therefore, exit the separator through the skim milk outlet which thus discharges 'homogenized' whole milk.

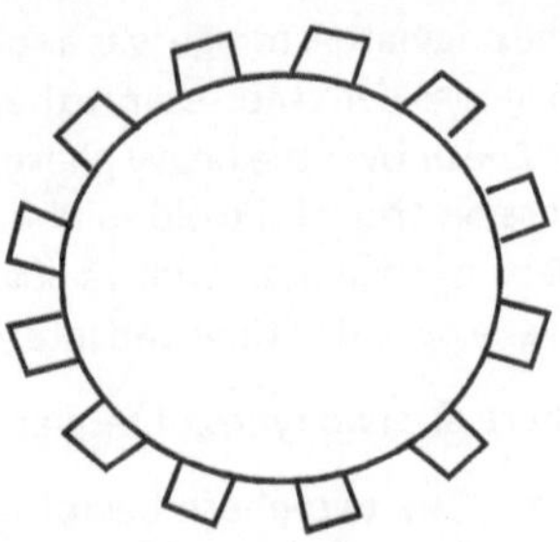

Fig. 5.9.2: Clarifixator disc

There is also a cream outlet through which the cream can be taken out when necessary.

When the cream / milk mixture passes through the set of separating discs, it is mainly the large fat globules that are separated while the smaller ones remain in the milk and go to the milk paring chamber from where they are pumped out by the milk parer. A certain amount of cream, therefore, constantly circulates within the bowl. Only when the fat globules in this cream (perhaps after repeated passage through the cream paring disc) have become sufficiently small, they leave with the milk. When equilibrium has been reached, a minute or two after the start, the milk leaving has the same fat content as that entering. The difference is that the size of the fat globules is considerably reduced. Furthermore, the milk has been efficiently purified.

Rate of Homogenization in Clarifixated Milk: The structural changes the milk is subjected to during passage through the homogenizing device, which in the clarifixator consists of the so-called cream paring chamber with stationary cream paring disc, have not yet been theoretically investigated. The clarifixator is about one-half as efficient as the pressure homogenizer. Because of its lower effectiveness clarifixation has not been used to any significant extent in the dairy industry.

5.9.3. Heat treatment of milk

Of all the steps involved in processing of milk, heating is by far the most important. Without heat processing the dairy industry would come to an abrupt halt. It is required by law that certain dairy products receive specified heat treatments. Other dairy products, such as concentrated and dry milk powders, gain their identity only through heat treatment. The objectives of heat processing may be summarized as follows: to meet public health requirements, that is pasteurization and sterilization, to remove water, to destroy enzymes, to facilitate mixing and blending processes, that is, ice cream mix and processed cheese, to achieve incubation temperatures, that is cheese and cultured dairy products, and to impart desirable properties.

In general, the main objective of heat treatment of milk is preservation. Keeping quality from a microbiological standpoint is the overriding consideration, although in the case of concentrated and dried products the effort may be toward preservation from chemical deterioration as well. This latter preservation is accomplished through removal of water (solvent) and is based on the principle that many chemical reactions are either slowed or completely inhibited in the absence of a solvent. Some other properties that may be imparted to dairy products as a result of heat treatment are: increased viscosity, reduced curd tension, resistance to oxidation, changes in flavour and colour, and alterations in protein stability.

The choice of heat treatment applied to milk depends on a trade- off between, first, the degree of microbial inactivation required to ensure safety and extend the shelf life by an acceptable factor and, second, changes in quality of the product; these two consequences of heating are usually, in effect, inversely correlated

Overall factors that should be considered in determining the heat treatment required for a particular product include:

- Post-heating growth potential of spore-forming bacteria. For example, low pH conditions or storage at low temperature suppress outgrowth of spore-forming bacteria; thus, products that include these additional hurdles , e.g. pasteurized or fermented milks, may not require as extensive heat treatment as higher pH products or products to be stored at room temperature.
- Consumer preference. For example, in some countries, such as Ireland and Australia, consumer preference is clearly aligned toward pasteurized milk, and the more strongly cooked flavours associated with UHT milk are undesirable.
- Target market. For example, the requirements for processing of infant formulae are among the most stringent in the dairy industry, due to the vulnerability of that group of consumers to food-borne illnesses.

Heat treatments applied to milk are generally defined by the maximum temperature of heating and the holding time at that temperature. The processes most commonly applied to milk and dairy products are summarized as follows:

Process	Temperature and Time	Microbiological Effect	Microbial Quality
Thermization	57-68 °C for 15 sec	Destroys psychrotrophs	3-4 log reduction in psychrotrophs
Pasteurization (LTLT)	63 ° C for 30 min	Destroys vegetative pathogens	Total plate count <1,00,000 cfu / ml
Pasteurization (HTST)	72-74 °C for 15-30 sec	Destroys vegetative pathogens	Total plate count <1,00,000 cfu / ml
Yoghurt mix heating	80-95 °C for 2-30 min	Destroys all pathogens and most spores	-
Forewarming	70-135 °C for 1 sec-5 min	Depends on treatment	-
High Temperature Pasteurization	120-130 °C for <1-5 sec	Destroys vegetative bacteria and most spores	-
UHT (indirect)	135-140 °C for <3-5 sec	Destroys all bacteria including spores	Total plate count <100 cfu / ml after 15 day at 30°C
UHT (Direct)	135-140 °C for <3-5 sec	Destroys all bacteria including spores	Total plate count <100 cfu / ml after 15 days at 30°C
In-container sterilization	115-120 °C for 10-20 min	- do-	-do-

5.9.3.1. Pasteurization

Pasteurization is the most important operation in the processing of milk. It involves heating raw milk to destroy pathogenic and spoilage microorganisms that may be present. The process is named after the French scientist Louis Pasteur who in 1864-65 demonstrated that heating wine at 50-60°C destroyed microorganisms responsible for abnormal fermentations. He made similar studies on beer and later reported that souring of milk was similar to spoilage of wine and beer; they all result from the growth of undesirable microorganisms. Commercial thermal processing of milk began in the late 1880s with one of the primary goals being the inactivation of *Mycobacterium tuberculosis,* the causative agent of tuberculosis in humans, which was endemic in the raw milk supply. Interest in minimizing the public health hazards associated with the consumption of milk grew steadily during the early 1900s; pasteurization was almost universally adopted by developed countries after the end of World War II. Having been used for more than 120 years, pasteurization has been, currently is and will probably remain the treatment of choice to render milk, cream and related products safe for consumption.

Pasteurization destroys all non-spore-forming pathogens and majority of potential spoilage organisms and helps in improving the shelf life of milk. The definition adopted by the International Dairy Federation (1980) states that "Pasteurization is a process applied to a product with the object of minimizing possible health hazards arising from pathogenic microorganisms associated with milk by heat treatment, which is consistent with minimal chemical, physical and organoleptic changes in the product." Pasteurization according to the Bureau of Indian Standards, refers to the process of heating every particle of milk at a specified temperature, holding the milk at such temperature continuously for specified period in a standard and properly operated equipment and immediate cooling in the same equipment after heating (IS 6397: 1992). The temperature of pasteurization should be such that it should have negligible effect or very little effect on colour, flavour, physicochemical properties and nutritive value of milk.

If the purpose of the heat treatment is exclusively to destroy pathogenic bacteria, then careful selection of time-temperature combinations will achieve the purpose without excessive destruction of the milk components. It is important to know that for any temperature above 63°C, different holding times may be specified to cause the needed destruction of pathogenic bacteria. Thus, at 63°C a holding time of 30 minutes is required for the certain destruction of the most resistant milk pathogen, *Coxiella burnetii*. However, as higher temperatures are chosen, the required holding time becomes less, and at 72°C, only 15 seconds of holding is required to destroy the organism.

Pasteurization of milk as defined by the US Code of Federal Regulations

63°C, LTLT (vat pasteurization)	30 minutes
72°C, HTST (high temp. short time pasteurization	15 seconds
89°C (higher heat shorter time)	1.0 second
90°C (higher heat shorter time)	0.5 second
94°C (higher heat shorter time)	0.1 second
100°C (higher heat shorter time)	0.01 second

By definition, pasteurized milk and fluid dairy products have received a heat treatment sufficient to minimize possible health hazards arising from pathogenic microorganisms associated with the raw product as well as adverse physical, chemical and organoleptic changes. All pasteurized dairy products that, by definition, are negative for alkaline phosphatase (a heat–labile enzyme) immediately after processing must be chilled rapidly and packaged without delay under conditions that minimize contamination.

The primary purpose of pasteurization is to reduce the number of bacterial pathogens in milk to levels that do not constitute a risk to human health. The process has been designed to destroy the most heat resistant non-spore forming pathogens found in raw milk including *Coxiella burnetii*, *Mb. tuberculosis* and *Listeria monocytogenes*. Other less heat-resistant pathogens of public health concern such as *Brucella, Staphyllococcus aureus, Salmonella, Campylobacter and Escherichia coli O157:H7*, are even more readily inactivated by pasteurization. However, thermoduric non-spore-forming bacteria (e.g. *Lactobacillus* and *Streptococcus*) as well as spore-forming bacteria (e.g. *Bacillus* and *Clostridium*) can survive pasteurization with growth of these organisms adversely affecting product quality during refrigerated storage.

Pasteurization tends to expel dissolved gases from milk; usually there is a loss of about 2.0 - 2.5 volume per cent of carbon dioxide, and this causes a decrease of about 0.01% in acidity.

Storage temperature has a vital role in determining the shelf life of heat-treated products. Ideally pasteurized milk should be kept at or below 4°C; if the storage temperature is raised to

10 °C, the shelf life is reduced by at least 50%. Zadow (1989) reported that shelf life is reduced to 50% by raising the temperature of the products by only 3 °C.

Methods of Pasteurization: There are three methods in use for pasteurizing market milk and cream:

1. Holding method
2. High-temperature short–time method
3. Ultra-pasteurization

Holding Method (LTLT): In holding / batch / vat pasteurization milk is heated to at least 63°C and held continuously at that temperature for at least 30 minutes and then immediately chilled in the same equipment to 5°C or less. Before continuous pasteurization systems became popular in 1940s, this method was most frequently used. This time-temperature treatment, termed low-temperature long-time (LTLT) pasteurization, was the first time-temperature treatment developed to render milk safe from microbial pathogens, including *Mycobacterium tuberculosis*, the most heat-resistant pathogen of major public health concern in milk. LTLT pasteurization remains the most economical of the three pasteurization processes available and is still used today, primarily by cheese manufacturers. This method is particularly suitable for small-scale batch operations where 3000 – 5000 litres of milk is to be processed at a time.

There are several types of equipment in use in which milk may be heated and held during the holding method of pasteurization. Vat and tank pasteurizers are by far the most common. Some types allow for the heating of the milk in the vat as well as the holding; but, in large volume operation, much time is saved by heating to the holding temperature by the flash method, with separate equipment, which raises the temperature in few seconds. With this arrangement the milk passes from the heater to the holder at a temperature of 63° C or above and remains in the holding vats at that temperature throughout the holding period.

The milk is heated to the required temperature and held there during the holding period, after which it is cooled with separate equipment. There are three types of vat pasteurizers in general use: coil, spray and jacketed vats with agitators.

The vat may be rectangular, but a vertical, cylindrical design is preferred. A typical jacketed vat type pasteurizer is shown in Fig 5.9.3. Double-walled vat is used for pasteurization. Indirect heating is done by circulating hot water in the jacket. The outer wall is insulated to reduce heat loss. In batch pasteurization heating is started when the batch of milk is in the vat or even before filling of the vat is complete. The heating water may be at 65-75°C and the time required to bring the milk up to the holding temperature commonly ranges from 30-45 minutes depending on the quantity of milk. When the temperature of milk reaches 63°C, the temperature of hot water is maintained at such a level that the temperature of milk in the vat remains constant for 30 minutes. The lid of the vat must be closed and the agitation must be continued to avoid surface cooling and pellicle formation. The heat exchange takes place through the wall of inner lining. Thereafter, it is chilled as quickly as possible either by circulating refrigerant / chilled water or through plate / surface chiller. Cooling the milk after pasteurization by circulating the refrigerant, in most cases cold water, through the jacket or, the vat may take long time.

Therefore, a separate small capacity surface, tubular or plate cooler may be used to rapidly cool the milk to the required temperature. This system also has the advantage that the vat will be quickly available for the next batch. From the point of energy utilization this is not an efficient system.

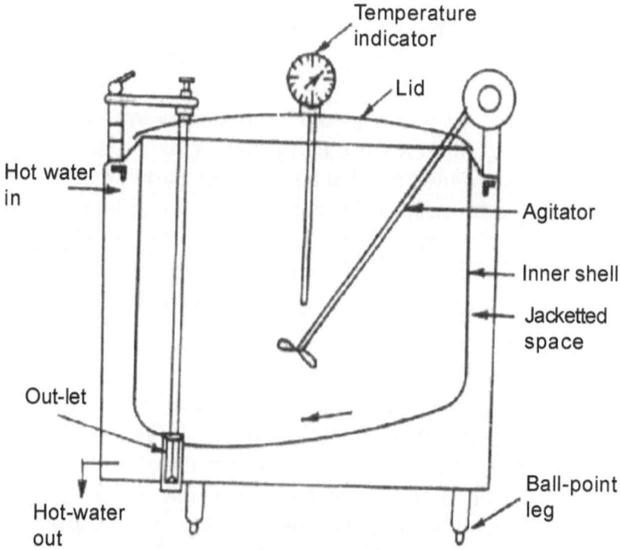

Fig. 5.9.3. Vat type pasteurizer

High-Temperature Short-Time Method (HTST): High-temperature short-time (HTST) pasteurization, a continuous process in which milk is held at not less than 72°C for a minimum of 15 seconds (or equivalent conditions at a higher temperature for a shorter time period) in properly operated equipment and cooling rapidly to 4°C is now a norm for processing fluid milk and cream. For milk products containing higher levels of milk fat or SNF, higher temperatures need to be employed for pasteurization depending upon the specific composition of the product.

Most vegetative bacterial cells are destroyed by both LTLT and HTST pasteurization. However, some thermoduric lactic acid bacteria and spore-forming organisms will survive, and this necessitates prompt chilling and refrigerated storage of the product to minimize the growth of psychrotrophic bacteria involved in spoilage. Milk continuously chilled to 4°C through regenerative chilling ensures maintenance of its nutritive value and original flavour.

Equipment: The milk may be heated by any method that raises the temperature rapidly to the required degree. Plate and double-tube equipment are commonly used when hot water is the heating medium. The plate type HTST equipment consists of following six parts: or section: float control tank, regenerative section, final heating section, holding tube, flow-diversion value, and final cooling section. These parts are connected with the necessary sanitary pipes and the automatic temperature-control instruments.

The raw milk usually flows by gravity from the storage tank to the float control tank, the top of which is below the level of plate heat exchanger. The milk is then drawn through the regenerator section by the timing pump, under a vacuum of 6 to 8 inches, and is heated to about 68-70°C by the hot pasteurized milk that flows in the reverse direction between the adjoining plates. In the pasteurizer milk must be heated by absorbing heat from a heating medium through the plates, with the medium being cooled concomitantly. Similarly, heat from the pasteurized milk must be transferred to cooling medium after reaching the pasteurization temperature. In a PHE, these two steps are conveniently combined and the pasteurized milk is used as a heating medium for the incoming cold raw milk with substantial saving of energy. This technique is called heat regeneration. In a pasteurizer, raw milk is heated in this manner by pasteurized milk from about 6°C to about 68-70°C; concomitantly, the pasteurized milk is cooled to about 10°C. The temperature of the milk thus preheated must be increased by only by 2-4°C (depending on the pasteurization temperature set-point) using steam or hot water in the final heating section, while in the cooling section the pasteurized milk must be cooled by only about 6°C (from 10 to 4°C). With a well-dimensioned regenerative section, it is possible to recover about 94-95% of the heat from the pasteurized milk. Milk is heated to nearly 80% of pasteurization temperature in the regeneration section.

Regenerative preheating of raw milk is usually divided over two to three sections of the PHE; milk between sections is at intermediate temperatures between 6 and 70°C. Milk at around 50-55°C is at the optimum temperature for treatment such as separation, clarification or homogenization as milk fat is in the liquid state. Incorporation of such processing steps into the pasteurization line avoids the need to heat milk separately to carry out these operations, making liquid milk processing more economical and reducing opportunities for contamination of the milk. Thus, milk can be routed out of the PHE between regeneration sections for treatment such as homogenization or standardization, before being returned to the PHE for completion of the pasteurization cycle. Milk may in theory exit the regeneration section for such parallel processing either while being heated (raw milk) or cooled (pasteurized milk). The former option is more common, as it avoids the risk of recontamination of pasteurized milk, which otherwise would have to be avoided by use of aseptic homogenization or separation systems.

Milk is then pumped under pressure through the final heating section, where the temperature is raised to 72°C by hot water that is at about 2-7°C above the temperature of milk and flows in the reverse direction between adjoining plates. Water is heated in separate heating and circulating unit then pumped through the heating section and returned to the hot water reservoir. A water to steam ratio of 2.5:1 and a temperature differential of 2-7°C between milk and hot water results in efficient heating and is least likely to cause defects in flavour of the product.

Milk then flows into the holding tube. The length and diameter of the holding tube are arranged to allow the passing through of the milk in 15 to 16 seconds at the capacity for which the equipment is designed. The diameter of the holding tube is 3.5-7.5 mm. It is designed so that the difference in temperature between the hottest and coldest milk in any cross section of the flow at any time during the holding period will not be greater than 0.5°C. The holding tube must have a continuous upward slope of not less than 0.1 mm / ft. This is to ensure that the holding tube will remain full and the air bubbles will not decrease the effective diameter of the tube. As the effective diameter decreases, the flow increases resulting in a reduced holding time.

A resistance thermometer (thermistor) monitors the temperature of milk, generally at the point of exit from the holding section. Less commonly, the thermistor may be located at the start of the holding section. The latter position allows more time for reaction to a drop in temperature, ensuring that no under- pasteurized milk can flow downstream for packaging, but does not account for the drop in temperature that can occur in an un-insulated external holding tube. The former position is thus more common, although a drop in temperature in the holding tube may be minimized by insulating the tube, or by heating the milk slightly above the set pasteurization temperature in the heating section. However, the latter option implies overheating of milk, with concomitant potential alterations to flavour and other properties.

The thermistor (which typically operates over the range 60-80°C) controls the action of the flow diversion valve (FDV), which is located downstream from the thermistor, either at the end of the holding section or, less commonly, after the cooling section of the pasteurizer. The function of the FDV is to prevent unpasteurized milk from reaching the packaging unit by returning milk to the balance tank should the temperature determined by the thermistor drop below the torget pasteurization temperature. The default, or fail-safe position on the pasteurizer FDV is the closed or divert position, and the valve opens only if and when the temperature exceeds the set-point. During operation, if milk temperature, as measured by the thermistor, falls below the set-point, a programmable logic controller (PLC) or similar device detects and records the decrease, often sounds an alarm for operators, and deactivates the FDV, causing the valve to close so that milk is diverted to the balance tank.

There is always a possibility of fractures or pinholes occurring in pasteurizer plates, which could lead to recontamination of pasteurized milk. To guard against this possibility, a booster pump may be fitted in the pipeline as it leaves the holding section to increase the milk pressure slightly (by about 0.01-0.02Mpa); should a pinhole then occur, the direction of leakage would be of pasteurized milk into raw milk, thereby precluding post-pasteurization contamination. A simpler means of protecting the pasteurized product is to increase the number of passes in the regeneration sections, thereby increasing the back pressure within the pasteurized milk section of the plant.

In the cooling section chilled water from an ice bank system of refrigeration, is circulated and returned to the chilled water reservoir. Chilled water to milk flow rate of 3:1 is normally maintained. Milk is cooled to a temperature of 4-6°C in the chilling section. The chilling section may also be provided with another section where the milk is partially cooled by water supply lines of the dairy plant and then passed to the chilling section. This reduces the quantity of refrigeration needed.

The chilled milk from the pasteurizer flows either to the intermediate storage tank or directly to a packaging unit. It is extremely important to avoid conditions that could introduce microorganisms in the pasteurized milk during processing downstream from the pasteurizer; it has been acknowledged that post-pasteurization contamination has in the past represented a significant influence on the shelf life and public health aspects of pasteurized milk. Such contamination may arise from intermediate storage tanks, pipelines, filling machines and packages.

The key operating parameters for a HTST pasteurizer are: plant capacity, temperature programme, regenerative efficiency, and the temperature of the heating medium and the cooling medium. During operation, the PHE may be controlled in a feed back loop by monitoring the temperature of the following fluids: milk in the heating section, milk leaving the cooling section, heating medium and cooling medium.

The shelf life of pasteurized milk is dependent on factors such as the microbial quality of the raw milk, the precise processing conditions used, post-pasteurization contamination and refrigeration temperature, but is generally about 10-16 days at 5°C (Kelly and O'shea, 2003).

Plate heat exchanger: Most of the HTST plants use plate heat exchangers (PHE) for regenerative heating, final heating and cooling. The plate heat exchangers consist of a number of thin stainless steel plates, sealed at edges with gaskets and also clamped tightly within the frame work of a press and a screw tightening device. The frame may contain several groups of plates, known as sections, in which different stages of treatments, such as preheating, final heat treatment and cooling take place. These stainless plates have been machined to fit snugly together, preventing leaks, and have been engineered so that milk will pass on one side of the plate while the heating or cooling medium flows in the counter-current direction on the other side the thickness of the plates has been maintained at a narrow tolerance to permit efficient heat transfer. The heat transfer area is determined by the number of plates in the pasteurizer. The heating medium may be steam or hot water, and the cooling medium may be cold water, brine, glycol or ice water depending on the desired outlet temperature of the product. The capacity of a milk pasteurizer depends on the size and number of plates, and can be as high as 1,00000 l/ h.

The plates are rectangular and are stamped from SS sheets type 320, normally 0.8-20 gauge. Normal gap between plates is 2.5-4.0 mm depending on the size of the pasteurizer. The plates are corrugated in a pattern designed to increase turbulence and, consequently, the efficiency of heat transfer. The plates are compressed together in the frame, but supporting points on the corrugations hold the plates apart so that thin, rectangular channels are formed between them. The liquids flowing in the PHE enter and leave these channels by openings at the corners of the plates, and varying patterns of open and blind openings route the liquid from one channel to the next. Gaskets (made from natural rubber, or more recently, from synthetic elastomers) around the edges of the plates and holes define the boundaries of the channels and prevent leakage. Though stainless steel is a relatively poor conductor of heat (about 10 BTU / hr / ft / °F) and it is difficult to weld during fabrication of equipment, it is used for heat exchangers because it is unreactive and easy to clean. In contrast, copper is an excellent conductor of heat (218 BTU / hr / ft / °F), yet it is not used in fabrication of heat exchangers because it catalyses the oxidation of fat in milk and thus produces off flavour.

Milk is introduced through a corner opening into the first channel of a section and flows vertically through the channel. It leaves at the other end through the openings at the opposite corner, and bypasses the next channel between plates. The heating or cooling medium is introduced at the other end of the section and passes in the same manner through inter-plate channels. Thus, milk has heating and cooling medium, in the respective sections, flowing countercurrent, on either side of it, separated by intervening plates.

For efficient heat transfer, the channels between the plates should be as narrow as possible; however, if a large volume of product has to pass through these narrow channels, both flow velocity and pressure drop will be high. Neither of these effect is desirable, and to minimize their significance the passage of the product through the PHE may be divided into number of parallel flows. One section of parallel flow is known as a pass, and passes in the PHE change the direction of flow a number of times. Within each section of the pasteurizer there are many passes, i.e. the direction of flow of product or heating / cooling medium is changed several times. Thus, the flow of the liquids through a plate heat exchanger is a counter-current and parallel.

Operation of Pasteurizer: Before starting the pasteurization, the plant should be sterilized properly by circulating chemical sanitizer, hot water at not less than 90°C for 10 minutes or by low pressure steam. After sterilization, the operation of the pasteurizer is regulated with water till stable water temperature conditions in the various sections are achieved. For this purpose the water is taken in the float control balance tank (FCBT) and circulated through all the sections of the pasteurizer and then returned. Hot water and chilled water from the reservoirs are also circulated. The temperature controls are properly adjusted while the water is being circulated; all pipe joints are inspected for leaks and tightened, if necessary. Air leaks in the raw-milk suction side will reduce the pump capacity and will result in over-holding, foaming of the milk, and consequent under-filling of the containers. When the proper temperatures are attained, the action of FDV is checked. The back pressure gauge is read and the required flow is adjusted in the flow controller. Then the water circulation is diverted to drain and milk circulation is started by taking it to the FCBT. The water is then forced out of the pasteurizer with milk, and the first few litres of milk are drawn off and separated because of their dilution with water.

Cleaning: The cleaning of plant is carried out immediately after the milk is pasteurized. The sequence of rinsing water and detergent solutions followed is as:

1. rinsing with luke-warm water and draining,
2. circulation of hot water at 65°C
3. circulation of lye at a concentration of 1.5% at a temperature of 70°C,
4. rinsing with luke-warm water and draining,
5. circulation of nitric acid / phosphoric acid solution, concentration not more than 0.5% at a temperature of 50°C,
6. rinsing with cold water and draining.

The recent trend in cleaning method is to hook up the plant to an automated Clean-in-place system which results in high cleaning efficiencies and also pasteurizers along with other processing equipment like homogenizer, cream separator and milk lines can be cleaned simultaneously. Separate tanks for holding rinse water and detergent solutions are used. The temperature of hot water and detergent solutions are maintained by steam coils and controlled by self-acting

... The inlet and outlet valves of the tank are connected to common inlet and outlet heade... s. Two pumps are used, one to pump the solution from the common intake line to the equipment and the second to return the solution from the equipment to the respective tanks through the common return line. All the valves are of pneumatic type and operated by compressed air supply lines. An electronic sequence timer and programmer operates the valves and pumps in a programmed and timed sequence to circulate the rinse water and detergent solutions in the sequence as mentioned before. In between circulations of the alkali and acid detergents a compressed air blows through a one-way solenoid valve which is introduced in the cleaning lines, for a few seconds, to avoid intermixing of traces of solutions.

Preventive Maintenance: Preventive maintenance will help to control damage, excessive wear and tear and occurrence of accidents. Preventive maintenance can be divided into two areas, (i) avoiding damage to the plant and equipment and(ii) observations and inspection of plant and equipment. Avoiding damage consists of basically the careful handling of machinery and equipment. The regular inspection of the plant and equipment is important as a part of preventive maintenance, and may include:

1. Periodical test may be made to check the flow rates of heating medium, cooling medium and milk.
2. The recording instruments such as thermometers, etc must be periodically checked for their accuracy.
3. Air operated instruments should be supplied with clean air.
4. The plate surfaces and gaskets must be checked during the cleaning of plants.
5. Filter cloth / filters must be changed at regular intervals.
6. The faces of the plate bar and tightening spindle should be lightly coated with grease.

Advantages of HTST Pasteurization

This system of pasteurization has certain advantages over the holding method. These have accounted for their wide adoption by dairy industry. The principal advantages are as follows:

1. Less floor space is required, because holding vats and separate coolers are not required.
2. With the plate equipment the capacity may be increased by increasing the number of plates and lengthening the holding tube without using additional floor space.
3. Labour may be better utilized with large installations by reducing the time required for cleaning and increasing the capacity of the equipment without lengthening the operations beyond the normal working day.
4. The milk packaging can start as soon as the pasteurization process begins, without the wait of 40 minutes to 1 hour required by the holding method.
5. The equipment, being completely closed, can be easily sterilized by pumping hot water or sterilizing solution through the system.

Methods of Sterilization

In-container sterilization in autoclaves, continuous sterilization and ultra-high-treatment (UHT) are used to sterilize milk and milk products in order to prevent microbial spoilage during storage. In addition, a more or less complete inactivation of enzymes as well as physicochemical changes of the constituents occurs during sterilization, depending upon temperature and treatment time. In order to retain as many as possible of the sensory and nutritive properties of the raw material, heating conditions can be selected by using kinetic data. Process conditions for continuous and in-container sterilization can be optimized by applying mathematical formulae which quantify the phenomena occurring during sterilization.

In-Container Sterilization in Batch Autoclave: Milk or milk products are processed in order to modify the constituents according to physical and biochemical long-life stability and to special product demands, e.g. colour, flavour and rheology. After filling into containers, the required microbiological effect for long-life stability is obtained by heating in batch autoclaves or continuously operating autoclaves. Conditions specified for in-container sterilization of milk include temperature from 105-120°C for 20-40 min. With this strategy, milk is prefilled into cans or bottles that are hermetically sealed, and then the milk is heated in an autoclave or a batch or continuous retort. The heat is transferred to food by means of hot water or condensing saturated steam via the container wall. Sterilization temperatures above 100°C are attained by pressures above atmospheric pressure in pressure vessels, so-called autoclaves. Usually upright or horizontal mantled cylindrical pressure vessels are used into which the containers to be sterilized are placed on racks, baskets or carriages. In batch autoclaves, short heating-up and cooling times are achieved by agitating of the content by means of rotation or swinging of the inserts with the containers from side to side. After raising the temperature and holding it for the required time, the cooling down period starts and the content of the autoclave is cooled by the circulation of water. In order to save energy in hot water operated autoclaves, the hot water is pumped into a storage tank situated above the autoclave and reused for the next batch. In practice, the containers are removed from the batch autoclave at a temperature of about 35°C, to enable the moisture on the surface to evaporate so that they are dry for labeling. Batch autoclaves are mainly used for small quantities and in processes where the type of product, container size and therefore the sterilization procedure has to be changed frequently. In-container sterilized milk products are less commonly manufactured than UHT products. The most common application of the process is in the manufacture of milk-based flavored beverages (e.g. coffee). In general, milk products processed in this manner are subject to more pronounced defects related to cooked flavours and the Maillard browning reaction than are products processed by other UHT strategies. In-container sterilized milk products have expected shelf life of a year or more with no refrigeration required.

In-Container Sterilization in Continuously Operating Autoclaves: For large throughputs, like production of sterile milk or condensed milk in bottles or metal cans continuous systems are used. One type of apparatus is the hydrostatic sterilizer which uses columns of water in order to counterbalance the pressure gradient between inside and outside of pressure sensitive packages during heating-up, sterilization and cooling down. The columns of water act as transit pressure valves for cans and bottles transported in pockets or recesses on continuous conveyor chains through the hydrostatic sterilizer.

Another continuously operating autoclave is only suitable for sterilizing products filled in cans. In this rotating autoclave, the cans are fed by means of a bucket wheel into a horizontal cylindrical pressure vessel. They are fed in at the circumference at one end and discharged at the other end. Within the vessel, a rotor rotates with continuous radial flanges at its circumference, between which the cans lie in rows. By means of guide bars on the stator, i.e. on the inner wall of the vessel, the cans are transported spirally through the vessel and thorough mixing of the contents of the cans are achieved depending on the consistency of the product

Sterilization of Milk: Milk is heated to 43°C and filtered or clarified to remove foreign matters. Following this milk is heated to 74-77°C and homogenized to prevent fat separation. The milk is canned and heated at temperatures between 105 and 120°C for 10-40 min through steam. The temperature of milk rises slowly on account of the slow heat penetration, especially when cans are not agitated in the sterilizer. Because of this and of the fact that bottles do not withstand sudden and extreme temperature changes, the milk must be sterilized by a time-temperature combination whereby the temperature is low and time rather long. This tends to give the milk a rather strong off-flavour and a brownish colour, especially if the bottles are not agitated in the sterilizer.

Sterilization of Condensed Milk: Fig. 5.9.4 demonstrates two variants of condensed milk manufacture. Up to the second step of standardization of the product, i.e. adjusting it to the desired final composition, the steps are comparable. Then, within the continuous flow sterilization process, the evaporated milk is homogenized before and after sterilization. There is an advantage in homogenizing after heating since it prevents or reverses protein-protein and fat globule-protein aggregation, which is not possible for in-container sterilized products, because the product is filled into separate containers before sterilization. A further advantage of the continuous process is that the product can be filled into flexible packages, which are not suitable for in-container sterilization. In the latter packages like metal cans, glass jars or bottles and plastic bottles are used.

Continuous Flow Sterilization: There are two systems used for continuous flow sterilization, viz. indirect heating in tubular or plate heat exchangers and direct heating by steam injection or infusion. Plants for continuous flow sterilization consist of four main sections. In the heating-up section the product is preheated and often held for certain time to denature the whey proteins in order to reduce fouling in the heating section and to prolong the heating time of the heating plant. In the heating section the product is brought up to sterilization temperature via indirect heating or direct heating. The holding time depends on public health aspects and on the requirement to reach commercial sterility. The product is held at required temperature in a tubular holding section. Heat regeneration with the incoming product or via an auxiliary water circulation in the cooling section allows a heat recovery of about 90%, and, if necessary, final cooling of the product with water. Homogenization is performed before and after sterilization. The first homogenization is applied to reduce the fat globule size to achieve the physical stability of the emulsified fat phase. The second homogenization step separates heat-induced protein-protein and fat globule-protein aggregates, which may also lead to physical instability during storage.

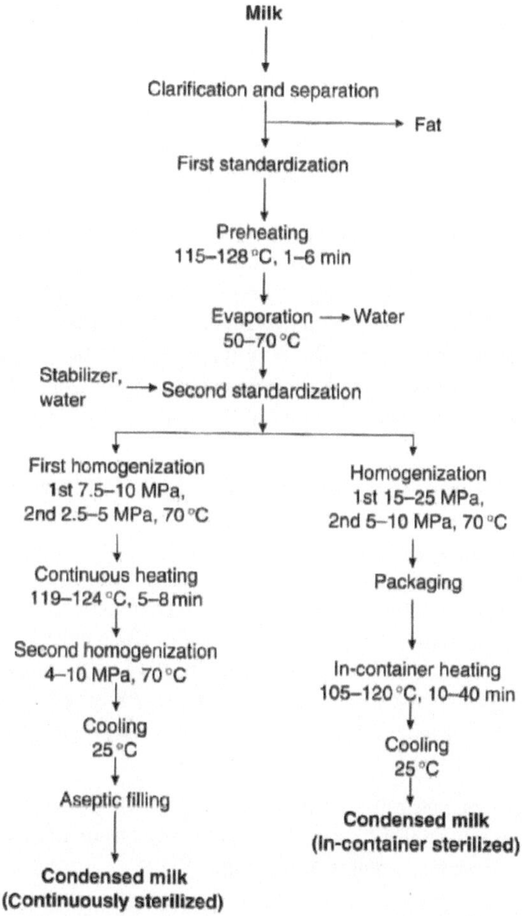

Fig. 5.9.4. Flowchart of continuously sterilized and in-container sterilized unsweetened condensed milk

Types of Sterilization Plants

Retort Sterilizers: Sterilizing retorts are either batch-type or continuous in operation. Batch-type sterilizers may be either vertical or horizontal. Horizontal retorts are easier to load or unload. They have facilities for agitating containers / cages. However, they require more floor space. Typically such horizontal retorts contain concentric cages. Cans are loaded horizontally into the annular space between the cages. When cages are full, the retort is sealed. The cages are supported by guide rails, which slowly rotate them. This stirring of the contents in cans facilitates proper heating. The continuous retorts are generally equipped with better controls. They cause very gradual change in pressure inside the cans. Thus products are heated more uniformly. Can seams are also subjected to less strain in comparison to batch process.

Continuous Sterilizer: Continuous sterilizers are of mainly three types: a) cooker-coolers, b) hydrostatic sterilizers, and c) rotary sterilizers. Cooker–coolers carry cans on a conveyor which pass through three sections of a tunnel. These sections are maintained at different pressures for preheating, sterilization and cooling. The hydrostatic sterilizer consists of a chamber equipped with provision for steam injection. The chamber that is partially full of water is connected to two water columns (12 to 18 meter tall, a barometric leg) which are used to adjust pressure in the chamber. If the height of the water columns is changed, the steam pressure changes and therefore the maximum attainable temperature also changes. For example to get a temperature of 116°C, a difference in height between the two water columns should be 10.7 meter while for attaining 121°C temperature in the chamber, the water column difference should be 13.7 meters. A conveyor with provision to accommodate cans of different sizes moves through the steam chamber carrying the food cans. The heating time could be regulated by varying the speed of the conveyor. Hydrostatic sterilizers are very flexible and suitable for large capacity plants. However, the size of structure and high capital costs are the major disadvantages of this system.

Continuous rotary sterilizer consists of several horizontal interlinked cylinders which allow for preheating, heating, pre-cooling and cooling in up to four continuous stages. The vessel has a spiral track on the inner wall. A spoke or reel within the centre of the cooker causes the cans to roll along the spiral track. Rotary valves used to interconnect the shells, maintain pressure in the heating and cooling sections. Sealed cans are introduced directly from the sealing machines. The contents inside the cans are mixed as cans travel along the helix and therefore enhance heat transfer and ensure least heat damage to the product. Cans coming out of the cooker are directly taken to labeling and palletizing machine. Rotary sterilizers are particularly suitable for processing of milk and milk based products, which are extremely heat sensitive and susceptible to browning.

Canning Process: Basic operations in conventional retorting / canning process include: preparation of the raw material, filling of the container, exhausting, sealing of container, sterilization, cooling of the cans, labeling and storage.

The preparation of raw material refers to washing, peeling, cutting, blanching, pre-cooking, etc in case of fruits, vegetables, meat, etc; and preheating, mixing, homogenization etc, in case of milk. Filling of containers can be carried out either manually or mechanically. Correct and accurate filling is important from economic standpoint as well as for prevention of entrapment of large volume of air / gas inside the can, which might decrease the intensity of heat treatment. Exhausting is an essential operation in the canning process and involves removal of air / oxygen from the container before it is closed. Removal of air ensures minimum of strain on the can seams or pouch seals through expansion of air during heat processing. Removal of oxygen is essential to prevent internal corrosion of the container through oxidation and creation of vacuum inside the container while cooling. Absence of oxygen inside the container also delays oxidative deterioration of the product besides destruction of ascorbic acid.

After exhaustion, containers are sealed. Depending on the type of containers (metal cans, glass bottles, flexible pouches); sealing machines are chosen. Glass jars are normally vacuum-sealed while tins are closed with a double sealing on the seal side and may also be vacuum-sealed.

Flexible retortable pouches are sealed by fusion of two thermoplastic materials [illegible]gh application of heat by heated plates or jaws.

Product in the closed container is heated in the sterilizer in an atmosphere of saturated s[illegible] or hot water or air-steam mixture. The sterilizing action of steam depends on its latent hea[illegible] evaporation as it condenses on the surface of the can. Saturated steam condenses readily an[illegible] is therefore an efficient sterilizing medium. Displacement of all air present in the retort by steam before the sterilizer is brought to the operating temperature is a very essential step. This is also known as venting. The purpose of this processing step is to maintain uniform steam-air mixture in the sterilizer and prevent under processing. Sterilization temperature-time combination in retort may vary from 110-130 °C for 10-30 min. Sterilized containers are then cooled and brought to room temperature for labeling and storage. Turbidity test developed by Aschaffenburg is conducted to ensure the sterility of the product. This is an indirect test and it measures denatured whey proteins. Complete denaturation indicates that the milk is adequately sterilized.

Flavour Quality of Sterilized Milk: Sterilized milk has a rich creamy appearance and a distinct cooked flavour (rich, nutty, caramelized). It is considerably browner in colour than the raw milk. The brown colour develops due to formation of coloured pigments resulting from interactions of free amino groups of proteins and aldehyde group of lactose through Maillard reactions. The intensity of cooked flavour and brown colour depends upon the severity of heat treatment. In-container sterilization causes loss of nearly half of the ascorbic acid (vitamin C) and sizable loss of thiamine (30-40%). Vitamin B_{12} is almost completely destroyed. Fat-soluble vitamin A, carotene, riboflavin and nicotinic acid are not affected. Biological value of proteins is only marginally affected. Sterilized milk cannot be coagulated with rennet unless calcium chloride is added externally.

Ultra-High Temperature Sterilization: Pasteurized milk is one of the most important components of market milk. However, maintenance of a cold chain, i.e. maintaining the temperature of milk at 4°C from the point of production till consumption is essential to prevent the spoilage of milk. Insurmountable difficulties have been encountered in the Indian context for maintenance of cold chain due to several techno-economic factors under the tropical climatic conditions. Furthermore, there is a worldwide concern for conservation of energy in processing and distribution of foods. All these factors have lead the planners to opt for UHT processing as national policy for market milk distribution. The first UHT commercial plant was commissioned at Surat (GCMMF) in 1982 followed by UHT plants at Indore (1984), Jaipur and Guntur (1985). For meeting the requirement of special packaging material for UHT milk, a Lamination plant was established at Itola, Baroda (Gujarat). Besides the Tetra Pak Packaging Systems, some of the UHT plants in India utilize pre-sterilised LDPE film imported from Finland (Sterilac, Finland).

Ultra-high temperature (UHT) treatment of milk is a continuous process aimed at producing a 'commercially sterile' product, that is, a product in which bacteria will not grow under the normal conditions of storage when packaged aseptically. It involves heating at a temperature higher than 130°C (usually 138-145°C) for a holding time of 1-10s (usually 3-5s).

...basic principle of UHT processing of milk is that, for the same bactericidal effect, high-...perature short-time heating, causes less chemical change than low-temperature long-time ...ating. Thus sterilization by UHT heating at ~ 140°C causes much less chemical change than ...atch sterilization in retorts at ~120°C.

The minimum time-temperature combinations for UHT heating are dictated by the need to destroy bacterial endospores while the maximum time-temperature combinations are those that cause the maximum acceptable amount of chemical damage, usually set at 3% destruction of the B vitamin thiamin. In practice, the lowest temperature used is that at which the spores are destroyed in a reasonable time (~135°C) while the upper limit is determined by the capability of the equipment (~150°C); very short holding times (fraction of a second) at elevated temperatures are practically impossible to achieve with current technology.

Nominal holding times are normally based on the average velocity of the particles in the product. Depending on the product and the dimensions of the holding tube, the velocity of the fastest particles can be several times that of the slowest particles. As a consequence, at time-temperature combinations at the lower limit of UHT processing, the fastest particle may receive insufficient heat while at time-temperature combinations at the upper limit, some particles may be overheated. The residence time distribution in the holding tube is particularly significant for the destruction of heat-resistant bacterial spores as the time taken for the fastest-moving spores to traverse the holding section can be much less than half that taken by the average particle, that is, the nominal holding time. Therefore, the length of the holding section of a UHT plant should be determined by the residence time distribution within the section and the decimal reduction time of heat-resistant spores.

In addition to heat treatment and aseptic packaging, UHT processing of whole milk also involves homogenization. When downstream of the sterilization step, homogenization must be performed aseptically. Homogenization reduces the average size of the fat globules in milk from ~3 μm to 0.5 μm and coats the new small globule with a membrane consisting largely of casein. This markedly reduces the rate at which the fat rises to the top of the milk during storage. Ideally, UHT milk should not develop a layer of fat on the top of the milk even after storage at ambient temperature for up to 9 months. In practice, many UHT milks develop a fat layer after storage.

The heating step in UHT processing usually involves superheated steam as the heating medium. As the temperatures used for UHT processing are higher than the boiling point of water (and milk), processing has to be performed under pressure (~0.4 MPa) to prevent boiling. The steam can be either mixed directly with the product (direct heating) or indirectly via metal tubes or metal plates (indirect heating). In recent years, combinations of both modes of heating have been introduced to take advantage of the benefits of both types.

Viscous products and products containing particulate matter have additional requirements over liquid such as milk in UHT processing. While some of these products can be processed by systems mentioned above, another form of heat exchanger, the scraped-surface heat exchanger, is used for this purpose. These are mostly indirectly heated although a variation utilizing direct steam heating is commercially available.

...ms utilizing steam are shown in Fig 5.9.5.

...are two types of sterilizing systems, indirect and direct.

...stems: In indirect type plant, product is heated by steam or hot water ... coming in direct contact. In indirect plant, rise in temperature is very gradual. T... e, heat load on the product is more. Changes in chemical quality are relatively more in indirect type than in direct type plants. There are three types of indirect heating systems: (a) Plate heat exchanger, (b) Tubular heat exchanger, and (c) Scraped surface heat exchanger.

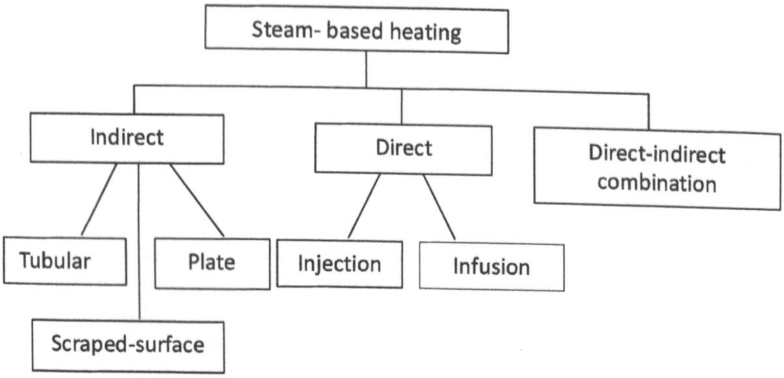

Fig. 5.9.5. UHT systems based on steam heating

Plate heat exchanger: This resembles plate heat exchanger of HTST plants. The principal differences between plate heat exchangers used for pasteurization duties and those used for UHT processes are that the latter must be able to withstand higher processing temperatures (135-150°C, as against 72-85°C), and that higher internal pressures must be withstood in a UHT heat exchanger. In plate heat exchangers, the heat transfer rate is high, due to large contact surface area, and high turbulence levels that can be achieved. High temperature processing generates high internal pressure. The gaskets are, therefore, made of heat resistant materials such as medium nitrile rubber or resin cured butyl rubber. A major advantage of this plant is, therefore, simple design and comparatively less cost. However, these are more easily fouled than tubular systems due to the narrow channels through which product flows.

Tubular heat exchanger: The most common type of UHT heating system uses the tubular heat exchanger. Different configurations of the heat exchanger are available, with the most common being the shell-in-tube and the concentric tube designs. The concentric-tube systems are formed by assembling two or three stainless steel tube lengths one inside another with a spacer, often a spiral wire, in each inter-tube space to maintain them concentric. Several such multiple tubes are bound together and placed into an outer cylindrical housing. Two tube heat exchangers are used for simple cooling and heating. In triple-tube heat exchangers, available heat transfer area is doubled. It is generally used in final cooling section. It is also suitable for processing of thick liquids, which generally reduces heat transfer rate. The product flows through the middle annular space. Heating or cooling medium passes through inner tube and outer annular space. In shell and tube type heat exchangers, 5-7 straight lengths of smaller tubes (10-15 mm internal diameter) are assembled in outer tube. The smaller tubes are connected to large outer tube at both ends by a manifold. The product passes through the smaller tubes. Heating or cooling medium passes through the space around them in a counter current flow. Tubular heat exchangers are mechanically very strong and can withstand even very high pressure generated during homogenization (200-300 bar). Therefore the need for acquiring an aseptic homogenizer to be placed after heating section is totally eliminated. Instead, the high pressure reciprocating pump of an ordinary homogenizer can be placed before the sterile section. The homogenizing valve can be put at any point on the downstream side (even after final heating section). The problem of product contamination arises from the homogenization pump and not the valve. Therefore, with tubular heat exchangers, the product can be homogenized before sterilization, after sterilization or on both the occasions. Fat-rich products like cream require homogenization after final heating to prevent re-association of fat globules due to high temperature processing after homogenization.

For UHT processing the product is pumped from the balance tank through the first preheating tubular heat exchanger section to give a homogenizing temperature of about 75°C at the homogenizer. It then passes through a second preheating section to give a temperature of 90-95°C at a holding section, a holding time of 60 s is recommended to reduce fouling on heat exchanger surfaces in the later stages of the process. It is known as a protein stabilization section as it causes denaturation of much of the whey protein β-lactoglobulin and so prevents it from being denatured and deposited on the walls of the subsequent heating tubes or plates. A final heating stage brings the product to final sterilization temperature of about 138°C, at which it is held for about 1.5 s in the holder. Regenerative cooling is utilized. A regeneration level of 90% or more can be obtained with this system. Regenerative heat exchange is through the closed water circuit which heats the product in heat exchanger sections. A restrictor provides the necessary back pressure in the sterilizer.

In indirect systems, the milk to be heated flows in the opposite direction to the heating medium (hot milk or steam). This minimizes the temperature differential between the two flows which in turn reduces the amount of fouling on the heat exchanger surface and allows longer operating times and better product quality. The temperature differential should be not more than 3°C.

Fouling or deposit formation is a major issue with indirect heating systems. The build-up of deposit restricts the flow of product through the tubes or plates and causes a decrease in pressure and a reduced transfer of heat from the heating medium to the product. This is more significant in plate than in tubular heat exchangers. Typically, this limits the run time in plate systems to 8-12 h before partial or complete cleaning is required to remove the deposit.

The product after sterilization is aseptically filled into appropriate sterile containers for non-refrigerated distribution and sale. UHT-sterilized milk products are considered shelf-stable, with expected shelf lives of 3 months to 1 year with no refrigeration required.

Scraped-Surface Heat Exchanger: Scraped-surface heat exchangers (SSHE) are used for high viscosity products for which alternative heat exchangers are impracticable. They use rotating mechanical scraper blades to continuously remove product from the heat- transfer surface and create turbulence to improve heat transfer. They operate with high temperature differential between the product and the heating surface and therefore have a high potential for burn-on on the heating surface. They have a relatively low energy efficiency compared with plate and tubular systems used for low viscosity products, as regeneration of heat is not possible with this system. The cost of processing is therefore very high. The SSHE units are very costly.

A variation of the scraped surface system (the Roto Therm™) utilizes a series of steam injectors along the scraped surface. In this system, the steam condenses and transfers its latent heat to the product. It also forms a film of water on the inside of the barrel which reduces burn-on and lubricates the surface. Processed cheese products are typical dairy products heated with this system.

Merits and Demerits of Indirect Heating System: It is simple in design and requires less pumps and controls. It can regenerate 90% of the thermal energy requirement. It does not require aseptic homogenizer, which is very costly. It does not require culinary steam and therefore special type of boiler. The indirect type plant is less noisy. It requires low initial capital and operational cost is also comparatively less.

In indirect type heat exchanger, the rate of heat transfer is low. More heat load results in less acceptable product quality. Deposit formation is more and therefore plant requires frequent cleaning. For removal of dissolved oxygen from milk, additional equipment 'deaerator' is required.

Direct Heating Section: There are two types of direct heating plants (a) Injection type and (b) Infusion type.

Injection type: Processing is through steam-into-milk arrangement. Steam injector is the heart of this plant. Pre-heated milk at 80-90°C enters the injector nozzles from out side. Steam at slightly higher pressure enters the injector from the other side. As the steam mixes with milk, steam condenses and the product is rapidly heated. Rapid condensation of steam prevents entry of air in holding tube. Air in holding tube results in improper heating. Back pressure is maintained on the discharge side. Back pressure ensures that product does not boil in holding tube. Boiling may result in fouling and improper heating of milk.

Infusion Type: In this system milk is heated by milk-into-steam arrangement. The processing unit consists of a chamber filled with pressurized steam. Milk enters the chamber from the top. There are two alternative arrangements for distribution of milk. In the first type, milk flows to a hemispherical bowl with loose circular disc closing the top. When the bowl is full, milk overflows and falls in droplets through the steam environment. In an alternative arrangement, milk flows through a series of parallel and horizontal distribution tubes. These tubes have slits along the bottom and milk flows like a thin film through the chamber. As milk reaches the bottom of the chamber, it is heated to desired temperature. This system is particularly suitable for thicker liquids and for liquids suspended with smaller chunks.

Merits and Demerits of Direct Heating Section: During processing in direct type heating systems condensing of steam coming into product contact results in dilution of the product. To remove this excess of water from the product, cooling is done in an expansion cooling vessel. In expansion vessel, along with the evaporating water incondensable gases and undesirable flavour volatiles produced during heating are also removed. The product therefore tastes better. Steam injection induces formation of casein aggregates, which give 'chalky' or 'astringent' mouthfeel to the product. Aseptic homogenizer, which can safely homogenize the product after final heating section, is generally preferred with direct heating sections to overcome such defects in the product.

The rate of heating is very high (takes less than 1 second to attain sterilization temperature). Thick / viscous liquid can also be easily processed. Deposit formation is minimum, hence plant can be operated for longer time without cleaning. Undesirable flavours are removed during flash cooling. Oxygen is removed during cooling, hence oxidized flavour defects are delayed during storage.

The cost of processing per unit volume of milk is high. Required additional equipment (vacuum expansion chamber and aseptic homogenizer) cost of plant is twice that of indirect type plant. Heat energy requirement is very high. Water and electricity consumption is high (25-50% more than in direct type). Requires culinary steam and hence a special boiler. Creates greater noise during operation.

Combined Direct-indirect Systems: Major equipment manufacturers have introduced systems incorporating both direct and indirect heating for producing UHT milk. The reason for this is to exploit the advantages of each system, in particular, the better flavour and superior bacterial spore destruction capability of direct heating (higher temperatures can be obtained without excessive chemical damage to the milk), and the higher heat-regeneration capacity of indirect systems.

The temperature profiles of the systems marketed by APV (High Heat Infusion) and Tetra Pak (Tetra Therm^R Aseptic plus Two) are illustrated in Fig 5.22 and 5.23, respectively. In both systems, the temperature rise achieved by direct heating is 20-30°C, compared with 60-70°C for the direct heating systems. They differ in sequence of heating and cooling steps. In the High Heat Infusion systems, the vacuum chamber is placed after preheating and before the high-heat sections, while in the Tetra-Therm^R Aseptic Plus Two system, it is placed after an initial cooling step following the high-heat (steam injection) section. The available data indicate that heat regeneration and the extent of chemical 'damage' to the milk in these combination systems are intermediate between the conventional direct and indirect systems. Up to 75% regeneration is claimed for the High Heat Infusion systems.

The discovery of very heat-resiststant bacterial spores in UHT milk in Europe was a major trigger for the development of these combination systems. The major organism of concern is *Bacillus sporo-thermodurans* which not only has a high thermal resistance (~150°C for 6 s required for satisfactory kill) but is also capable of growth in the temperature range for mesophilic bacteria. The high temperature (up to ~150°C) that can be achieved by the direct heating is more likely to destroy the spores of such an organism than is the highest practical temperature possible with indirect heating.

The Microflora and Enzymatic Activity of Heat-Treated Market Milks-Influence on Quality and Shelf Life

Food product shelf life is the length of time that a food can be kept under practical storage conditions and still retain acceptable quality characteristics. These characteristics include sensory appeal (odour, flavour texture and physical appearance) and product safety (Muir, 1996). The initial quality and shelf life stability of heat-treated market milks is dependent on a) the microbiological and enzymatic quality of the raw milk and other ingredients used in manufacturing, b) the heat resistance and activity of intrinsic and microbial enzymes associated with the raw milk, c) the types and initial numbers, and potential growth of microorganisms that survive the heat treatment processes, and d) the incidence, types, and growth of microorganisms that re-contaminate the product after the heat treatment (post-pasteurization contamination). In general, obvious sensory defects related to microbial growth do not occur until bacterial populations exceed 10^6- 10^7cfu / ml, although the actual defects encountered are dependent on the types and activity of the microflora present (Patel and Blankenagel, 1972; Muir, 1996).

Pasteurized Milk: Pasteurization by either LTLT or HTST method is sufficient to destroy non-spore-forming pathogens likely to be present. Bacteria commonly isolated from pasteurized milk are usually the same types of bacteria that are found in raw milk. Bacteria found in pasteurized milk originate from a) thermoduric organisms present in the raw milk, b) raw milk contact with contaminated handling and processing equipment, and c) post-pasteurization contamination. Unless temperatures and times higher than the minimums for pasteurization are used, however, a group of bacteria known as thermodurics survive. These are mesophilic organisms that grow in the range of 20-45°C and include species of Micrococcus, Microbacterium, Bacillus, Enterococcus, Streptococcus, Arthrobacter, Lactobacillus, and Clostridium. Thermoduric mlcroorganisms generally grow slowly in milk at 5° C and usually cause spoilage problems only if present in large numbers. However, they do contribute to numbers of bacteria determined by the plate-count procedure and so, if present in large numbers, could cause milk to exceed the established bacterial standard, which, for pasteurized milk, is 50,000 cfu / ml (PFA).

Another group of bacteria which can be found in pasteurized milk are thermophilic. These bacteria can grow at pasteurization temperature. These include spore-forming *Bacillus spp. such as B. stearothermophilus, B. thermoacidurans, B. calidolactis.*

Not all thermoduric strains of bacteria are capable of reproducing in pasteurized milk under conditions of refrigerated storage. Small numbers of bacterial contaminants of this nature are unlikely to cause product spoilage within a typical fluid milk product shelf life. However, psychrotrophic strains of *Bacillus, Micrococcus, Enterococcus, Corynebacterium, Microbacterium, Arthrobacter*, and *Lactobacillus* have been identified. Strains of *B. cereus* (and the closely related *B. mycoides*) have been implicated as the cause of "sweet curdling" of milk and "bitty" cream. Although commonly present in milk, *B. cereus,* a potential foodborne pathogen, may not grow as well at lower refrigeration temperatures (<5° C) as other *Bacillus spp* such as *B. polymixa* and *B. circulans.*

Psychrotrophic gram-positive organisms other than *Bacillus spp* also may be responsible for limiting the shelf life of pasteurized milk. The presence of gram-negative spoilage organisms, particularly *Pseudomonas spp*. are the primary contributors to the psychrotrophic spoilage of pasteurized milk. Although milk spoilage is most commonly attributed to the presence of high numbers of *P. fluorescens*, strains of *P. fragi, P. putida* and *P.maltophilia* are also common. Defects associated with the growth of *Pseudomonas* include fruity, bitter, rancid, and unclean off-flavours as well as coagulation of the milk proteins. Other psychrotrophic gram-negative bacteria that grow and cause spoilage in pasteurized milk include strains of *Alcaligenes, Flavobacterium,* and *Enterobacteriaceae*.

Because gram-negative coliform bacteria do not survive pasteurization treatments, the presence of these organisms in pasteurized products is used by the dairy industry as an indication of the possibility of post pasteurization contamination. Coliforms are defined as aerobic and facultative anaerobic, gram-negative, non-spore-forming rods that are able to ferment lactose with the production of acid and gas at 32 or 35° C within 48 hrs. Coliform bacteria isolated from milk and milk products include species of *Escherichia, Enterobacter*, and *Klebsiella* and selected strains of other fermentative bacteria. Currently, the legal limit for coliform in pasteurized milk is 10 / ml.

Numbers of psychrotrophic contaminants occurring in freshly pasteurized milk can be very low, perhaps below detection limits by conventional enumeration methods, i.e., <10 cfu / ml (Douglas et al., 2000). However, the ability of these organisms to reproduce at refrigeration temperatures can allow them to grow during storage. Cousin (1982) describes generation times for some psychrotrophic milk contaminants of less than 6 h at temperatures less than 7°C. Given these kinetics, if one bacterium were to reliably double every 6 h, bacterial numbers could exceed 10 million after 7 days. Thus even low levels of post-pasteurization contamination can dramatically influence product shelf life.

In general, post-pasteurization contamination contributes the majority of the microorganisms that contaminate and spoil pasteurized milk, thus, elimination of contamination sources can dramatically influence process product shelf life. To illustrate HTST product shelf life was extended from <7 days to >21 days following identification and elimination of a single point source of *Pseudomonas* spp contamination in a product filling unit (Ralyea et al., 1998).

Ultra-pasteurized Milk: The primary objective of ultra-pasteurization processing is the elimination by heating of virtually all microorganisms present in raw milk. The heating process may not inactivate heat-stable enzymes, however, and these enzymes can contribute to product deterioration during storage. Sources of heat-stable enzymes in raw milk include gram-negative psychrotrophic organisms and indigenous enzyme systems, including plasminogen and plasmin. To date, the influence of heat-stable enzymes on ultra-pasteurized milk quality has not been well documented; however, refrigerated storage of these products may help reduce enzymatic degradation of the products during product shelf life. In general, the optimum activities of the majority of heat-stable enzymes that have been studied are above refrigeration temperatures, generally ranging from 30-45° C, with reduced or limited activities below 7° C (Mottar, 1989).

Microbial numbers in ultra-pasteurized milk are controlled by a) microbial destruction from ultra-pasteurization heat treatment, b) sterilization of milk contact surfaces, and c) application of disinfection strategies to ultra-pasteurization milk packaging materials. In general, ultra-pasteurization milk packaging equipment is enclosed to protect the product from environmental contamination. The air within the filling equipment is usually treated by high-efficiency particulate air filtration to reduce the presence of airborne contaminants. Immediately prior to filling, packaging materials are typically disinfected with hydrogen-peroxide, heat, ultraviolet light, or a combination thereof. Effective application of these combined strategies can render the milk product virtually free from microbial recontamination. Prevention of product contamination by potential spoilage microorganisms can allow refrigerated product shelf life of 30-90 days and more. However, any deficiencies in the sanitation process could allow post-processing contamination, which could result in product spoilage similar to that seen in conventionally pasteurized milk.

UHT Sterilized Milk: Microbial control strategies for UHT milks are similar to those described for ultra-pasteurization processing, except that the products are aseptically packaged in sterilized packaging materials in a sterile environment to yield commercially sterile products. Product spoilage due to post-processing contamination is prevented by adherence to and documentation of scientifically established processing parameters with properly operated equipment and reliably sealed containers. If the sterility of the system is compromised at any point during processing, the process must be shut down and the equipment cleaned and sterilized before processing is resumed.

Effect of UHT Treatment on Nutrients: Lactose can isomerizes to lactulose in heat-treated milk. Lactulose isomerization is catalyzed by free amino groups of casein and is strictly dependent on time of heating, heating temperature and pH. Normally, lactulose does not occur in fresh milk and highly pasteurized milk, but only in UHT and sterilized milk. Lactulose content is therefore considered a suitable indicator of heat treatment. Recently, it has been proposed to stipulate a lactulose content of less than 600 mg / l for UHT milk and more than 600 mg / l for sterilized milk (IDF, 1991).

During storage, lactulose concentration in UHT milk can either decrease (via beta-elimination to galactose, tagtose and formic acid) or increase (via lactose isomerization), the former process being more temperature dependent than the latter. Light did not affect lactulose concentration during milk storage at 18°C for 115 days(Andrews, 1989).

UHT processing does not cause reduction in biological value of proteins. There is only small loss in available lysine (6-7%). UHT processing changes the casein micelle structure. This slows rennet action during cheese manufacture. Serum proteins are denatured (direct processing – up to 50-75%, indirect processing up to 70-90%). Denatured serum proteins interact with casein and increase casein micelle size. This reflects more light and UHT milk appears whiter. The brightness of colour of UHT milk is greatly influenced by storage conditions. The rate of decrease in whiteness is higher at storage temperatures above 20°C.

Heat treatments might also negatively affect the nutritional quality and, in particular, protein digestibility. Efigenia and coworkers (1997) evaluated the effect of heat treatment on milk nutritional quality for samples of raw, pasteurized, domestic boiled and UHT milk: fat, protein, and N contents were not significantly modified by any of these treatments. Protein efficiency ratio, digestibility and *in vitro* liver protein synthesis, studied by feeding trials in rats, were unaffected by heat treatments, with the exception of a lower rate of protein synthesis in the liver of rats fed with boiled milk

Effects of heat treatment on protein digestibility and lysine availability of pasteurized milk (72 or 85 °C for 15 sec) and UHT milk (140 °C for 3 sec or 130°C for 10 sec) were also studied. Lysine loss was the highest in UHT milk and correlated with heat severity, although the degree of lysine loss was not sufficient to affect milk nutritional values. In *vitro* protein digestibility was highest in milk pasteurized at 72 °C. Results suggested that in severely heated milk samples, lysine availability and protein digestibility decrease simultaneously.

Milk contains enzymes that have the ability to catalyze specific chemical reactions. In milk both endogenous and exogenous enzymes are present: endogenous enzymes are mainly hydrolases (lipase, the heat- stable plasmin and alkaline phosphatase, destroyed by minimum pasteurization temperatures), and exogenous enzymes, generally heat stable, are produced by psychrotrophic bacteria. As expected, enzyme activities can be considerably affected by thermal processing.

There is no physical or chemical change in milk fat. The total mineral content also does not change during UHT processing. The vitamin content of UHT milk is comparable to pasteurized milk. Losses in B-complex vitamins are not more than 10%. Study of vitamin B_1 (thiamine) in milk subjected to different heat treatments (pasteurization at 75, 82 and 89°C, direct and indirect UHT) showed similar results: significant loss of vitamin B_1 due to heat treatment was not observed. Heat treatment causes slight or no variation in riboflavin content (B2), and no significant difference in riboflavin content can be detected between raw and UHT milk samples. Folic acid and ascorbic acid are destroyed up to 15% and 25%, respectively. Fat soluble vitamins A, D, E, and K are not affected by UHT processing. The beta-carotene content of milk is unaffected by UHT processing. Tocopherols (vitamin E) are sensitive to oxidation, heat and light, but usully or small losses of alpha-tocopherol are observed after UHT treatments (Vidal- Valverde, et al. 1993). Alpha-tocopherol losses from 3-14% were observed in UHT milk after 1 month of storage at 30°C, losses increasing with longer storage time. In a recent study, no losses of alpha-tocopherol and retinol in UHT milk at 8°C, a temperature typical of home refrigerator, which stresses the importance of storing UHT milk refrigerated (0-4°C) after opening. The extent of losses of water soluble vitamins is shown in the Table 5.9.6.

Table 5.9.6. Losses of vitamins in milk by different heating procedures (Renner, 1981).

	Losses (%)				
Heating procedure	Vit. B1	Vit. B2	Vit. B12	Folic acid	Vit. C
Pasteurization	10	0-5	10	5	5 - 15
UHT treatment	5-15	10	10-20	10 -20	10 -20
Sterilization	30-40	10-20	80-100	40-50	30-50

UHT milk, either freshly prepared or stored has slightly cooked flavour. The cooked flavour is due to the release of –SH (sulphydryl) groups from the denatured serum proteins. The direct UHT process is claimed to give a better flavour due to the vacuum flash down. After UHT treatment it has been also reported that direct UHT milk stored at 5° C was the only product comparable to the pasteurized milk and that too for a storage period of not exceeding 8 weeks. Stale or oxidized flavours occur due to formation of aldehydes and ketones.

Maillard Reaction: The most studied chemical reaction of heat-treated milk is, undoubtedly, the Maillard reaction, in which amino groups (mainly casein-bound lysine residues) and reducing sugars (mainly lactose) are the main reactants. The Maillard reaction consists of several steps, strictly dependent on temperature, pH, water activity, and type of sugar and amino group involved.

In the early stage of Maillard reaction, condensation of the reactive free amino group of lysine with the free carbonyl group of lactose occurs, via formation of the Schiff's base, which is subsequently transformed via the Amadori rearrangement into the Amadori product (ε-deoxyketosyl compounds). In milk this Amadori product is lactosyl-lysine (bound to protein).

The initial stage of Maillard reaction has important nutritional consequences: formation of lactosyl-lysine represents a considerable loss of biologically available lysine. The amount of lysine loss in Maillard reaction has been proposed as a marker of the severity of heat treatment.

The Maillard reaction, on severe industrial treatments, can carry on with the Amadori product undergoing a cleavage, leading, through different pathways, to many reactive compounds. In the final stages of Maillard reaction, polymeric reactions lead to brown pigments (melanoidins), responsible for food odors and flavours.

Changes in UHT Milk during Storage: Chemical, physical and sensory changes in stored UHT milk are dependent on storage temperature. Changes are rapid if storage temperature exceeds 30°C. Separation of the fat layer adversely affects the shelf life of UHT milk. It has been reported that homogenizing milk after or before heating produces milk of similar microstructure that forms cream layers of similar thicknesses during storage. Nevertheless, it was recommended that UHT milk be homogenized before treatment with high temperature, to avoid use of aseptic homogenizers. Browning reaction between protein and lactose progresses during storage. At higher storage temperature (>30°C) UHT milk may become little brown after 3-4 months In contrast to in-container sterilized milk, it may develop certain defects during storage (bitter and rancid off-flavour, gelation, coagulation of milk proteins) without concomitant growth of spoilage organisms. These defects are generally believed to be due to surviving enzymes. Certain psychrotrophic bacteria including pseudomonads and spore forming bacilli produce proteases and lipases during storage of raw milk at temperatures as low as 4 °C. Some of these enzymes being extremely heat resistant withstand to a large extent the UHT process. These proteases are hundred times more heat resistant than the bacterial spores. Extensive proteolysis and other physico-chemical changes occurring as a result of interaction of proteins and salts during storage may cause thickening or sweet curdling also referred as age thickening (gelation) after longer storage (more than 6 months). Gelation is caused by modifications of casein micelle aggregation, producing a three dimensional network. The mechanism is not completely known, but it is probably due to proteolysis induced by either heat-resistant native proteinases (plasmin) or microbial proteinases. While plasmin, a native alkaline serine proteinase, is almost completely inactivated by the UHT process, its precursor, plasminogen, is particularly resistant to heat. Plasminogen is converted to plasmin by an activator whose activity increase after heat treatment (Datta and Deeth, 2003). Usually plasmin attacks beta-casein and alpha-2-casein, while the microbial proteinases prefer to attack κ-casein. Note that as little as 1 ng of bacterial proteinase / ml is sufficient to cause gelation of UHT milk during storage. Lipase surviving UHT treatment act on lipid fraction. Short and medium chain fatty acids are released. Short chain fatty acids, particularly butyric acid contribute to the development of rancid flavour in the product. Air in the product or in the packet reacts with unsaturated fatty acids. This auto-oxidation reaction causes formation of aldehydes and ketones. These compounds cause oxidative rancidity (flavour defect) in the product. The cooked flavour in UHT milk disappears in first few days and milk tastes best after this period. Few weeks after this, depending on the temperature of storage, oxidized flavour defects appear which become more pronounced with progressive storage. In milk stored for considerable period of time, which could be 3-4 months at >30°C, stale flavour is a common defect. Several compounds that are formed during the progress of Maillard reactions in stored milk are associated with the appearance of this defect. Sometimes coconut-like flavour defect also appears in UHT milk stored for longer periods. Compounds such as ä-dodecalactones are responsible for this. To minimize the risk of processed product defects associated with heat resistant microbial enzymes, Burton (1988) suggested maintaining raw milk bacterial numbers <$5x10^5$ cfu / ml prior to processing.

5.9.3.3. Thermization

Thermization is the generic description of a range of subpasteurization heat treatments of milk which reduce markedly the number of spoilage bacteria with minimum collateral heat damage to milk components and do not cause changes in flavour. Originally thermization was developed as a heat treatment of milk before cheese making. Thermization at 57-68°C for 10-20 s was aimed at destroying the adventitious bacterial flora and providing a suitable environment for the multiplication of lactic acid bacteria introduced in starter cultures. In the 1970s, when the cold storage of raw milk became a widespread practice, a concept was developed to extend the keeping quality of raw milk by its thermization on delivery to dairy plants or between collections on farms. The thermized and promptly cooled milk could be cold-stored for an additional three days because thermization reduces markedly the heat-labile psychrotrophic microflora responsible for spoilage at low temperatures (spoilage without souring). Those microorganisms produce at low temperatures heat-stable proteinases, lipases and phospholipases. The natural antimicrobial system in milk (i.e., the lactoperoxidase-thiocyanate- hydrogen peroxide system) is unaffected by thermization. Extension of the keeping quality allowed dairies to be closed over weekends. Thermization at 62-68°C for 15 s is practiced widely. The treatment can be conveniently performed in a plate heat-exchanger designed for the pasteurization of milk using a standard 15 s holding time.

Heat treatment at subpasteurization temperatures (55-65°C for 20 s to 10 min) has been introduced to prolong the shelf-life of cultured milk products such as yoghurt and quarg cheese.

Extracellular proteinases and lipases produced by pseudomonads during cold storage of milk survive UHT sterilization but are less heat stable at 55-65°C than at temperatures >70-80°C.

Low temperature inactivation (60°C for 5 min or longer) has been proposed to inactivate these enzymes before or after UHT sterilization of milk.

Inactivation of Heat-Stable Proteinases and Lipases: Heat treatment at 50-70 °C inactivates to various degrees, proteinases and lipases from pseudomonads and several other species of psychrotrophic microorganisms. The most efficient low temperature inactivation was found for *pseudomonas* proteinases in the temperature range ~ 50-60°C and for *pseudomonas* lipases at 60-70°C.

UHT sterilized milk produced from raw milk containing > 10^6 bacteria per ml by heating at 140°C for 5 s had a shelf life, due to defects caused by lipolysis or proteolysis, 3-8 times shorter than that of milk which was first UHT sterilized and then held at 60°C for 5 min.

Effect of Thermization on Microbial Quality of Cold-Stored Milk: Psychrotrophic pseudomonads account for ~10% of microflora of fresh milk, but they become the dominant microorganisms in raw milk stored in farm tanks at 4-5°C for 60-72 h; the most frequent isolate after that period is Pseudomonas fluorescens. A rapid increase in bacterial population is noted between 2nd and 3rd day of storage. Thermization reduces lactoperoxidase activity only slightly and apparently has little effect on the natural lactoperoxidase-thiocyanate-hydrogen peroxide anti bacterial system in milk. This system is most effective in promptly cooled milk during a short period of storage. Pseudomonas species are markedly more heat-labile than *Listeria* spp. or bacterial and indigenous enzymes. Decimal reduction times (D values) for *Pseudomonas* spp. indicate that thermization should reduce these microorganisms by several log. Treatment at a temperature of 60-63°C gives at least a 4-log reduction of *Salmonella* spp. and a 2-log reduction of *Listeria monocytogenes.* Thermoduric or spore-forming psychrotrophs grow markedly slower at <7°C than *Pseudomonas* spp. provided that recontamination after thermization is avoided, thermized milk has markedly better microbial quality after 3 days of cold storage than milk which has not been thermized. The effect of thermization on keeping quality during subsequent cold storage depends clearly on the temperature of thermization and the microbial quality of raw milk before thermization. Alternative to thermization may be cold storage at a very low temperature (not higher than 2°C) which is expensive and / or purging the milk with nitrogen or CO_2.

Activation of Spores: Thermization at 65°C for 10 s may be sufficient to stimulate the germination of *Bacillus cereus* spores. Activated spores may germinate after 6 h at 10°C. If post-thermization contamination is avoided, the vegetative cells which have developed from germinating spores during cold storage between germination and pasteurization may be destroyed effectively by pasteurization and the resulting quality of the pasteurized milk may be improved.

Effect on Cheese Yield: Thermization of milk has very little effect on the renneting properties of milk. Thermization of milk on farms or in dairies increases cheese yield primarily because the treatment reduces and even reverses, at least partially, low temperature dissociation of â-casein and calcium from casein micelles. A reduction of cheese yield of 35% due to bacterial proteolysis is observed for milk of very poor microbial quality, containing 10^7 psychrotrophs ml^{-1}.

Cheddar cheese produced from milk thermized at 65°C for 15 s and stored for 3 days at 4-5°C had better quality than cheese produced from the same milk thermized at 55°C for 60 s or from control unthermized milk that had been cold stored for 3 days and then pasteurized. Addition of selected lactic acid bacteria, which do not grow below 7°C, to thermized milk before cold storage and pasteurization resulted in improved renneting properties of the milk and in cheese of improved quality, provided that the milk before thermization was of reasonably good microbial quality.

Long cold storage of cheese made from unpasteurized milk is mandatory in some countries. During storage of some cheese varieties at 2°C for not less than 60 days, many pathogens die off. The combination of thermization of cheese milk and cold storage of some cheese is considered to be a safety precaution equivalent to the pasteurization of cheese milk.

Thermization of Cultured Dairy Products: The main spoilage microorganisms in cultured products are moulds and yeast, and their usual sources are fruits added to yoghurt or other fermented milks. Either the activity of rennet used in the production of quark or the activity of heat-resistant proteinases from psychrotrophic microflora may also contribute to the development of bitter taste. Spoilage occurs due to 'post-acidification' or 'over-acidification' by starter microflora during storage.

Thermization of cultured milks may be performed before or after packing. To avoid recontamination before packing, heat treatment is combined with aseptic or hot filling. Thermization of fermented products requires scraped-surface heat exchangers. Hydrocolloids are usually added to thermized cultured milk to improve the consistency of the final product.

Thermization of yoghurt and quark reduces the number of both the lactic acid bacteria and contaminants. Although lactic acid bacteria, especially in yoghurt, are more resistant than yeasts, moulds and coliforms, their viable count after thermization is reduced substantially. Measurable post-acidification did not occur in thermized yoghurt or quark after storage of these products for 2 months at 20°C. Quark that contained experimentally added proteinase from *Ps. fluorescens* and was thermized at 55°C for 6 min had a markedly better taste and less proteolysis than the unthermized control after storage at 7°C for 5 weeks. Proteinase from *Pseudomonas* was inactivated due to self-hydrolysis or to aggregation with casein at both pH 6.6 and 4.5. Thermization also reduced proteolysis in quark without added *Pseudomonas* proteinase.

Although thermization achieves its goal, i.e. extension of the shelf- life of cultured dairy products, its rationale is often questioned. The importance of viable bacteria is emphasized in standards and regulations for yoghurt and other fermented milks. The viable microflora assures maintenance of all probiotic properties of these products. Some properties, like the enhancement of lactose hydrolysis in the digestive tract, are similar for viable and non viable cultured milk, but stimulation of the immune system by probiotic cultures has been observed with viable bacteria only.

The preparation of attenuated starters is usually accomplished by adjustment of cultured milk to pH 7.0 and heat treatment at 60-68°C for ~15 s. Attenuated starters contain heat- damaged or killed cells of lactic acid bacteria but about 20- 50% of proteolytic enzymes in the bacterial cells remain active and participate in cheese ripening. A larger amount of attenuated starter than normal starter can be thus added to accelerate cheese ripening or to obtain more piquant cheese.

5.9.3.4. Forewarming

The term forewarming, or preheating, is employed largely in connection with the manufacture of condensed and evaporated milks. Forewarming enables introduction of the milk into the vacuum pan at a temperature well above the boiling point inherent within the pan, thus facilitating removal of water. In addition, it imparts to milk certain qualities that are manifest in the finished evaporated milk as satisfactory protein stability and viscosity properties. In general, temperatures from 88° to 100°C are employed in forewarming. There currently is a trend toward preheating above 100° C. The time employed for holding milk at the forewarming temperature will depend upon the temperature used, the stability of the milk, the type of forewarming equipment used, and the degree of concern that the manufacturer may have for colour and flavour of the finished evaporated milk. A 10-minute holding period seems ample to insure uniform temperature in a hot-well of milk. When forewarming temperatures are substantially elevated, some compensation by reduction of the holding time is usually made.

Forewarming applied to milk not subsequently concentrated lowers its heat stability. Forewarming continues to cause lowering in heat stability of milks that are concentrated up to a 13% nonfat- solids. If a milk is further concentrated to 14% or more solids-not-fat, its heat stability is markedly increased by a proper forewarming treatment. Thus there is a critical solids level, about 13.5%, below which forewarming of raw milk decreases stability and above which it raises stability. Hence, forewarming is an important manufacturing step in the evaporated milk industry, where a milk of at least 18% solids-not-fat is to be produced.

No heat stability test is known which, when used on raw milk, will accurately predict the stability of its concentrated product. It is, therefore, not possible to predetermine the forewarming to apply to a fresh milk, so that after concentration it will respond to a sterilization process by producing a required body. The evaporated milk industry determines heat stability and regulates the body of the finished product by making pilot-batch tests and by addition of stabilizing salts. Tests to determine approximate heat stability, such as alcohol, phosphate, or protein stability test are sometimes used on raw milk. A decision as to the optimum forewarming conditions is usually made on the basis of the behaviour of the milk received the previous day.

Marked variations in stability occur with variations in forewarming temperature and time. Rapid improvement in resistance of the concentrate to heat coagulation is brought about by increasing forewarming temperature. Milk to be concentrated and sterilized as evaporated milk is usually forewarmed in a hot-well by direct steam injection to raise it to 95°C where it is held for 10-20 minutes. The stability thus imparted to the milk will usually enable it to withstand heat sterilization as a 26% solids as evaporated milk. Greater heat stability can be obtained by the use of high temperature forewarming carried out by injecting steam directly into the milk, or by forcing the milk through a pressure-heating system, usually in the form of tubular heater. As the temperature of forewarming is raised, shorter holding times are necessary to attain heat stability. For the manufacture of 3:1 sterilized milk of 35% solids content, a high-temperature forewarming treatment within the range of 115°C for 2 minutes to 138°C for 15 s will usually be required. The forewarming of sweetened condensed milk must be conducted differently from that of evaporated milk.

The rapid decrease in the heat stability of milk with increasing concentrations makes it impractical to attempt to sterilize a product which has been concentrated to a ratio substantially higher than 3:1 (27% nonfat-solids). In commercial practice evaporated milk concentrated 2:1 can be sterilized under several temperature-time combinations, such as 115°C for 16 min, 130°C for 2 min, and 140°C for 3 s. Milks concentrated to 3:1 can sometimes be adjusted by forewarming and salt-balance procedures so that they will withstand a heat necessary for sterilization.

For manufacture of sweetened condensed milk, the raw milk should be forewarmed at a lower temperature than that for manufacture of evaporated milk to avoid age thickening. Although forewarming at 71°C gives a low-viscosity product, this temperature does not effectively destroy many bacteria, yeasts, moulds and enzymes, the presence of which often cause body and flavour defects during storage. It is commercial practice to forewarm the milk at about 82°C. This yields a product that has sufficient viscosity to retard separation of fat and crystallized lactose during storage, but will not gel when held at room temperature or lower for several weeks. When high-temperature short-time heating equipment is available, forewarming at 115°C for less than 1 min may be used to produce low-viscosity sweetened condensed milk for shipment to warm climates.

From a practical standpoint there seems to be no question that the extent of forewarming treatment can be a factor in the colour and presumably the flavour, of evaporated milk. The tendency is for successive heat treatments of milk to have cumulative effects. Milks that have been rigorously forewarmed (in excess of about 100°C for 10 minutes) will show a greater degree of browning with a given concentration and sterilization process than milks receiving more moderate forewarming. For unconcentrated skimmilk sterilized at 120°C for 20 minutes, the first additive effects of forewarming (100°C) on colour were noted between 15 and 30 minutes holding time (22). Pilot-scale experimentation with a milk supply will ordinarily reveal a forewarming treatment that is sufficient to impart desired properties of body and protein stability to an evaporated milk and yet will have no additive effect on colour.

5.9.3.5. Condensing

The purpose of the condensing operation is the removal of water. For all practical purposes, heating under vacuum is the sole means employed in the dairy industry. Concentration by mechanical removal of ice crystals or sublimation of ice, although feasible in other segments of the food industry, has never proved practical in application to milk. With the widespread use of multiple effect evaporators for condensing milk, it is not possible to specify precisely the degree of heat treatment to which milk may be subjected in the condensing operation. In some of the low temperature evaporators the heating effect is essentially nil. In a single effect vacuum pan the evaporating temperature usually ranges between 43° to 55°C. Though milk may be exposed to only slightly elevated temperatures during condensing, the significant factor to remember is that application of heat is essential to the operation, either in the process of forewarming or within the pan to facilitate evaporation.

Drying: The purpose of drying milk and milk products is to remove virtually all the water in them with a minimum amount of irreversible physical and chemical change. Of the various processes that are used to dry milk, spray drying is by far the most important. Lesser quantities of milk and other dairy products are roller dried. Spray drying consists of atomizing concentrated milk into a stream of hot dry air. The moisture-laden air is continuously replaced in the drier and the dehydrated particles of milk are usually removed through the combined effects of gravity and dust collection systems. In the roller process for drying milk, the concentrated milk is deposited in a thin film on a metal drum heated with steam. During the course of one revolution of the drum the milk film is deposited, dried and removed from the drum surface by an appropriately placed knife edge. Double drums placed with extremely small clearance and rotating counter to one another are used more frequently than a single drum.

It is very difficult to assess the effects of heating on milk during the drying process. The fact that the milk is in a progressing state of concentration suggests that some of its constituents may be rendered more liable to the effects of heat, whereas others may be stabilized. Moreover, the cooling effects of evaporation must be taken into account. In spray drying the length of time that dried milk remains in the drier is a factor, but in the roller process the speed of the drum will determine how long the milk film is in contact with the heated metal surface. In spray drying, air inlet temperatures ranging from 71° to 177°C may be employed and in atmospheric drum – drying processes temperatures of 90° to 132°C are used. The precise temperature conditions vary with the particular drying equipment.

Current trends toward use of minimum heat treatment in the processing of milk have focused interest on the actual temperature that a particle of dry milk achieves during the spray drying process. There is no simple method of measuring the temperature of such a minute particle. It has been postulated that the temperature of the particle never exceeds the exhaust air temperature of the drier. Measurement of temperatures at the surface to which the dried particles fall appears to confirm this postulation. However, it can readily be seen that with driers operating at an air inlet temperature of 150°C and an exhaust temperature of 71°C, the maximum temperature achieved by the particle can be very significant from the standpoint of heat damage.

In general, atmospheric roller drying of milk is more problematic regarding heat damage than is the spray drying process. Roller- dried milks frequently contain burnt particles. Not only is the overall potential for heat damage in milk by the process greater than with spray drying, but extreme care must be taken to avoid uneven deposition and removal of the milk film. Although roller drying under vacuum overcomes these difficulties and, indeed, yields a much better dried product, the process has not been widely adopted by the industry.

5.9.4. Homogenization

Homogenization has become a standard industrial process, universally practiced as a means of stabilizing the fat emulsion against gravity separation. Gaulin invented the process in 1899. Homogenization is a mechanical process in which milk is forced through a homogenization valve under a very high pressure. The milk is thus deflected at right angle through a narrow opening of about 0.1 nm (100 μm). As the milk comes out of this valve opening, there is sudden drop in pressure and the milk is subjected to impact against an impact ring. This complete process results in disruption of fat globules leading to decrease in the average diameter (typically from 0.2 - 2 μm) and an increase in the number and surface area of fat globules.

Homogenization with reference to milk / dairy applications thus refers to a mechanical process that is used to reduce the size of fat globules such that milk fat does not rise to form a cream layer during storage of milk. Although homogenization renders fat globules uniformly disrupted in the body of the milk, upon prolonged storage it does not remain completely dispersed.

Definition of Homogenized MILK: United State Public Health Service has proposed one of the most comprehensive definitions for homogenized milk. This has been most widely accepted and referred definition. It states that "homogenized milk is milk which has been treated in such a manner as to ensure break –up of the fat globules to such an extent that after 48 h of quiescent storage no visible cream separation occurs in the milk and the fat percentage of the milk in the top 100 ml of milk in a quart bottle (946 ml), or of the proportionate volumes in containers of other sizes, does not differ by more than 10 per cent of itself from the fat percentage of the remaining milk as determined after thorough mixing."

Theories of Homogenization The principle underlying the process of homogenization is to subject the fat globule to enough severe conditions, which disrupts it into smaller fat globules. The newly formed fat globules are maintained in dispersion for sufficient time to allow milk fat globule membrane (MFGM) to be formed at the fat-serum interface. The following theories have been proposed to be responsible for the entire phenomenon.

Shearing or Grinding: As milk is passed at high pressure (velocity ~200-300 m s^{-1}) through the homogenizer valve (100 μm gap), fat globules undergo shearing action. The shear between fat globules and the surface of the homogenizer wall coupled with wire drawing effect results in elongation of the fat globules which progressively becomes unstable. These phenomena result in subdivision of fat globules. Furthermore, the difference in velocity of faster moving serum phase at the center of the liquid stream causes the fat globules to grind against each other. The turbulence created by the difference in velocity and eddy currents of the liquid add to the shear effects and thus enhances the process of disruption of the fat globules.

Exploding: This theory suggests that during homogenization, there is a build-up of tremendous pressure. When this pressure is suddenly released, the internal pressures within the fat globules pull the globule apart with exploding effect. This results in disintegration or subdivision of fat globules into smaller globules.

Splashing / Shattering: As the high homogenizing pressure is attained in the homogenizer, the homogenizing valve releases the highly compressed milk at very high velocity. The liquid suddenly strikes a retaining wall/ perpendicular surface. This causes splashing or shattering effect on the fat globules resulting in breakdown of globules into smaller sizes.

Acceleration and Deceleration: This theory relates sudden change in velocity of milk as it passes through the homogenizer to the homogenizing effect. When milk enters the homogenizing valve, velocity of milk changes from almost static to very high velocity. As it comes out of the valve, there is a sudden deceleration at a rate at which it was accelerated. This sudden change in velocity results in shattering effect leading to the division of the fat globules.

Cavitation: It is postulated that as the milk passes through the homogenization valve, the initial homogenization pressure decreases sharply due to sudden increase in velocity of milk. Depending on the back pressure that exists outside the homogenization valve, the pressure can drop to as low as the saturated vapour pressure of liquid. This leads to formation of vapour bubbles due to cavitation. Cavitation generates shock waves, which could be in excess of 1600 kg / cm^2 in intensity. Due to overlapping of these shock waves, disintegration of fat globules may occur.

These theories of the mechanism of high pressure homogenization have been presented over the years. For an oil-in-water dispersion like milk, when most of the droplets are less than one μm (10^{-6}m) in diameter, two theories have survived. Together they give good explanation of the influence of different parameters on the homogenization effect. The theory of globule disruption by turbulent eddies ("microwhirls") is based on the fact that a lot of small eddies are created in a liquid traveling at a high velocity. Higher velocity gives smaller eddies. If an eddy hits oil droplet of its own size, the droplet will break up. This theory predicts how the homogenizing effect varies with the homogenizing pressure. This relation has been shown in many investigations.

The cavitation theory, on the other hand, claims that the shock waves created when the steam bubbles implode disrupt the fat droplets. According to this theory, homogenization takes place when the liquid is leaving the gap, so the back pressure which is important to cavitation is important to homogenization. This has also been shown in practice. However, it is possible to homogenize without cavitation, but it is less efficient.

Process Requirements: The physical state and concentration of the fat phase at the time of homogenization contribute materially to the size and dispersion of the ensuing fat globules. Homogenization of cold milk, in which the fat is essentially solidified, is virtually ineffective. Processing at temperatures conducive to the partial solidification of milk-fat (i.e. 30-35°C) results in incomplete dispersion of the fat phase. Homogenization is most efficient when the fat phase is in the liquid state and in concentration normal to milk. Products of high fat content are more likely to show evidence of fat clumping, especially when the concentration of serum proteins is low with respect to the fat content. Cream with higher fat content than 12% cannot normally be homogenized at the normal high pressure, because clusters are formed as a result of lack of membrane material (casein). A sufficiently good homogenization effect requires about 0.2 g casein per g of fat.

High-pressure homogenization procedures cause the formation of small fat globules. The dispersion of the lipid phase increases with increasing temperatures of homogenization and is commensurate with the decreasing viscosity of milk at higher temperatures.

Homogenization temperature normally applied are 55-80°C, and homogenization pressure is between 10 and 25 MPa (100-200 bar), depending on the product.

Single-stage and two–stage homogenization: Homogenizers may be equipped with one homogenizing device or two connected in series, hence the names single-stage homogenization and two stage homogenization.

In single-stage homogenization the whole pressure drop is used over one device. In two-stage homogenization the total pressure is measured before the first stage, P_1 and before the second stage, P_2. The two stage method is usually chosen to achieve optimal homogenization efficiency.

Best results are obtained when the relation P_2 / P_1, is about 0.2.

Single-stage homogenization may be used for homogenization of:

- Product with low fat content,
- Products demanding high viscosity (certain cluster formation)

Two-stage homogenization is used primarily to break up fat clusters in:

- Products with high fat contents,
- Products with high content of dry matter,
- Products where a relatively low viscosity is required,
- Optimal homogenization (micronization).

Design and Operation of Homogenizers: There are several types of homogenizer valves and therefore, design of homogenizers varies depending on manufacturers. However, many homogenizers used in the dairy industry have been developed based on the principles introduced by Gaulin. Homogenizers essentially consist of two components, a piston pump to generate high pressure and a homogenizing valve.

The homogenizer pump is generally a positive displacement pump with at least three and sometimes five or seven pistons, which operate consecutively to generate steady pressure. Single piston pumps generate pulsating output with fluctuating pressure thereby resulting in poor homogenization. The pump block is generally made of stainless steel, possibly with some components made of ceramic materials but the piston seal rings are of a soft composite material.

Homogenizer valves, used for milk may be either a 'poppet type' or 'ball type'. A poppet design has a relatively large contact surfaces and provides close fitting seals. If maintained properly, 'poppet' valves give better performance with low viscosity liquid milk. 'Ball' valves can exert greater pressure on the much small seal and are, therefore, suitable for high viscosity liquids or suspensions with smaller particles.

Milk from high pressure manifold enters into the center of the valve seat. The internal diameter of the valve seat is smaller than the manifold. As it passes into the narrow gap between the fixed and the adjustable faces of this valve, milk velocity gets accelerated. The gap is maintained against the feed pressure by a counter force exerted by an adjustable heavy duty spring. Shear effects result from the high velocity gradients between the liquid and the surface of the homogenizing valve. Turbulence also results from the high velocity of the liquid in the valve, causing eddy currents within the flow. Liquid which passes across the valve at about 200-300 m s^{-1} suddenly drops in pressure to below saturation vapour pressure. This permits microscopic bubbles to form for a few microseconds before collapsing. The high velocity jet of milk then impinges on a perpendicular impact ring. These effects contribute to the disruption of the fat globules. Homogenizer valves are made of very tough corrosion resisting alloys such as stellite. Better resistance to corrosion can be achieved by using tungsten carbide and ceramic valves, which are used by many manufacturers in modern homogenizers.

As the fat globules are subdivided into smaller globules, there is increased surface area of the newly homogenized fat globules. The original milk fat globule membrane (MFGM) material is not sufficient to cover this. Proteins, particularly casein micelles migrate from serum phase to form new membrane material with the existing MFGM. This may result in sharing of the casein micelles and therefore some aggregation of fat globules could take place thus defeating the purpose of homogenization. A second stage homogenization, therefore, becomes essential at reduced pressure (almost 20% of 1st stage pressure (175 kg / cm^2 or up to 35 kg / cm^2). This enables aggregated fat globules to be disrupted for formation of stable emulsion of finely dispersed fat globules.

The pump piston has been a source of problems since they need to move through seals that must be capable of resisting both high pressure and microbial colonization. Pressures up to 20MPa are common for milk homogenization but may be up to 30 MPa for other applications. In most homognizers, chevron seals made from relatively soft composite materials are used, held in place by a threaded sleeve so that wear can be taken up and leakage minimized. Piston movement should be sufficient to ensure that the seals are wetted by the cleaning and disinfecting agents. A fine water feed onto the piston provides lubrication and reduces wear; in hard water areas, care must be taken to avoid a build-up of water scale. Where aseptic processing is required, the water lubrication must be replaced by a steam box or equivalent disinfection system.

High Pressure Homogenization Technology: With significant improvement in understanding of machine design, material strength and fluid mechanical knowledge, homogenizers with higher pressure capabilities have been developed. Such high pressure homogenizers could be operating based on two principles: a) conventional valve type homogenizers operating at a far higher pressure, b) micro-fluidization based on the principles of collisions between high speed liquid jets.

Advantages

1. Uniform distribution of fat, no cream line formation.
2. Whiter, more appetizing colour
3. More full- bodied flavour, better mouth feel,
4. Softer curd, more digestible
5. Reduced sensitivity to fat oxidation,
6. No churning of fat during milk transportation,
7. Faster coagulation in the manufacture of rennet cheese,
8. Better stability of cultured milk products.

Disadvantages

1. Homogenized milk cannot be efficiently separated,
2. Somewhat increased sensitivity to light- sunlight and fluorescent tubes- can result in 'Sunlight flavour',
3. More sensitive to lipase attack, leading to rancidity in milk,
4. Low thermal stability of milk, especially in case of single- stage homogenization, high fat content and other factors contributing to fat clumping.
5. Low suitability for production of semi- hard or hard cheeses,
6. Homogenization offers possibility of incorporation of foreign fat into milk.

References

Andrews, G. 1989. Lactulose in heated milk. Bulletin of the International Dairy Federation, 238:45.

Burton, H.1988. Ultra–Temperature Processing of Milk and Milk Products, Elsevier Applied Science, London,

Data, N. and Deeth, H.C.2003. Diagnosing the cause of proteolysis in UHT milk. Lebensmittel, *Wissenschaft and Technologie*, 36:173.

Deeth, H.C. and Datta, N. 2003. Heating systems. *Encyclopedia of Dairy Sci.* Vol, IV, pp 2642.

Efigenia, M., Povoa, B. and Moraes–Santos, T. 1997. Effect of heat treatment on nutritional quality of milk proteins. *International Dairy Journal*, 7:609.

International Dairy Federation (IDF), 1991. B-Document ,198.

Mathur, H. 2007. Prospects and opportunities: *Dairy India*, ed., 6, pp 43.

Mottar J.F. 1989. In Enzymes of Psychrotrophs in Raw Food. R.C. Mckellar, ed., CRC Press, Boca, Raton, FL., pp.227.

Muir, D.D. 1996. *J.Soc. Dairy Technol.*, 49(1), 24.

Patel, G.B. and Blankenagel, G. 1972. *J. Milk Food Technol.* 35: 203.

Pizzoferrato, L., Aromolo, R, Bruschi, L. Manzi,,P. and Quattrucci, E. 1993. In *vitro* protein digestibility and lysine availability in milk and dairy products. In: Proceedings of Bioavailability, 1993: Nutritional, chemical and Food Processing Implications of Nutrient Availability; Part I, Ettlingen, pp. 78.

Raleay, R.D., Wiedmann, M. and Boor, K.G. 1998. J Food Prot., *Protein digestibility* 61: 1336.

Renner,E. 1981. Proc. of Seminar on U.H.T. Processing, Aus. *Soc. of Dairy Technol, Tech. Publ.* No. 26: 47.

Stepaniac, L. and Rukke, E.O. 2003. Thermization of milk. *Encyclopedia of Dairy Sci.*, Vol. IV. pp: 2619.

Zadow, J.G. 1989. Extending the shelf life of dairy products. *Food Australia*, 41: 935.

6

Membrane and Alternate Technologies

Membrane technology is a proven separation method used on the molecular and ionic levels. Since the beginning of the 1970s, this technique has been adopted by the dairy industry. Membrane separation is widely used in dairy processing plants to perform an ever-increasing range of duties, e.g. pre-concentration, partial demineralization, protein separation, bacteria removal, brine clarification and waste water recycling. Representing one of the great technological developments occurring within the dairy industry during the second half of the twentieth century, progress was driven initially by the transfer of know-how gleaned from the application of cellulose acetate-based reverse osmosis (RO) and ultrafiltration (UF) membranes in other industrial sectors to whey processing. Later, new membrane materials and engineering designs were built on this initial achievement and opened up further opportunities for the application of the full spectrum of membrane separation systems that also includes Nan filtration (NF) and cross-flow microfiltration The integration of these unit operations into traditional dairy processes has led to the development of innovative ingredients as well as improvements in yield, efficiency and product quality. R & D work indicates potential RO application for concentration of milk for products like khoa, condensed and dried milk products and of UF application for the manufacture of shrikhand, paneer, chana and cheese. Application of these processes permits higher energy saving, higher yields and superior product quality compared to traditional processes of thermal evaporation.

The membrane processes have certain in-built merits as follows:

- Membrane technologies are perhaps the first continuous molecular separation processes that do not involve either a phase change or inter-phase mass transfer.
- Energy requirements of the membrane processes are very low compared to other processes such as evaporation, freeze concentration and freeze-drying.
- Membrane processes can be operated at ambient temperature, thus, oxidative degradation or heat damage problems common to evaporation processes are avoided resulting in better nutritional and functional properties.

- There is minimum change in pH and ionic strength of the feed used.

Range of Membrane Processes: Membrane filtration is subdivided into four classes according to the molecular size of the retained solutes, however, no sharp demarcation boundaries exist between these classes and usually there is an overlap between the molecular sizes that can be separated by these processes.

- Ultrafiltration (UF)
- Reverse osmosis (RO)
- Micro filtration (MF)
- Nan filtration (NF)

6.1. Ultrafiltration

Ultrafiltration (UF) can be defined as a pressure driven membrane process that can be used in the fractionation, purification and concentration of the substances, having a molecular weight between 10^3 to 10^6 Daltons. It consists merely in pumping the feed solution under pressure over the surface of a suitably supported membrane of the appropriate chemical nature and in the optimum physical configuration. In the UF process, the pressure gradient across the membrane would force the solvent and smaller species through the pores of the membrane, while the larger molecules would be retained. The retained phase 'retentate' or concentrate as it is referred to, will thus be enriched in the retained macromolecules, while the permeate stream will be depleted of the macromolecules. The retentate, of course, will contain some of the permeate solutes also.

Macromolecular material such as protein (and fat if present) is readily recovered from solutions such as whey while lower molecular weight material (lactose, minerals, other solutes and water) permeate the membrane. In the dairy industry, traditional application of UF is in the separation and fractionation of individual milk proteins from lactose and minerals in whey. Significantly the permeate stream is 'sterile' due to the retention of microorganisms. The pore size of membranes used range from 100A° to 1,000 A° and operating pressure range fro 10 to 200 psig.

The UF process has been successfully applied in the manufacture of Feta and Cheddar cheese. It has also been used on pilot scale in the manufacture of shrikhand, chana and paneer. In case of chana, application of UF facilitates recovery of proteins, thus enhancing the yield from about 15.4% (by traditional method) to 18.3%. Likewise, in the manufacture of shrikhand, the application of UF also permits the recovery of whey proteins, which are otherwise lost in the whey. The yield is enhanced by 23% than that of the traditional process. The technological feasibility of the UF application in paneer manufacture has also been demonstrated. With UF process, the yield of pander increases by 33%than that by the traditional process. Other industrial application includes enzyme recovery in various operations, e.g. lactose hydrolysis by soluble lactase preparation

UF in the Process

Connection of the Module: UF plants can be used for both batch and continuous production:

Batch Production: Plants for batch production are mainly used for filtration of small amounts of product, e.g. in laboratories and experimental plants. A certain amount of the product to be filtered is kept in a buffer tank. The product is circulated via this tank and through the UF membranes until the required concentration is obtained.

Continuous Production: The product to be concentrated is pumped through the plant, which consists of several sections – filtration takes place in several stages – and leaves the plant at the required concentration. The holding time for the product in the plant is only a few minutes. The capacity of the plant can be increased by connecting modules in parallel or in series.

Specific load on a membrane: The productivity of a UF plant is mainly determined by the specific load on the membrane, expressed in l / m^2 per hour. This affects the physical data of the product, for example density and viscosity. The specific load on a membrane is in the range of 25–50 l / m^2 per hour.

6.2. Reverse Osmosis

The name 'Reverse Osmosis' (RO) is derived from the word, osmosis, the natural phenomenon which provides water to plant and animal cells to support life.

Normal osmosis takes place when water passes from a less concentrated solution to a more concentrated solution through a semi-permeable membrane (Fig. 6.2.1). A certain amount of potential energy exists between the solutions on each side of the semi-permeable membrane. Water will flow because of this energy difference from the less concentrated to the more concentrated solution until the system is in equilibrium. The addition of pressure energy to the concentrated solution will stop the transport of water across the membrane when the applied pressure equals the apparent osmotic pressure between the two solutions. The apparent osmotic pressure is a measurement of the potential energy difference between the two solutions.

As more pressure is applied to the more concentrated solution as shown in Fig. 6.2.2, the water will begin to flow from the concentrated solution to the less concentrated solution. The rate of water transport is a function of pressure applied to the concentrated solution, the apparent osmotic pressure (i.e. the difference in the absolute osmotic pressure of each solution), and the area of the membrane being pressurized. The absolute osmotic pressure is the potential energy difference between any solution and pure water.

Thus in a normal osmosis solvent passes from the solvent side of the membrane to the concentrate side thus diluting the solution and at the same time setting up a pressure. If an external pressure greater than the osmotic pressure is applied on the concentrate side, the process may be reversed, and solvent will be pushed out of the concentrate back into the solvent side. This is the principle of Reverse Osmosis (RO). On this principle has been built a technology for concentrating solutions or for purifying solvents by controlling either the concentrate or the filtrate according to the product required. Reverse osmosis can be used for either purification or concentration. Production of pure water is an example of purification in which the contaminated water passes through the membrane and pure water is recovered as permeate. For concentration, the components retained by the membrane constitute the product, and permeate, usually water, is discarded. Concentration is a more difficult process, since it intensifies all the problems of concentration polarization by the nature of the process. The tight nature of the membrane calls for the highest operating pressure compared to the other membrane separation processes. The pore size of the membrane used range from 1 to 10 A° with operating pressure of 1500 psig.

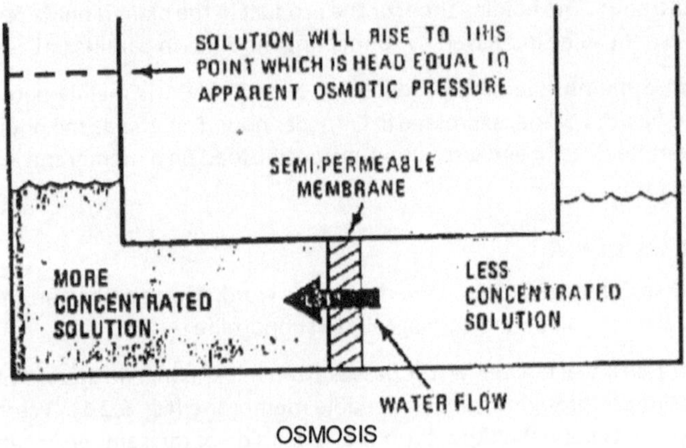

Fig. 6.2.1. Illustration of osmosis phenomenon

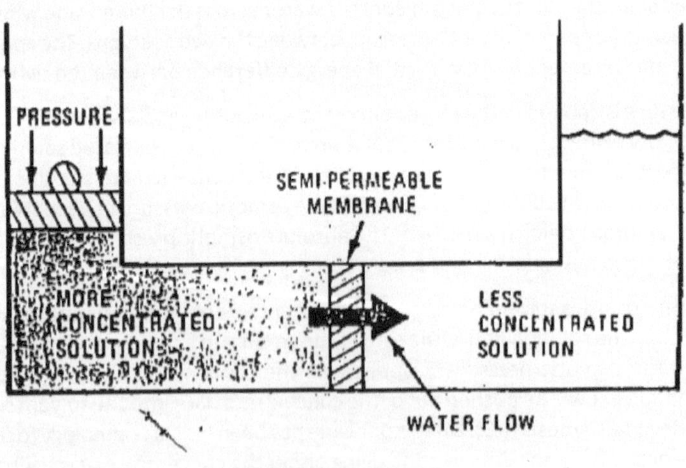

Fig. 6.2.2. Illustration of osmosis phenomenon

Considerable pressure is required to reverse the transport phenomenon (osmosis) that prevails when water migrates across semi-permeable membranes in order to equilibrate the osmotic effect created by the solutes present in the solution on the other side of the barrier. The effect is demonstrated classically when water and sucrose solutions are separated by a semi-permeable membrane. Hence, whey, with its relatively high content of lactose (~5.0%) was originally seen as an appropriate medium for the application of RO technology as an economical means of dewatering.

The RO membrane has special structure. Low molecular molecules will be separated and the active filter layer must therefore be designed for this purpose. The membranes used are called diffusion membranes. They are unsymmetrical or have extremely thin, symmetrical layers. There is no membrane that can separate all materials and only allow the solvent to pass. The efficiency for desalination is 87– 99%, depending on the filter material used. The difference between the separation efficiency for a UF membrane and an RO membrane is shown in (Fig 6.2.3).

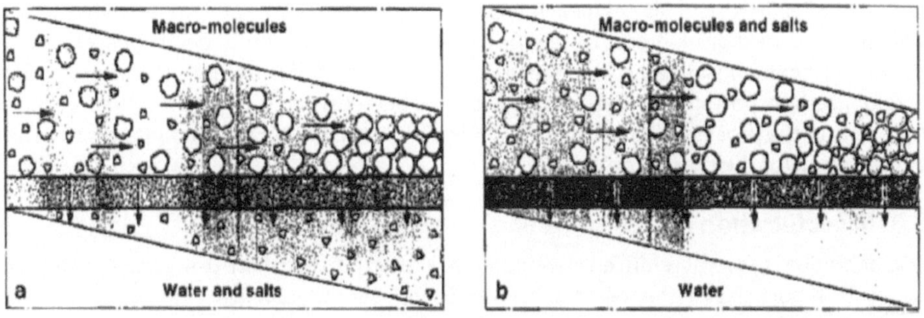

Fig. 6.2.3. Difference between the separation in a UF membrane (a), where salts can pass through the membrane, and in an RO membrane (b), where salts are also separated

The concentration of a product is limited by technical and scientific factors. The osmotic pressure is the limiting factor. It increases with the increased product concentration. This can be illustrated by an example from desalination of seawater which, with a salt content of 3 – 5%, has an osmotic pressure of 24 bar. The osmotic pressure increases to 48 bar if 50% of the water is removed. In practice this pressure increase limits the yield to approximately 75% as increased concentration results in too high a pressure load on the membrane and a steep increase in the power consumption. The membranes do not have a 100% degree of separation and the filtrate will therefore contain a certain amount of dissolved substances. For a certain separation efficiency of the membranes the amount of dissolved material in the filtrate is always directly proportional to the content of dissolved material in the initial solution in this case the seawater. This means that the content of dissolved material in the filtrate will increase if the concentration is carried out too far.

Pretreatment of the raw material is necessary in order to obtain the longest possible operating times. The pretreatment removes all suspended and dissolved substances that can disturb the process. Particularly small protein molecules and other colloids from a gel layer on the membrane surface and reduce the flow of filtrate through the membrane. Calcium deposits on the membrane surface also have an adverse effect on permeability.

In skim milk or whey, the osmotic pressure is around 0.7 MPa, a pressure that must be exceeded in RO before permeate (i.e. essentially water) will flow through the membrane. However, when milk or whey is concentrated by RO or evaporation to 25% total solids (commonly referred to as retentate), the osmotic pressure increases to 2.7-3.5 MPa. Thus, the osmotic effects of increasing lactose and mineral concentration in RO retentate limit both permeate flux and maximum concentration achievable. During the course of RO, component transport occurs by diffusion through the membrane or essentially through the thin layer of the membrane which is semi-permeable and the porous remainder of the membrane is merely a support. The rate of transportation is proportional to the solubility of the component in the membrane and to its effective diffusivity. Factors diminishing the effective pressure difference during operation include the increasing concentration gradient near the membrane's surface as well as the likelihood of gel layer formation.

The most effective use of RO has been made in concentration of whey to produce whey powder. Milk intended for khoa manufacture may be partially concentrated by RO before heat application. There has been considerable interest in utilizing RO for reducing the bulk of raw milk to economize transportation. Extensive studies have been carried out on the techno-economic feasibility of the process as a means of concentration. Various operating parameters have been standardized for the process optimization.

6.3. Microfiltration

Microfiltration is a pressure-driven membrane separation process which uses porous membranes with cut-off pore sizes in the region of micron (10^{-6}m), allowing passage of proteins but retains fat globules, microorganisms and somatic cells. In literature, the term 'cross flow' or 'tangential flow' microfiltration has been used to signify that the fluid flow is tangential to the membrane surface and perpendicular to the permeate flow through the membrane so as to counteract the formation of deposit layers. In this process, typical operative pressures are somewhat lower and fluxes about 1 order to magnitude higher than for the classical UF. The process may also be described as a 'loose UF'. The pore size of the membrane ranges from 0.1 to 10 micron and operating pressure from 1 to 25 psig.

The emergence of micro filtration (MF) as a potential commercial process is drawing the attention of engineers and scientists all over the world. Microfiltration offers great developmental possibilities for the dairy and food industry. Application of the uniform trans membrane pressure concept and the use of ceramic membranes have resulted in a number of successful MF processes. The main advantages of the processes involving MF are improvement of the bacteriological quality and the extension of the shelf life of pasteurized milk while maintaining the characteristic fresh taste. Cheese production without nitrate addition, purification of brine, standardization of protein content and modification of the ratio of casein to ß- casein in cheese milk are some other MF applications of interest. The production of native phosphocaseinate on MF of skim milk provides an alternative substrate for the development of new processing technologies such as in the manufacture of yoghurt, cheese or process cheese analogues.

The development of new ceramic membranes has been a major breakthrough in making MF an acceptable industrial separation technology in the dairy and food industry. The ceramic membranes with a highly permeable support and a multi-channel geometry as also high stability to heat acid and alkali, have opened up novel applications of MF technology. In the range of membrane processes, MF fits between the tangential flow ultrafiltration (UF) and the traditional particle filtration based on perpendicular flow using filters of varying porosity. MF is a pressure driven membrane process usually operating at trans-membrane pressures of less than 1 bar. It is used in the separation of suspended particles in the range of 0.05 to 10μm. A wide range of MF membranes is now available with pore sizes varying from 0.1 to 1.4 μm.

A significant development in the MF technology has been the introduction of uniform trans-membrane pressure (UTP) concept. In this case the space on the permeate side of the module which is normally empty is filled with plastic beads (approx. 2 mm dial). An additional circulation pump is provided within the permeate collection and removal operation. The permeate is circulated at high speed, concurrently with the retentate to obtain UTP all over the membrane area. This ensures the prevention of any secondary layer formation on the membrane surface which may change the sieving characteristics of the membrane. The fouling is limited and MF operational times are higher.

The emergence of MF as a means of bacteria and spore removal from milk has generated much interest about the alternative technologies for the manufacture of quality dairy products. Possible applications include shelf-life extension of liquid market milk, production of cheese with minimal risk of blowing and without nitrate addition and purification of brine. The feasibility of removing bacteria by MF appeared remote until the development of Membralox multichannel 1.4μm membrane, which proved to be suitable for debacterisation of skim milk with only minor losses in solids-not-fat (Jost and Jelen, 1997). The difference existing in size distribution between casein micelles and the microorganisms most frequently encountered in milk has led to the development of 'Bactocatch' process by Tetra Laval group (Larsen, 1996). In this process skim milk is circulated under pressure along a ceramic MF membrane (Pore size 1.4 μm) at a temperature between 20 to 55°C. The average TMP is 0.55×10^5 Pa. Transmission rates of total solids, protein, fat and cholesterol are respectively 99.5, 99, 63 and 85% when concentration factor is equal to 20. The system is capable of removing 99.5% of all the bacteria in the skim milk. The bacteria concentrate is mixed with the cream which is used for standardizing the cheese milk and this mixture is heated to 130°C for 4 s in the UHT equipment. Finally, the permeate and the cream/retentate mixture are re-mixed and when the milk reaches renneting temperature it is led into the cheese vats (Kessler, 1997). The number of anaerobic spores in cheese milk is reduced significantly without sacrificing the properties of coagulation (Samuelson *et al.*, 1997).

6.4. Nanofiltration

Like RO from which it evolved, NF is also a pressure driven membrane separation process which is capable of reversing the osmotic effects of liquids. In addition to dewatering/concentration, NF membranes are also partially permeable to mineral ions and other low molecular weight constituents so that the occurrence of some demineralization represents a further bonus in certain processing application. NF membranes are usually fabricated as thin film composites by forming, for example, a polyamide layer on a microporous polysulphone support to give a surface which is rich in carboxylate groups.

At the time of its introduction to the dairy industry during the 1980s, a variety of terms were used to identify this membrane process, e.g. 'loose' RO, 'leaky' RO, as well as a proprietary term, Ultra-Osmosis. NF is now the adopted nomenclature since separation of solutes occurs in the nanometer (10^{-9} m) range. A size exclusion range of 10-100 Dalton suits the permeation of water, mineral ions and low molecular weight nitrogenous compounds. However, some lactose is also lost. The main emerging application for the dairy industry is in partial demineralization of whey and UF permeate from milk or whey thus solving the problem of waste disposal and lactose recovery. Effectiveness of NF is also in terms of the removal of mineral ions that contribute significantly to the osmotic pressure in process fluids. The operating pressure employed are generally lower than the pressure used by RO due to the larger pore size of the membranes, which is sufficient to retain most of the lactose. In this manner, the process could also be viewed as an ultra-tight UF as well as loose RO. The theoretical basis for the mass transfer mechanism appears to be a mixture of diffusion and pore flow. The pore size of the membrane range from 10 A° to 100 A° and operating pressure is 300 psig. The temperature tolerance of NF membranes may vary depending on the make but the usual range is 5-50°C while the operating pH range is 3-11; however, certain NF membranes have been reported to operate over a much wider pH and temperature ranges.

Table 6.4.1. Comparative characteristics of different membrane processes

Membrane process	Pressure (bar)	Pore size(μm)	Function
Reverse osmosis (RO)	30-60	10^{-4}-10^{-3}	concentration of solutions by removal of water
Nanofiltration (NF)	20-40	10^{-3}-10^{-2}	concentration of organic components by removal of part of monovalent ions like sodium and chlorine (partial demineralization)
Ultrafiltration(UF)	1-10	10^{-2}-10^{-1}	concentrat ion of large and macro-molecule
Microfiltration (MF)	<1	10^{-1}-10^{1}	removal of bacteria, separation of macro-molecules

Structure of Filtration Modules: The membranes in the dairy industry are built in different ways by different manufacturers. They may be of different configurations, viz.:

Design	Typical application
Spiral-wound	RO, NF, UF
Plate and frame	UF, RO
Tubular, based on polymers	UF, RO
Tubular, based on ceramics	MF, UF
Hollow-fibre	UF

The following points must be considered when modules are designed:

- They must be designed for efficient cleaning,
- The ratio between installed filter surface and the volume of the pressure chamber should be advantageous,
- Replacing the membranes should be economical.

Plate and frame design: These systems consist of membranes sandwiched between membrane support plates which are arranged in stacks, similar to ordinary plate heat exchangers. The feed material is forced through very narrow channels that may be configured for parallel flow or as a combination of parallel and serial channels. A typical design is shown in Fig. 6.4.4.

A module is usually divided into sections, in each of which the flow between pairs of membranes is in parallel. The sections are separated by a special membrane support plate in which one hole is closed with a stop disc to reverse the direction of flow, giving serial flow between successive sections. Modules are available in various sizes.

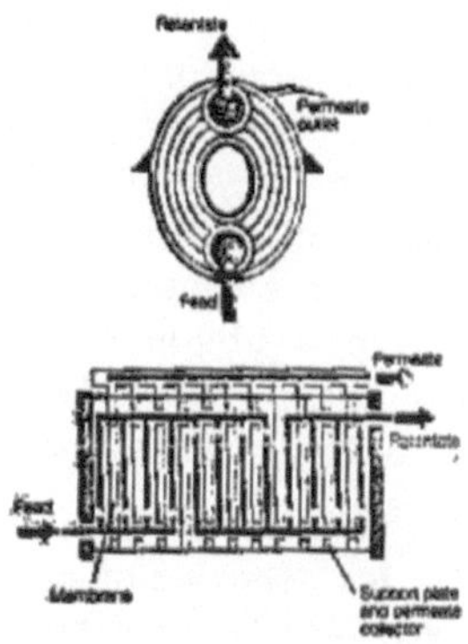

Fig. 6.4.4. Plate and frame

Membrane material: typically polymers.

The advantages of these membranes are: (1) economic in energy consumption, intermediate between spiral wound and tubular systems, (2) operating mainly in laminar flow, (3) fairly good performance with viscous solutions, (4) low hold-up volume, (5) minimum floor space requirement and (6) replacement of membrane on site is relatively easy. The disadvantages are: (1) fairly difficult to clean and (2) susceptible to plugging.

Tubular design - *polymers:* The system made by Paterson and Candy International Ltd, PCI, is an example of tubular systems used in the dairy industry. The PCI module for UF is illustrated in Fig. 6.4.5. The module has 18x12.5 mm perforated stainless steel tubes assembled in a shell-and-tube-like construction. All 18 tubes are connected in series. A replaceable membrane insert tube is fitted inside each of the perforated stainless steel pressure support tubes. Permeate is collected outside of the tube bundle in the stainless steel shroud. The module can readily be converted from UF to RO.

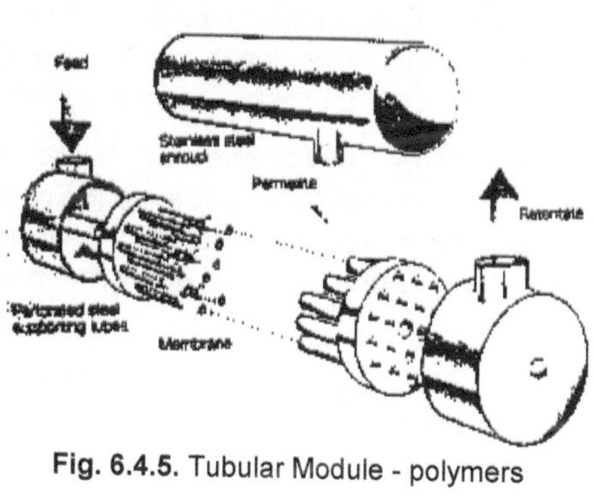

Fig. 6.4.5. Tubular Module - polymers

Tubular design - *ceramic:* A tubular concept with ceramic membranes is steadily gaining ground in the dairy industry, especially in systems for reduction of bacteria in milk, whey, WPC and brine.

The filter element, Fig. 6.4.6 is a ceramic filter manufactured by a French company, SCT (Societe des Ceramiques Techniques/ Ceraver).

The thin walls of the channels are made of fine-grained ceramic and constitute the membrane. The support material is coarse-grained ceramic. In MF for bacteria removal the system is fed with skimmilk (with whole milk, the fat would also be concentrated, which is not wanted in applications for bacteria reduction). Most of the feed (about 95%) passes through the membrane as permeate, in this case bacteria-reduced skim-milk, the retentate, some 5% of the feed, is bacteria-rich skim-milk.

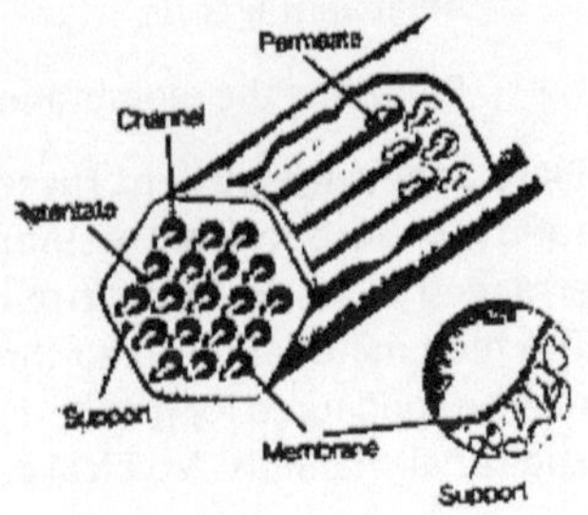

Fig. 6.4.6. Tubular design - ceramic

The filter elements (1, 7 or 19 in parallel) are installed in a module. Fig. 6.4.7 shows a module with 19 filter elements, one of which is exposed to the left of the module. For industrial purposes two modules are put together in series, forming a filter loop together with one retentate circulation pump and one permeate circulation pump.

Depending on the required capacity, a number of filter loops can be installed in parallel.

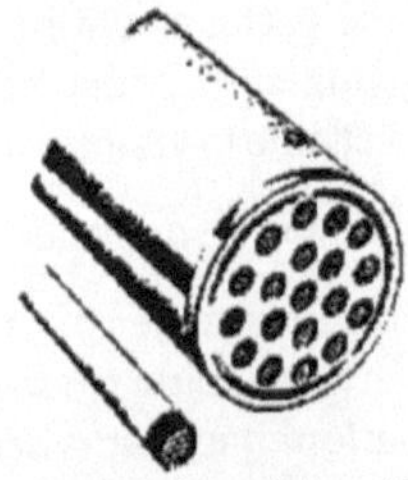
Fig. 6.4.7. A module with 19 filter elements

The feed is pumped into the modules from below at a high flow rate. The very high transmembrane pressure (TMP) at the inlet quickly causes clogging of the membrane. This shows conventional cross-flow microfiltration. Experience shows that a low transmembrane pressure gives much better performance, but in conventional cross-flow microfiltration a low transmembrane pressure occurs only at the outlet, i.e. on a very small part of the membrane area.

A unique Uniform Transmembrane Pressure (UTP) system has been introduced to achieve optimum conditions on the entire area. The patented system involves high-velocity permeate circulation concurrently with the retentate inside the module, but outside the element. This gives a uniform TMP over the whole of the membrane area, with optimum utilization of the membrane.

The latter system is possible because the space between the elements inside the module, i.e. on the permeate side, is normally empty, but in the UTP version it is filled with plastic grains. The high-velocity circulation of permeate causes a pressure drop inside the channels. The pressure drop on the permeate side is regulated by the permeate pump and is constant during operation of the plant.

The advantages of this system are: (1) capable of handling feed stream with fairly large suspended particles (maximum particle size 10% Of the tube diameter), (2) easy to clean by standard CIP system and (3) individual membrane tubes can be easily replaced on site. The disadvantages are: (1) need efficient pumping system to generate high velocity (>10,000 Reynolds Number) and (2) high pressure drop.

Spiral - wound design: As the spiral-wound design differs from the other membrane filtration designs used in the dairy industry, it calls for a somewhat more detailed explanation.

A spiral-wound element contains one or more membrane "envelopes", each of which contains two layers of membrane separated by a porous permeate conductive material. This material, called the permeate channel spacer, allows the permeate passing through the membrane to flow freely. The two layers of membrane with the permeate channel spacer between them are sealed with adhesive at two edges and one end to form the membrane "envelope". The open end of the envelope is connected and sealed to a perforated permeate collecting tube. The envelope configuration is illustrated in Fig. 6.4.8.

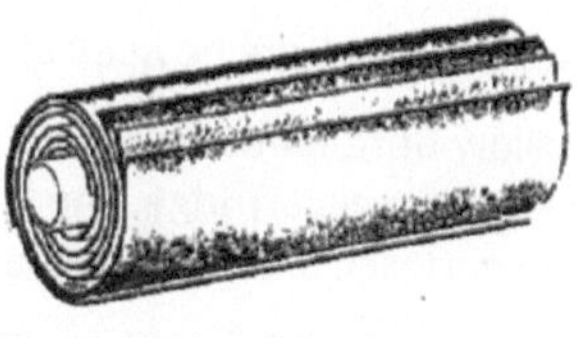

Fig. 6.4.8. Envelope formation of the spiral-wound filter design

A plastic netting material, serving as a channel for the flow of feed solution through the system and known as the feed channel spacer, is placed in contact with one side of each membrane envelope. Due to the netting design the feed spacers also act as turbulence generators to keep the membrane clean at relatively low velocities.

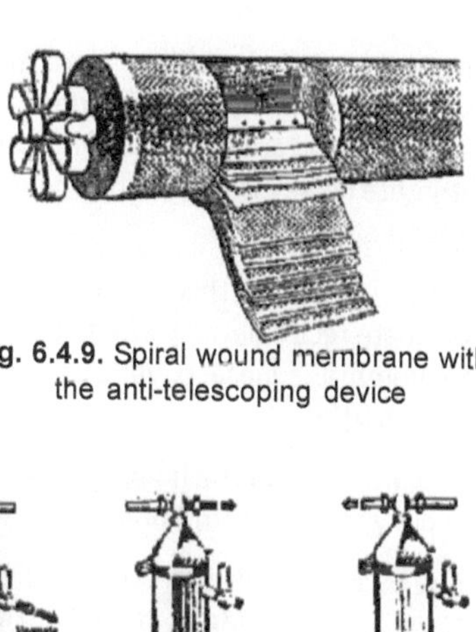

Fig. 6.4.9. Spiral wound membrane with the anti-telescoping device

The entire assembly is then wrapped around the perforated permeate collecting tube to form the spiral-wound membrane. Spiral-wound membranes are equipped with an anti-telescoping device between the downstream ends of the membrane elements to prevent the velocity of treated fluid from causing layers to slip. A spiral-wound assembly with the anti-telescoping device is shown in Fig. 6.4.9.

Several elements normally - three- can be connected in series inside the same stainless steel tube as shown in Fig. 6.4.10.

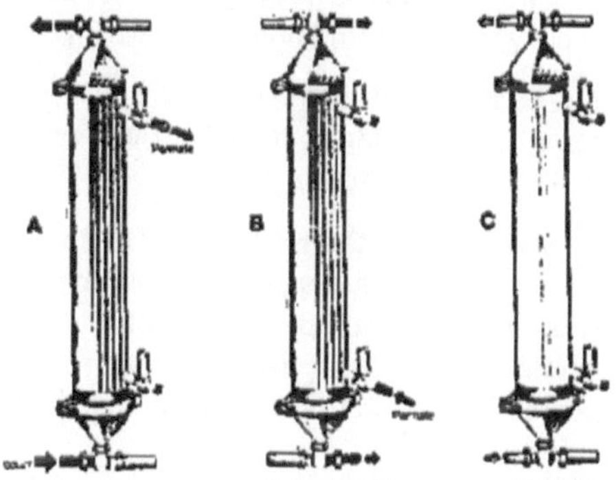

Fig. 6.4.10. UF cartridge during filtration (A) backflushing (B) and cleaning (C) Membrane and permeate spacer material: polymer.

The advantages of the system are: (1) compact, high surface area per volume, minimum floor space required, (2) minimum energy consumption, (3) low capital and operational cost and (4) low hold-up volume. The disadvantages are: (1) difficult to process fluids which are high on suspended solids, (2) high pressure drop, difficult to operate with high viscous solutions, (3) mesh spacer creates dead spots in the flow which may retain particles and (4) faulty membrane elements require charging the whole module.

Hollow-fibre design: Contrary to other types of membranes, UF with the hollow-fibre membrane requires a low hydrostatic pressure. Pumps, valves and pipes, well known to the dairy industry, can therefore be used in a plant. The hollow-fibre membrane is built up from a synthetic polymer and can therefore be used at temperature up to 75°C and within a wide pH range.

Hollow-fibre modules are cartridges which contain bundles of 45 to over 3000 hollow-fibre elements per cartridge. The fibres are oriented in parallel; all are potted in a resin at their ends and enclosed in the permeate collecting tube of epoxy.

The membrane has an inner diameter ranging from 0.5 to 2.7 mm, and the active membrane surface is on the inside of the hollow fibre. The outside of the hollow-fibre wall, unlike the inner wall, has a rough structure and acts as a supporting structure for the membrane. The feed stream flows through the inside of these fibres, and the permeate is collected outside and removed at the top of the tube.

The build-up of the hollow-fibre module results in a very high structural stability. The active membrane surface on the inside of the hollow-fibre has a thickness of 0.1 μm which gives a low filtration resistance. During filtration the product is pumped through the hollow fibres and retentate flows inside. The permeate passes through the membrane and is drained through the support structure.

A special feature of this design is its backflushing capability, which is utilized in cleaning and with permeate recirculated through the outer permeate connection to remove product deposits on the membrane surface. Various modes of operation of a hollow-fibre module are illustrated in Fig. 6.4.10.

In a plant many of the hollow fibres are combined in bundles to form cartridges and embedded in epoxy resin at both ends. Each cartridge has two supply and two filtrate connection.

UF plants are built with separately, or several in parallel, mounted cartridges. A plant with hollow fibre cartridges, pumps, valves, pipes, connections and control equipment is called a membrane separator.

The advantages of the system are (1) high surface area per volume, (2) low hold-up volume, (3) fair resistance to blockage of the flow channel, (4) improved cleanability by back- flushing and (5) low energy consumption. The disadvantages are: (1) fibres are susceptible to plugging at the cartridge inlet, (2) low maximum pressure followed, (3) connection of several elements is limited to parallel configuration and (4) difficult to maintain high flow with high viscous solution in low cartridges.

6.5. Membrane Materials

The use of the membrane technique has spread by leaps and bounds over latter years. The reason is the development of new membranes. The first membranes were made of cellulose acetate. They had some disadvantages and the use of these membranes was limited. The most important disadvantages were poor mechanical and thermal strength and they were not resistant to lye and acid during cleaning.

The previous disadvantages disappeared to a great extent when plastic materials, in the form of different polymers, were used.

The following demands are placed on membranes for dairies:

- They must manage high permeate flows
- They must have a high selectivity
- They must have good chemical and bacteriological resistance
- They must be resistant to detergents and disinfectants
- They must be cheap

Some of these demands cannot be combined in any membrane today. The membrane must therefore be selected for the application in question, see Table 6.5.1.

Table 6.5.1. Different membranes and their characteristics

Characteristics	Materials in the membranes		
	Cellulose acetate	Synthetic polymers	Inorganic Colloids
Structure	Unsymmetrical / Symmetrical	Unsymmetrical	Symmetrical
Max. Temperature	30-35°C	Up to 120°C	140°C
pH range	3-8	1-14	0-14
Cleaning	Enzymatic	Chemical	Chemical
Chlorine resistance	50 ppm	3000 ppm	300 ppm
Resistance to organic solutions	Poor	Good	Good

The transition from earlier cellulose acetate to polymeric membranes has played a significant role in providing the dairy industry with protein separation processes that are operationally robust and hygienic. A variety of polymers may be used, but the more commonly used membranes are constructed of either a polysulphone (PS) and polyethersulphone (PES) active layer deposited on a more porous PS support. Other polymers in use include polyvinylidene fluoride (PVDF) and polyacrylonitrile (PAN). Modifications to the surface layer of membranes have also been suggested in order to improve performance with more difficult products. Although identified more closely with microfiltration duties, membranes constructed of inorganic materials, such as zirconium oxide and alumina, are also available in UF specification.

Membrane Structure: The membrane structure – the composition of the membrane depends to a great extent on the material. Symmetrical and unsymmetrical membranes are available.

Unsymmetrical membranes: The unsymmetrical membranes are formed with a 0.2 to 1 mm thick polymer layer which has been "moulded" on a porous support. The support does not affect the material transport through the membrane. This membrane structure is obtained by means of phase inversion of a polymer solution mixture and coagulation in a coagulating bath.

Suitable polymers are, among others, cellulose acetate, polyamide, polysulphone and polyacrylic nitrile/polyvinyl chloride. The separation of material only takes place at the "active" surface and the UF is therefore regarded as a surface-filtration process.

Symmetrical membranes: In the symmetrical membranes the filter layer continues through the entire cross section of the membrane. In this process, deep filtration, the material is separated inside the membrane. This membrane type is also made by means of phase inversion.

The volume flow is inversely proportional to the thickness of the membrane. The filtrate flow rate through the unsymmetrical membrane is therefore higher than through the symmetrical membrane. This explains the dominating position of the unsymmetrical membrane within UF.

Separation limits for membranes: The separation limit for a membrane is determined by the lowest molecular weight that can be separated. The membrane can have a definite or a diffuse separation limit. Membranes with a definite separation limit separate everything with a definitely lower molecular weight, whilst membranes with a diffuse limit will let some material with a higher molecular weight through and stop some with a lower molecular weight.

The separation accuracy for a membrane is determined by pore size and pore distribution. The definition that the molecular weight determines the separation limit should be regarded with certain reservation as the shape of the separate particles also has an influence. A spherical particle is easier to separate than a chain-formed particle.

6.6. Process Engineering Aspects

Material transport through the membrane: The most important characteristic of a UF membrane is the flow rate, expressed as l / m^2 per hour.

Factors that affect the separation capacity:

For UF, as for all the filtration processes, certain resistances must be overcome:

- The membrane resistance: This is characteristic for each membrane and is determined by the following factors:
- The thickness of the membrane
- The surface area which consists of pores
- The pore diameter
- The transport resistance: This occurs when the separated material is deposited on the filter surface. The layer causes the actual filter resistance and it is often described as a secondary membrane. This secondary membrane causes reduced flow through the filter, changes the separation ability and the bacteriological standard after long periods of stand-still.

Build-up of the secondary membrane: High-molecular material will deposit on the membrane surface during filtration. This is caused by the high filtrate flow rate in UF processes and on the laminary flow close to the membrane surface. Material will therefore concentrate on the membrane surface, so called concentration polarization. Part of this material will diffuse outwards in the layer. The secondary membrane increases in thickness until there is a balance between the amount of material supplied to the layer by means of convection and the amount that diffuses out of the layer.

Affecting factors: Three different factors affect the result – the flow velocity, the length of the membrane and the product concentration.

***Flow velocity**: The flow profile close to the membrane surface changes when the flow velocity increases. The laminar layer becomes thinner and the transport of the separated material more efficient.*

The possibility of increasing the flow velocity is often limited by design, product and production factors.

Membrane length: Fig 6.6.11 shows how material is deposited along the length of the membrane. It is apparent that the thickness of the secondary membrane increases as the permeate flow velocity slows down because of friction and the increasing thickness of the laminar layer.

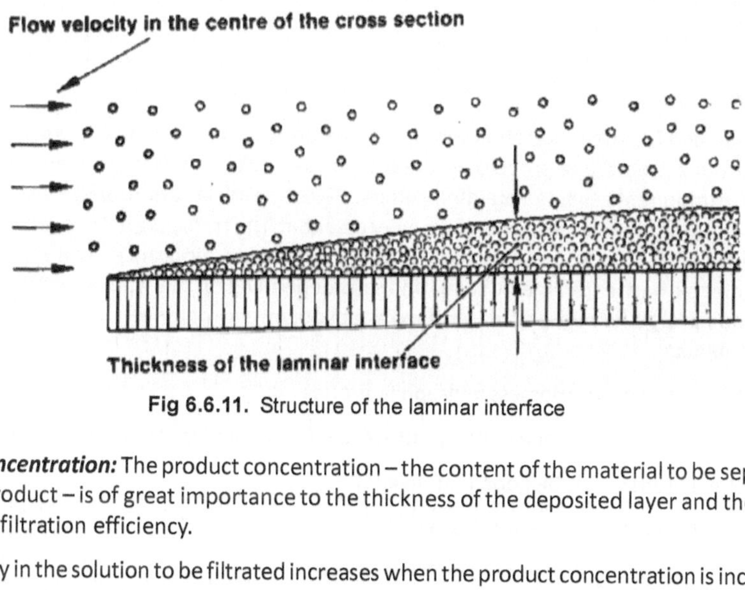

Fig 6.6.11. Structure of the laminar interface

Product concentration: The product concentration – the content of the material to be separated from the product – is of great importance to the thickness of the deposited layer and therefore also to the filtration efficiency.

The viscosity in the solution to be filtrated increases when the product concentration is increased.

The low–molecular ingredients in the product are of minor importance to the formation of the secondary membrane. One exception is the salts that act as complex formers. They are found in milk in the form of calcium ions and they can, amongst other things, determine the formation of the protein micelles in the milk. This is only of importance when the protein concentration is high, for example skim milk.

Fig 6.6.12 shows that a fixed hydrostatic pressure means a constant filtration velocity. The reason is the difference in concentration between the interface of the secondary membrane and the product concentration. The balance that has been achieved between the convective feed transport of material and the amount of material that diffuses from the layer does not change because of an increase in the product pressure. Such an increase results in a short increase of the permeate flow rate through the membrane, but at the same time the amount of material supplied to the layer through the membrane will increase by means of convection. This results in a corresponding increase in the thickness of the secondary membrane and in the diffusion of the material from the layer. The balance has, in a short time, been restored.

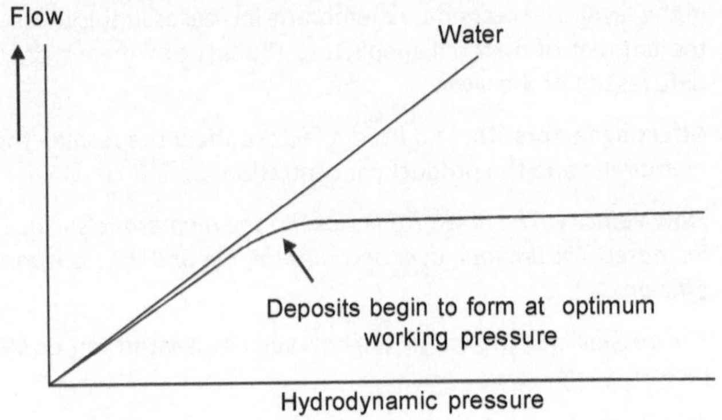

Fig. 6.6.12. The flow rate as a function of the hydrostatic pressure for water and for a macro-molecular solution respectively

Operation and Maintenance of Membrane Filtration Systems: Membrane is considered to be the heart of a membrane process because it acts as a selective barrier permitting passage of certain components, while retaining others. Selection of an appropriate material for the manufacture of membrane is, therefore, very essential. The transport properties of the material should be such that water can pass through with little hindrance, while presenting an un-permeable barrier to organic solids and salts depending on the type of membrane process. To provide a large flow rate of water (flux) a real polymeric material must meet the following requirements:

- The material must possess hydrophilic groups.
- Ions and non-hydrogen bonding substances must not enter the membranes.
- The material must be good film maker.
- It must have high swelling characteristics.
- The membrane should have high wet strength.
- It must exist in extremely thin layer so that it offers least resistance to passage of water.

In addition to these basic requirements, the rejection or retention coefficients and compatibility of membrane material towards temperature, pressure and pH are also important considerations (Roberts, 1994). The efficiency and economy of a membrane system depend largely on the flux rate and life of the membrane which are affected by different factors (Cheryan, 1998, Dharam Pal, 1993).

Factors Affecting Flux and Efficiency

- The operating parameters
- Pressure
- Feed concentration
- Temperature
- Velocity / flow rate
- Concentration polarization
- Fouling of membranes
- Cleaning and maintenance of membranes

Pressure: Flux for a particular membrane is directly proportional to pressure of the feed solution and inversely proportional to the viscosity. The osmotic pressure and the membranes are the major flux limiting factors with RO. In UF and MF applications, the osmotic pressure of retained solutes are negligible and the major resistance to flux are the membrane, concentration polarization and associated boundary layer and fouling. Thus, the direct relationship between applied pressure and flux holds true only when (a) the pressure is low, (b) at low feed concentration and (c) at high feed velocities. Under all these conditions, the concentration polarization is negligible.

Feed Concentration: The flux decreases exponentially with increasing feed concentration. When the concentration of solutes at the membrane and in the bulk is the same, the flux is zero. It is, therefore, always beneficial to use feed with low solids.

Temperature: In general, higher temperature will lead to higher flux in both pressure-controlled and mass transfer-controlled regions. This assumes that there are no other heat induced effects occurring simultaneously, such as salt precipitation, protein denaturation or other fouling phenomenon, that may confound the interpretation of the data. In the pressure-controlled regions, temperature favourably affects viscosity. The elevated temperature also increases the diffusivity. In general, it is best to operate at the highest possible temperature consistent with the limits of the feed and membrane.

Velocity (Flow rate): This is the velocity of the feed or retentate stream flowing tangentially or across the membrane. This turbulence, whether produced by stirring or pumping of the fluids has a major effect on flux in the mass transfer region. By increasing the velocity the accumulated solids near the membrane surface are swept away and the turbulence reduces the thickness of boundary layer, thereby maintaining the flux.

Concentration Polarization: Concentration polarization occurs due to the convective movement of solids towards the membrane during processing. The rejected solids accumulate on the surface, causing a steep concentration gradient of solute within the boundary layer. This causes a back transport of retained solutes back to the bulk solution due to diffusion (Fig 6.6.13).

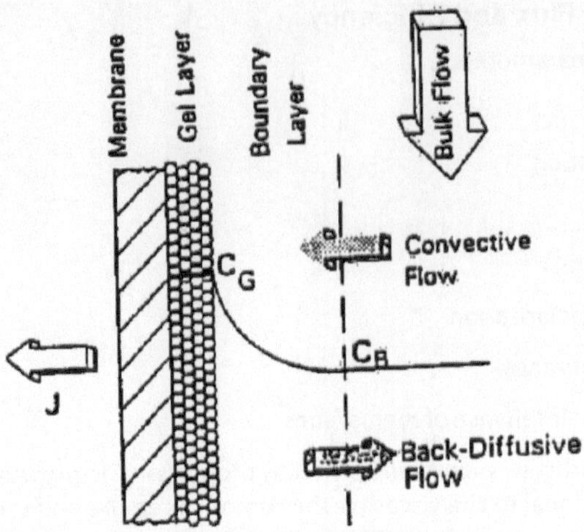

Fig. 6.6.13. Illustration of concentratin polarization

Eventually a steady state is reached where the two phenomena- the connective transport towards the membrane and the diffusive transport away from the membrane balance each other. Soon the solute concentration in the concentration polarization layer reaches a maximum commonly known as the "gel concentration". It is due to this consolidated gel layer on the membrane that flux become independent of pressure. At this stage increasing the trans-membrane pressure nearly results in a thicker layer. After a momentary rise, the flux will drop back to the previous value. Thus flux in the mass transfer controlled region will be controlled by the efficiency of minimizing boundary layer thickness, and enhancing the rate of back transfer of polarized molecules (Cheryan, 1998).

Membrane Fouling: The fouling of membranes is another major limiting factor in membrane processing. Contrary to CP, which is considered a time-dependant, reversible process, fouling is an irreversible phenomenon. During fouling, flux drops with operating time, usually rapidly in the initial stages and slowly in later stages. Fouling is generally attributed to:

- The accumulation or adsorption of macromolecules or colloidal particles, such as proteins, lipids, microorganisms and/or inorganic salts, on the membrane surface.
- The precipitation of permeable solutes, such as sugars and salts, due to overcrowding within the membrane pores.

The fouling of membranes not only reduces the flux but also makes the cleaning operation more difficult and expensive. The rejection properties of the membrane are also altered due to the formation of this secondary layer.

The fouling problem can be alleviated by proper: (1) selection of the membrane and plant design, (2) pretreatment of the feed, and (3) cleaning of the membrane. In fact, the pretreatment of the feed plays an important role in reducing fouling problems, and differs from feed to feed.

In addition to CP and fouling, changes in membrane properties, either due to compaction or chemical deterioration, are also responsible for a decline of flux. The compaction of membranes generally takes place due to faulty operating conditions (high pressure and temperature), and the use of strong cleaning solutions is responsible for chemical deterioration.

Cleaning and Maintenance of Membranes: The most important consideration in cleaning and maintenance is never to allow the feed constituents to dry out on the membrane surface. While deciding on the cleaning schedule for membrane, the nature of the feed constituents that foul the membrane, and the recommendations of the membrane and detergent manufacturers should be kept in mind. The following general procedure can be adopted for routine cleaning of a membrane.

- After the processing is complete, the feed stream is flushed out from the whole plant with water. The highest temperature of wash water compatible with the membrane should be used. Flushing is stopped when clear water starts coming out of the system.
- Then a commercial detergent solution is circulated through the plant. The dfferent types of acid and alkali detergents are available in the market compatible with different types of membranes. The detergents are circulated one after the other. The addition of a sequestering agent, e.g. hexa-meta-phosphate, to cleaning detergents is very beneficial. In the case of CA membranes and excessive fouling of PS and TFC membranes, the use of a proteolytic enzyme is essential.
- After each circulation of detergent, the whole system is thoroughly rinsed with hot water.
- To ensure proper cleaning, the flux rate with water under standard conditions is tested. If the water flux is lower than the initial flux, step (2) is repeated.
- The membrane is sanitized and stored in 0.5% formaldehyde solution. It is never allowed to remain dry.

6.7. Electrodialysis

Electrodialysis is a separation process in which membranes are used to remove ionic species (electrically charged) from non-ionic species. Electrodialysis is employed in dairy industry to demineralize whole whey and other milk derivative solutions. Electrodialysis may be defined as the transport of ions through membranes as a result of an electric driving force. The membranes used have anion and cation exchange functions respectively, which gives the electrodialysis process a capability to reduce the mineral content of a process liquid e.g. seawater or whey. It consists of a number of compartments separated by alternate cation and anion exchange membranes which are spaced about 1mm or less apart. The end compartments contain electrodes. When electric current passes through solution compartments and membranes, cations tend to migrate towards the negatively charged electrode (cathode) and anions tend to migrate towards the positively charged electrode (anode). The cations and anions in one set of solution compartments can pass freely through the cation and anion exchange membranes that are the walls of this first set of compartments. However, once the cations and anions are in the second set of solution compartments (the alternate compartments) cations are blocked from further transfer because the anion exchange membranes will not allow their passage, and anions are blocked similarly from further transfer because they are blocked by cation- exchange membranes. An ion-depleted solution can be withdrawn from the first set of compartments; an ion-enriched solution can be withdrawn from the second set of compartments.

Membrane Process: Ion exchange membranes can be characterized as an ion exchangers in film 0.2-0.5 mm thick. The active groups are chemically bound to a matrix plastic material, for example, a co-polymerisate of styrene/divinyl benzene. The cation function often comes from sulphonic acid groups linked to the matrix. Similarly mostly quarternary amine groups are used to obtain the anion function.

To understand what occurs in the membrane it can be characterized as a three-dimensional network which is penetrated with many pores in which the functional groups act as carriers of cations and anions diffusing from the product channel to the salt – collected liquid. Anions entering a cation membrane are rejected electrostatically and vice versa. The diffusion of ions within the membrane, reinforced with applied voltage, is the rate limiting mass transport step of the electrodialysis process which leads to a concentration polarization effect at the membrane surface. The selectivity of ions is determined by the equilibrium constant for the fixation of the respective ion to the functional group. Monovalent ions (Na^+, K^+, Cl^-) are more loosely bound to the functional groups than multivalent ions. This means that, due to retardation of multivalent ions, the monovalent ones are favoured in demineralization, using electrodialysis.

Membrane – stack construction: Between the membranes there are sheet flow spacers of porous polyethylene (net structure) which give the membranes mechanical support and a good flow distribution pattern. The electrode chambers are placed at the outer ends of the membrane stacks, which often contain 100–200 individual flow compartments. Platinized titan is often used for the anode, and stainless steel for the cathode.

The electrode chambers are connected to rinse systems which free these solutions from aggressive compounds, formed during the electro-dialysis process, which may harm the anode compartment. The electrode chambers are isolated from the rest of the electrodialysis stack by neutral membranes.

The electrodialysis plant: A pipe system for a two-membrane stack system. The stacks are connected in series with internal circulation over each stack. The salt-up taking process water must continuously be renewed with a feed-and-bleed system. It also needs continuous acidification with hydrochloric acid in order to compensate for alkalinization during the process. The process water requires preheating to operating temperature. 2–5 m^3 of water per m^3 of whey (6% DM) is used, depending on the demineralization rate.

The electrodialysis plant can be run either continuously or in batches. A batch system, which is often used for demineralization rates above 70%, can consist of one membrane stack over which the process liquid, e.g. whey, is circulated until a certain ash level is reached. This is indicated by the conductivity of the process liquid. The holding time in a batch system can be as long as 5–6 hours for 90% demineralization at 30–40° C. Preconcentration of the whey to 20–30% DM is desirable with regard to capacity utilization and electric power consumption. The whey concentrate should be clarified before entering the electrodialysis unit.

The high process temperature is risky as bacteriological growth can take place in the product. A bacteriostatic compound such as hydrogen peroxide is therefore often added to the whey, when allowed. The process liquid is heated during the process and a cooling stage is therefore needed in order to maintain the process temperature. In a continuous plant, consisting of five membrane stacks in series the holding time can be reduced to 10–40 minutes. The maximum demineralization rate of such a plant is often limited to about 60–70%. In relation to capacity the installed membrane area is much larger in a continuous plant than in a batch plant.

An electrodialysis plant can easily be made automatic and supplied with a programmed CIP system. The cleaning sequence normally includes water rinse, cleaning with an alkaline solution (max. pH 9), water rinse, cleaning with hydrochloric acid (pH 1) and a final water rinse. A typical cleaning time is 100 minutes.

A typical industrial electrodialysis stack for demineralization of whey employ about 200 pairs. Each membrane has an effective area of 0.5 m^2, giving a total of 50 m2 per stack. An actual process for demineralization by electrodialysis begins with pasteurization of whey and concentration to 28% TS. Concentrated whey is clarified to remove any soluble proteins and fines and then passed through the electrodialysis stack. For batch operation, process times of 3.5-6.0 h are typical, depending on operating temperature (35-45°C) and for continuous operation, a short residence time (10-30 min) is required at low temperatures (12-20°C). After demineralization, whey is further concentrated by evaporation to 55% solids and spray dried.

Power supply and automation: DC-current is used in the electrodialysis plant. The current should be possible to regulate in the range 0–185A and the voltage 0–400V. Flow rates, temperatures, conductivity, pH of process water and product, product inlet pressure, pressure difference between the stacks and current, as well as voltage over each membrane stack are monitored and controlled during production.

Limiting factors in electrodialysis: A major limiting factor for using electrodialysis in dairy processing is the cost for the replacement of membranes, spacers and electrodes, which constitute 35–40% of the total running costs in the plant. The need for replacement is caused by the fouling of the membranes, which in turn is caused by:

- Precipitation of low-soluble calcium phosphate on the cation membrane surfaces,
- Deposition of proteins on the anion exchange membrane surfaces

The first problem can be handled by proper flow design over the membrane surface and regular acid cleaning.

The main factor reducing the life length of the anion membranes is the protein deposits. The background of this problem is as follows: At the normal pH of whey, the whey proteins can be regarded as large negative ions (anions) and move as such under the influence of the electrical field in the stack. These molecules are too large to pass through the anion exchange membranes and consequently deposit in a thin problem layer on the faces of the anion exchange membranes in the whey compartments. Techniques such as polarity reversal can be used to dislodge these deposited materials from the membrane.

Although frequent high-pH cleaning removes most of the deposits, disassembly of the stack for manual cleaning is recommended with two to four weeks' intervals.

The processing cost of electrodialysis depends very much on the demineralization rate. Increasing the capacity in steps from 50% to 75% to 90% doubles the processing cost per step. This means that it is four times as expensive per kilo of product solids to demineralize to 90% than to 50% and this is due to the reduction in plant capacity when working with 90% demineralization.

The operating costs of a demineralization plant are costs for water treatment, electrical energy, chemicals and steam. A great part of the operating costs is for waste water treatment. During production lactose leaks through the membranes at a rate of 7–10% at 90% demineralization. The phosphate removed from whey is also collected in the waste stream. The cost of electric energy is 10–15% of the processing cost, whereas the chemicals uses in the process, mainly hydrochloric acid, constitute less than 5%. The costs for steam used for preheating of the product and the cooling costs for the control of the process temperature are 10–15%, depending on the demineralization level.

Electrodialysis is best for demineralization levels below 70% where it is very competitive compared with ion exchange.

Non-thermal Processes

The major technologies that are employed to preserve the quality and ensure microbial safety of foods include heat processing, chilling, freezing, drying, curing, fermenting, acidifying, use of chemical preservatives and aseptic packaging. These processes either inactivate the microorganisms and enzymes or slow down or prevent the growth of microorganisms or restrict their access to food products. Recently, there has been an increasing interest in the alternate technologies primarily because of severe effects of heat on food components and cost.

Consumers always look for quality in foods. There is an increase in demand for minimally processed food products with little heat induced changes in nutritional and organoleptic properties. Such a demand has promoted the development of various non-thermal processes of food preservation during the recent years. These methods include high pressure technology, utilization of electric and magnetic fields, ionizing radiation, microwave radiation, light pulses, ultrasound, Laser (light amplification by simulated emission of radiation) and Maser (microwave amplification by stimulated emission of radiation), hurdle technology, bio-preservatives and lytic enzymes. Such methods may be applied singly or in combination or in association with less intense thermal treatment to extend the shelf life of liquid milk.

For the newer technologies of food preservation, it is important that they deliver not only the promised improvements in quality but also an equivalent, or preferably enhanced level of safety compared to the processes intended to be replaced.

High Pressure Processing: The application of high pressure, rather than heat, to food enables destruction of microorganisms without causing significant changes to the colour, flavour and nutritional attributes of the food. In this way, the food can be preserved in the safe state but still have many of the attributes of a fresh product. In addition, high pressure can cause rheological changes in food which result in beneficial sensory and structural effects.

The potential of high-pressure treatment of food was first recognized by Hite in 1899 who investigated it as an alternative method for pasteurization of milk. However, it attracted little attention until it was 'rediscovered' in the 1980s. The first food produced commercially by this technology appeared on the market in Japan in 1990. They included yoghurts, fruit jellies, salad dressings and fruit sauces. Several other pressure-treated foods are now manufactured, including pressure-'pasteurized' milk, but the total amount remains relatively small.

The Process: Typically, high-pressure processing is performed at 300-1000 MPa at room temperature for 2-30 min. During pressurization, an increase in temperature (up to 3°C for each 100 MPa) occurs due to adiabetic heating; a corresponding decrease occurs during depressurization. These changes can be minimized by temperature control of the high-pressure equipment by circulating water.

During high-pressure processing, the pressure is instantaneously and uniformaly transmitted in all directions, regardless of shape or volume. Consequently, the food is treated evenly throughout and no particles escape the treatment. This contrasts with processes involving heating where different parts of the food can be heated at very different rates.

High pressure disrupts noncovalent bonds but has little effect on covalent bonds. Thus, the large bio-molecules such as proteins, nucleic acids and poly-saccharides, which depend on noncovalent bonding such as hydrophobic interactions and hydrogen bonds to maintain structure and function, are most affected. On the other hand, smaller organic molecules such as those responsible for colour, flavour and nutrients (e.g. vitamins) in which covalent bonding is the dominant or only type of bonding are not affected, or affected very little by the pressure- treatment. The low temperature at which high-pressure treatments are performed ensures little or no heat-induced change in these components.

Equipment and Operation: A typical high-pressure system consists of a high-pressure vessel with closure, a pressure generation system, a temperature control device and a material handling system. The pressure vessel in many cases is an alloy-steel cylindrical vessel of high tensile strength. Once loaded with food packages and closed, the vessel is filled with pressure transmitting medium. In most isostatic pressure applications, it is simply water mixed with a small percentage of soluble oil for lubrication and anticorrosion effects. Liquid food can be compressed directly in the pressure vessel, eliminating the use of a pressure transmitting medium. High pressure is generated by direct or indirect compression, or heating of the pressure medium.

The pressure treatment can be performed in batch or semicontinuous operations. In batch operations, a pressure chamber containing the liquid or solid food is pressurized for a given holding time and then decompressed. A variation of the batch method is the pulsed high-pressure process where the pressure is raised and lowered repeatedly at intervals of several minutes. In semicontinuous processing, several vessels are connected in series, while some are under constant pressure, others are being pressurized, unloaded or loaded. This minimizes the operation time and allows a portion of the energy contained in the vessel under pressure to be used to pressurize another vessel, thus reducing operating costs. A continuous system suitable for liquid foods such as milk and fruit juice has been reported, but only on a research scale (Data and Deeth, 2003).

Microbial Effects

Vegetative Organisms: A major function of high –pressure processing of food is destruction of microorganisms. When a microbial cell is subjected to high pressure, the following detrimental changes take place:

1. Cell membrane are destroyed via irreversible changes to the structure of the membrane macromolecules, particularly proteins.
2. The homogeneity of the intermediate layer between the cell wall and the cytoplasmic membrane is disrupted.
3. Membrane ATPase is inactivated.
4. The nucleic acids and ribosomes involved in the synthesis of proteins are disrupted.

The result is permeabilization of the membranes and concomitant leakage of the contents of the cells and organellese, with eventual death of the bacterial cell.

In general, Gram-negative bacteria are inactivated at a lower pressure than Gram-positive bacteria, and rod-shaped bacteria are more sensitive to pressure than cocci. The pressure sensitivities of yeasts are reported to be intermediate between these two bacterial groups. Bacteria in the stationary phase are more resistant than those in the early log phase of growth, due to a transition of the vegetative organisms into a dormant condition.

The bactericidal efficiency of high pressure can be increased by combining it with heat or other 'hurdles' as well as other energy forms such as ultrasound, shear, electromagnetic fields or high-voltage pulses. Concomitant treatment of foods with chemical agents such as ethanol, lysozyme, chitosan, and sorbic and benzoic acids enhance the effect of pressure on microorganisms, and allow the use of lower pressures, lower temperatures or shorter application times to be used to achieve inactivation. The medium containing the bacteria can also affect the bactericidal efficiency. For example, *Listeria monocytogenes* is more susceptible in buffer solutions than in milk as proteins, carbohydrate and fat seem to protect the bacterial cells.

Bacterial Endospores: The antibacterial effect of high-pressure processing is limited in that it can not destroy bacterial endospores. Because of this limitation, it cannot be used for processing sterile products, and all pressure treated foods have to be kept refrigerated. However, high pressure can stimulate germination of bacterial spores which enables the resulting vegetative form to be destroyed. Some variations of the standard single- pressure treatment, such as repeated cycling between high and low pressure, 'pulsed' or 'oscilatory' pressurization, and combined high pressure and high temperature, enhance the sporicidal effect of high pressure.

Effect on Bacterial Flora and Keeping Quality of Milk: Hite in 1899 observed 5-6 log reduction in the number of microorganisms when milk was treated at 680 MPa for 10 min at room temperature. Subsequent reports have supported these observations, all finding a small proportion of the bacterial population which could not be inactivated under normal high-pressure operating conditions. These resistant organisms are mostly sporeformers. It has been concluded that to achieve the shelf life of thermally pasteurized milk of 10 days at 10 °C, a pressure treatment of at least 400 MPa for 15 min or 500 MPa for 3 min is required.

While a reasonable shelf life of milk may be obtained with pressure treatments of 400 or 500 MPa, some strains of the pathogenic bacteria *Listeria monocytogenes* and *Staphylococcus aureus* are quite pressure-resistant and may not be sufficiently inactivated. Some mutant strains of *E. coli* are particularly barotolerant being only reduced 2 log at 600 MPa for 30 min. It has also been suggested that high-pressure treatment might sublethally injure a proportion of cells which then could grow slowly at refrigeration temperatures. The risk of the presence of barotolerant pathogenic bacteria in milk must therefore be considered before this technology is adopted for producing pasteurized milk.

Chemical Effects: High-pressure processing of food differs from heat processing in the chemical effects produced. The pressure-induced effects are mostly concerned with secondary and tertiary structural changes in large molecules. Consequently, enzymes and polysaccharides in an aqueous environment undergo reversible or irreversible conformational changes resulting in denaturation, dissociation, aggregation or gelation. By contrast, the heat-induced breaking of covalent bonds in both small and large molecules causes changes to colour, flavour and other sensory properties which are not observed with pressure treatment.

Changes to the water component by high-pressure processing have significant direct and indirect relevance to foods. The changes include: reduction of volume, which at high pressure can be substantial, e.g. 15% at 600 MPa, reduction in the freezing point of water and decrease in pH.

Moderate pressure (<150 MPa) favours dissociation of oligomeric proteins, while pressures higher than 150-200 MPa induce unfolding of proteins and reassociation of subunits from dissociated oligomers. For example, below 150 MPa, β-casein is reversibly dissociated whereas at higher pressures, a temperature-dependent reversible reassociation occurs. Significant tertiary structure changes are observed beyond 200 MPa. However, reversible unfolding of small proteins occur at higher pressure (400-800 MPa). Secondary structure changes occur at very high pressures (>700 MPa) and lead to non-reversible denaturation. No changes in covalent bonding (including disulphide bridges) have yet been observed in the pressure range studied.

The effects of pressure on casein micelles depend on the pressure and temperature. Under the least sever conditions, such as pressures ~230 MPa or higher pressures at low temperatures (~20 °C), casein micelles are reduced in size and free casein (particularly κ- and α-casein) and small casein clusters (perhaps only two or three molecules) are released. This causes a decrease in turbidity and whiteness, and an increase in viscosity of milk. Under more sever conditions, such as 400 MPa at 50-60 °C, micelles are increased in size.

Whey proteins can undergo partial, but fully reversible, unfolding of their native molecular structures under suitable pressures (100-300 MPa). Denaturation of β-lactoglobulin commences at ~150 MPa and increases with increasing pressure and temperature. Almost complete denaturation has been reported at 750 MPa at 30 °C for 30 min, or 450 MPa at 60 °C for 15 min. Alpha-lactalbumin and immunoglobulins are more resistant to denaturation by pressure than β-lactoglobulin.

Solutions containing whey proteins increase in viscosity and turbidity when subjected to pressure. These changes are due to denaturation of the β-lactoglobulin, which undergoes polymerization reactions through disulphide linkages to form protein aggregates, and concomitant increase in water-binding capacity; this phenomenon can be used to advantage in yoghurt manufacture. Solutions of whey protein isolate and whey protein concentrate undergo gelation at high concentrations (>10%) under high pressures (>400 MPa).

Milk enzymes vary in their sensitivity to high pressure. For example, phosphohexose isomerase, γ-glutamyl transferase and alkaline phosphatase in milk are partially inactivated at pressure greater than 350, 400 and 600 MPa, respectively, and almost completely inactivated at ~550, 630 and 800 MPa, respectively. The effect on alkaline phosphatase is of interest in milk processing because of its universal use as in internal indicator of effective pasteurization. Since its complete inactivation, if feasible, occurs at very high pressures, alkaline phosphatase is unlikely to be appropriate as an indicator of effective 'pasteurization' by high-pressure treatment.

Crystallization of fat can be accelerated, enforced or initiated because of the shift in the phase transition temperature caused by application of high hydrostatic pressure. As a consequence, high pressure treatment reduces the ageing time of ice cream mixes and enhances the physical ripening of cream for making butter.

The fat globule size distribution and flow behaviour of pasteurized liquid cream are not significantly modified by high-pressure processing at 450 MPa and 25 °C for 15-20 min or 10 °C for 30 min. Some fat globule aggregation occurs at 40 °C but physical stability remains unchanged. With UHT-sterilized cream, treatment at 450 MPa induces fat globule aggregation and increases viscosity, whether carried out at 25 °C for 15-20 min, or at 10 or 40 °C for 30 min. The aggregation which may be caused by the effect of high heat treatment on the milk fat globule membrane, is partly reversed during chilled storage.

Effects on Dairy Products and Processes

Yoghurt: pressure treatment (PT) at 200-300 MPA for 10 min at 10-20 °C can be used to control post-acidification of yoghurt, without decreasing the number of viable lactic acid bacteria or modifying the yoghurt texture. Treatment at higher pressures destroys the lactic acid bacteria. Above 400 MPa for 15 min *Lactobacillus delbruekii subsp. bulgaricus* is inactivated whereas *Streptococcus thermophilus* is more resistant but loses its acidifying capacity.

Yoghurt made from milk treated at 600 MPA for 15 min shows different rheological properties and gel microstructure than conventional yoghurts. The PT yoghurt gels are less continuous with larger interstitial spaces which may cause the gel to flow or break at lower deformation. Although β-lactoglobulin is associated with the protein network in the PT gels, the long- range â-lactoglobulin bridges found in the corresponding heat-treated yoghurt gels are not present. This makes the yoghurt less firm and cohesive, which significantly affects the mouthfeel.

Rennet Coagulation and Cheese Yield: High-pressure treatment of milk (e.g. 300 MPa for 30 min) decreases the coagulation time, and increases the curd firming rate, curd firmness and curd yield during cheese manufacture. The last is due to denaturation of β-lactoglobulin and incorporation with the casein curd which promotes moisture retention and hinders syneresis.

Cheddar cheese manufactured from high-pressure treated (three 1-min cycles at 586 MPa) milk is not significantly different in sensory quality to that made from HTST- pasteurized milk. However, the pressurized milk cheese has a higher moisture content which causes pasty and weak texture defects. The higher moisture content of the pressurized milk cheese suggests that pressure treatment may be useful in the manufacture of reduced fat cheese, for improving texture which is usually very hard.

Generally, pressure treatment of low-fat milk prior to cheese making improves cheese texture and overall acceptability. Cheese made from HTST- pasteurized, pressurized milk has been reported to be significantly more tasty than that made from either pressurized or HTST-pasteurized milk. Protein breakdown is faster in cheese made from pressurized milk, which leads to a softer texture; this has been attributed to a higher level of residual rennet.

While a small number of coliforms can survive pressure treatment of milk, much lower numbers, or none at all, can be isolated from the pressurized milk cheese. This may be explained by the recovery of sublethally injured cells in the pressurized milk during the enumeration procedure and the death of the injured cells in the cheese during storage.

Proteolysis of Whey Proteins: In making modified milk for infants, β-lactoglobulin can be selectively eliminated from whey protein concentrates by hydrolysis with thermolysin at elevated hydrostatic pressure. Alpha-lactalbumin is resistant to hydrolysis due to the presence of four disulphide bonds. When the thermolysin digestion is performed under high pressure, β-lactoglobulin is hydrolyzed faster and more completely than at atmospheric pressure, but there is no effect on α-lactalbumin. In this way, milk resembling human milk, which contains α-lactalbumin but no β-lactoglobulin, can be obtained.

Application in Dairy Processing: to date, there has been very limited commercial use of high-pressure treatment of milk and milk products. However, the technology and associated processing equipment have now been developed to the stage where it is feasible to establish processing plants. Milk treated in this way can be used for either manufactured products, such as yoghurt and cheese, or for the liquid milk market. Other liquid milk products such as cream and ice cream mix, used in the production of butter and ice cream, respectively, could also be treated to advantage. Pressure treatment of manufactured products such as yoghurt and cheese could be used to produce effects not achievable by alternative means.

Milk treated at pressure of up to 500 MPa for a few minutes has been shown to have a shelf life of at least equivalent to that of HTST- pasteurized milk. Most vegetative cells, including non-spore forming thermodurics, can be eliminated. However, the nature of the bacteria remaining after such treatments, which limit the shelf life of the product, requires further investigation. Furthermore, the conditions necessary to achieve an equivalent bactericidal effect in modified milk products and products with high solids contents have not been well defined.

The difficulty of destroying bacterial spores currently limits the bactericidal applications of high pressure to those presently covered by pasteurization. However, the combined use of pulsed-pressure treatment and temperature shows considerable promise for eliminating both spores as well as vegetative cells. If this promise is fulfilled, it may be possible to produce pressure-sterilized milk with a fresh milk taste, quite different from UHT milk with its distinctive heated flavour.

An advantage of high pressure over heat treatment (and other alternatives such as pulsed electric field technology) is the even and instant distribution of the energy (pressure) throughout the product. This ensures the absence of dead spots and localized over-processing which are a problem in other treatments.

6.8. Pulsed Energy Technologies

Pulsed energy technologies for treatment of foods utilize high energy levels in short bursts or pulses (microseconds to milliseconds) with the expenditure of average power consumption. The energy is initially generated as electrical energy and accumulated in a storage capacitor. The accumulated electrical power (many megawatts) is discharged almost instantaneously in the form of high–energy electric field pulses (pulsed electric field technology), high intensity light pulses (pulsed light technology) or high intensity magnetic field pulses (oscillating magnetic field technology). The electronics that drive the dose-generating devices for each of the technologies are similar.

These pulsed energy technologies offer alternatives to traditional heat treatments for the production of safe, nutritious foods with fresh-flavour characteristics. To date, they have found little commercial application in the dairy industry but show considerable potential for adoption in the future.

Pulsed Electric Field Technology: Pulsed energy field (PEF) technology has the potential to replace or at least complement, the traditional thermal processes for the pasteurization and sterilization of liquid milk products. Since PEF operations are performed under mild conditions, often at ambient temperature, the technology offers considerable consumer benefits in terms of better quality (flavour, colour) and comparable or better safety than corresponding thermally processed products. It may also offer processors benefits in terms of lower operational costs than thermal processes.

The application of pulsed electric fields with high field strengths for killing microorganisms, is gaining popularity as one of the promising non-thermal methods alternative to conventional pasteurization of milk. This method does not produce undesirable changes in taste and flavour of milk and does not form deposits of salts and proteins on heat exchange surfaces. In addition, the PEF treated milk remains fresh with satisfactory shelf life at ambient temperature.

Equipment: The essential components of a PEF processing system are (1) a high-voltage power supply (~30 kV); (2) an energy storage capacitor; (3) a pulse generator and switching system; (4) a treatment chamber, containing two electrodes, through which liquid food is pumped; (5) a cooling system; (6) a unit of control and monitoring of voltage, current and electric field strength; and (7) a product delivery and packaging system.

Energy from the high voltage power supply is stored in the capacitor, and discharged almost instantaneously at high levels of power. While the discharge is extremely fast (1-30 μs), the time between discharges is comparatively long (1 m s to seconds). The number of pulses can vary from 10 to 100. Total treatment times are generally less than 1 s. The strength of the electric field which passes through the food is directly proportional to the voltage supplied across the electrodes, and inversely proportional to the gap or distance between the electrodes. PEF technology utilizes electric field strengths of 10-50 kV cm^{-1}. When applied as pulses, the disadvantages of continuous high-voltage current treatments, electrolysis and ohmic heating, are minimized.

The design of the treatment chamber is critical to the efficacy of this technology. It is essential that a uniform electric field exists throughout the cell so that there are no 'cold spots' and no area which promote electric breakdown of the food product. The electrodes are usually 3-5 mm apart but several different treatment cell designs have been developed and patented. Common configurations are parallel plate, cofield, collinear and coaxial. Some have specific characteristics such as a conical shape electrode and insulators to prevent gas depositing within the treatment volume which can lead to electrical breakdown of the food. Some systems operate under pressure to prevent such gas development. Multiple treatment chambers can be used to eliminate the effect of non-uniformity of electrical field strength within individual chambers.

Bactericidal Effects: The most important aspect of PEF technology in the treatment of liquid milk products is the effect on bacteria. Most vegetative cells can be destroyed by the technology but bacterial spores are much more resistant.

When high voltage is applied to a liquid containing microbial cells, a transmembrane potential is induced across the membrane of the cell. When this exceeds a critical value, about 1 V, electroporation occurs, that is, pores form in the cell membrane. As a consequence, the content of the cell is released and the cell dies. Pores, which are either predominantly hydrophobic or hydrophilic, are formed by the electrical breakdown of lipid layers. Hydrophilic pores conduct current, resulting in localized joule heating which causes changes in the liquid crystalline structure of the lipid layer in the cell membrane. This impairs the semi-permeability of the membrane and increases its permeability to ions. If the pores exceed certain radius, they cause mechanical breakdown of the membrane.

Microorganisms are more sensitive in the log phase of growth than in the stationary phase. Studies on the effect of the composition of the medium have shown that fat protects microorganisms against electric pulses. For example, destruction of bacteria in milk containing 3.5% fat is less than in milk with 1.5% fat. Similarly, higher electric field strengths are required to destroy bacteria in a xanthan gum solution than in a saline solution. This is attributed to the protective effect of the gum afforded by interaction between the polymer chains of the gum forming a network of molecular aggregates around the microorganism. Another important factor is the presence of air in the medium being treated. For this reason, some treatments are performed under vacuum.

Bacterial endospores, such as those formed by *Bacillus* and *Clostridium* species, are more resistant than vegetative cells to many food preservation treatments, and PEF is no exception. There are several reports of PEF being ineffective against endospores. The reason for the greater resistance of spores to PEF is that the electrical conductivity is considerably lower in endospores than in vegetative cells, due to the low water content and relative immobility of ions within the spore core. It has been suggested that spores are more susceptible to PEF at the time of germination and outgrowth. However, germination is not initiated by PEF. Therefore, processes capable of inducing germination (e.g. treatment with high hydrostatic pressure, heat or ultrasound) may enhance the effectiveness of PEF in inactivation of spores.

Effect on Enzymes: PEF has a variable effect on enzymes with some being partially or completely inactivated (e.g. milk plasmin), some being stimulated (e.g. lysozyme and pepsin) and some being unaffected (e.g. pectinesterase). The effect also varies with electric field strength, pulse width and treatment time. Significant enzyme inactivation generally requires the higher electric field strength than destruction of vegetative cells.

In dairy processing, it is of interest that milk plasmin (alkaline protease) which is resistant to heat treatments, even UHT, is largely inactivated by PEF. However, alkaline phosphatase and lipase which are completely inactivated by HTST pasteurization are only partially inactivated by PEF.

Mechanisms proposed for the inactivation of enzymes by PEF include alteration of secondary and tertiary structures of the protein and oxidation of key components of the enzyme. In the case of enzymes present in microorganisms, localized joule heating of cell membrane components due to PEF may cause thermal denaturation of membrane bound enzymes. Stimulation of some enzymes may be caused by creation of more active sites or increasing access to existing sites.

Application in Dairy Processing: Milk has been subjected to PEF in several studies and the results are reasonably consistent. Most report 4-5 log reductions of non-sporeforming bacteria. Typical conditions used are 50-55°C at 20kV cm^{-1}; lower reductions are observed at lower temperatures (20-40 °C). PEF treatment, without pasteurization, can achieve a safe product (the bacterial count of raw milk inoculated with 10^8 cfu ml^{-1}Listeria spp. was reduced to ~10^1cfu $ml^{-1,}$ i. e the level of spores in the raw milk before inoculation, by treatment at 60°C; the corresponding thermal effect is 1-2 log reduction) and up to 14 days extension of shelf life. Little or no change in flavour, colour, lipid oxidation, alkaline phosphatase activity, bovine serum albumin, fat globule membrane, casein micelles or coagulation properties have been observed. However, a reduction in vitamin C in milk treated with PEF has been observed. PEF-treated yoghurt containing yeast (10 cfu ml^1), which can reduce its shelf life, had no detectable yeast after storage for 30 days at 7-9 °C.

Pulsed High-Intensity Light Technology: Broad-spectrum white light in intense, short-duration pulses is capable of reducing the microbial load on surfaces and transparent fluids. The spectrum of light used is from ultraviolet (UV) to near infrared (NIR), with 70% between 170 and 2600 nm. A typical spectrum is: 25% UV, 45% visible, 30% IR. Significantly, it includes the UV wavelengths 200-300 nm which are filtered out by the atmosphere; these are important for killing some microorganisms. The intensity of the pulses, or fluence, is 0.01 to 50 J cm^{-2}, about 20,000 times intensity of sunlight at the surface of Earth. The duration of pulses ranges from 1μs to 0.1 s and the frequency of the flashes applied is in the range of 1 to 20 s^{-1}. A high level of microbial inactivation requires only a few flashes so the treatment time is typically less than 1 s. The normal light energy required in a treatment is 6 J cm^{-2}, for example, 2 pulses of 3 J cm^{-2} per pulse; an excessive treatment uses 10 pulses. Use of light pulses with a relatively high UV content minimizes the total fluence necessary to achieve the desired microcidal effect.

Generation of a Light Pulses: A pulsed light unit consists of two main parts: the power unit which generates high voltage, high-current electric pulses; and the lamp unit which consists of one or more inert gas (xenon) lamps. The high-voltage, high current pulses energize the lamp unit and the high current passing through the gas emits an intense pulse of light. The flashing frequency is selected according to the application.

Effect on Microorganisms: High-intensity pulsed light is more bactericidal than continuous UV light, but the UV content of the pulses is important. It has a broad spectrum microcidal effect and destroys bacteria resistant to other agents such as heat, H_2O_2 and gamma radiation, bacterial endospores (e.g. *Bacillus* spp.) and mould spores (e.g. *Aspergillus niger*). For example, *Bac. cereus* and *Aspergillus spores*, inoculated onto packaging material at up to 10^3cfu cm^{-2} were destroyed by a single light pulse of intensity 2 J cm^{-1}.

The most effective application of this technology is in the destruction of bacteria on surfaces. On smooth, nonporous surfaces, light pulses can cause a 9-log reduction of vegetative organisms. By contrast, on porous and complex surfaces such as plastic packaged cheese and meat, reductions of $\leq$ 3 log are observed. For example, a 1.5-log reduction was observed when curds of commercial dry cottage cheese inoculated with *Pseudomonas* spp. were treated with light pulses of 0.5 ms duration and total energy of 16 J cm^{-2}; no effect on the taste of the cheese was noted.

When the light absorption coefficient of a surface is low, an absorption-enhancing agent is required. The enhancing agent may be applied by spraying, dusting or vaporizing the agent onto the surface. Carotene, red dye no. 3, lime green, black cherry and cooking oil can be used as absorption enhancing agents. Such agents increase the photothermal and photochemical reactions on the surface which affect microorganisms.

A further surface application for pulsed light treatment in the dairy and other food industries is in sterilization of the surfaces of preformed packages or packaging material used in the fabrication of the food packages, such as those used for extended shelf life (ESL) and UHT dairy products. A process for sterilization of the continuous roll paperboard material used for aseptic cartons has been described and patented.

Pulsed light can be used for fluids provided they are transparent to light at the wavelengths supplied. In fact, the technology is successfully used commercially for drinking water. For satisfactory disinfection, it is preferable for the fluid to have a transparency to UV light and for at least half of the incident light at 260 nm to be transmitted through 0.25 cm of the fluid.

Microorganisms are inactivated by a combination of photochemical and photothermal mechanisms. The biological effect of UV wavelengths contained in the pulsed light spectrum is through absorption by conjugated double bonds in proteins and nucleic acids. Inactivation of enzymes, which is due to photochemical effects, may also contribute to the effect of pulsed light on microorganisms.

Oscillating Magnetic Field Technology: High-intensity oscillating magnetic fields (OMF) can inactivate microorganisms in foods. However, while there is research and commercial interest in this technology, there is less published information on it compared to other two pulsed technologies mentioned above. Oscillating magnetic fields used are of 5-50 Tesla (T) (50-500 kilogauss (kG) intensity, a frequency of oscillation of 5-500 kHz and total exposure time 25 μ s to 100 m s for 1-100 pulses. Frequencies higher than 500 kHz are less effective for microbial inactivation and generate heat in the food. Food to be treated is typically contained in a plastic package; metal packages can not be used.

The most important requirement for the application of this technology is that the food material must have high electrical resistivity, greater than 1-2.5 Ω m. since most dairy products have resistivity higher than 2 Ω m., this technology is applicable to these foods. The magnetic field intensity applied depends on the electric resistivity and the thickness of the food being treated; the lower the electrical resistivity and the greater the thickness of the food material, the higher the intensity of magnetic field required.

Inactivation of microorganisms by OMF is attributed to the coupling of the energy into the magnetically active parts of large critical molecules such as DNA where separation of charge constitutes a dipole. The amount of energy per oscillation which can be coupled to one dipole in the DNA is 10^{-2} to 10^{-1} electron volts in a magnetic field of intensity of 5-50 T. When several dipoles in the DNA molecules are activated in an OMF, sufficient local energy may result in the breakdown of covalent bonds with eventual inhibition of growth and reproduction of microorganisms.

At a maximum log reduction of about 2, this technology currently has little to offer to the dairy industry over existing or other emerging preservation technologies. Developments in the technology can be expected to improve its efficacy and renew interest in its application to preservation to dairy foods.

6.9 Microwave Processing

Microwave heating is a novel method that offers technique of heating requiring neither conduction nor convection. This greatly reduces the need for long conduction lags, that is generally associated with traditional processes. It also eliminates the formation of hardened crust during heating. Microwaves generate heat within the food rapidly raising the temperature to the desirable extent. The increasing consumer demand for convenient and safe food products of high nutritive value and organoleptic quality has resulted in growing usage of microwave technology both at home and in commercial applications. The process has been generally successful for low and intermediate moisture products. The use of microwaves offers a number of advantages over conventional method of heating. The increasing demand of the consumers for kitchen convenience and time saving in domestic heating applications has made microwaves a household term. It has also gained favour with certain segments of the food processing industry.

Microwaves cover the broad range of radio frequencies from 300 MHz (million cycles per second) to 300 GHz (billion cycles per second). Microwaves are produced by vacuum tube devices called magnetrons which convert the 50 Hz electric current into microwave power usually at 915 MHz or 2450 MHz. Microwaves are reflected by metals, transmitted by electrically neutral materials such as glass, plastics, ceramics and paper and absorbed by electrically charged materials. The application of microwave energy for heating has achieved substantial importance, in recent years, due to the well known advantages, which derive from the rapid and direct transfer of heat to the material (volumetric heating), the more even temperature distribution throughout the product and the absence of the contact with hot surfaces which avoids overheating of the product. The use of continuous microwave systems for heat treatment of milk reduced the total number of bacteria without causing extensive whey protein denaturation. The inclusion of a holding phase to maintain the time and temperature conditions achieved in the microwave oven provided the conditions required for proper pasteurization of milk.

Mechanism of Microwave Heating: Microwaves deeply penetrate into the product and as they penetrate, the energy they carry is converted to heat, actually by its own constituents (water and salts) and by the mechanisms of polar and ionic orientation. When an electric field is applied, the polar water molecules which are present in random orientation attempt to line up with the electric field. When the field is removed, the molecules tend to return to random orientation. When the electric field is alternated rapidly, millions of times per second, kinetic energy of high speed oscillating water molecules is expended to generate heat. Ionic orientation occurs when ions in solution move as an electric field is applied. Kinetic energy is imparted to the ions by the electric field so that when the field is alternating rapidly heat is generated.

Lethality of Microwaves: There is no substantiated mechanism for the interaction of microwaves with microorganisms other than the thermal effect. Studies involving laboratory scale continuous flow microwave heating systems have shown that the total microbial count of milk could be drastically reduced and alkaline phosphatase inactivated without causing extensive whey protein denaturation. However, microwave heating may not completely eliminate pathogenic bacteria present in milk. Studies on inactivation of milk borne pathogens like *Listeria monocytogenes, Salmonella typhimurium, Staphylococcus aureus and Escherichia coli* indicated that microwave processing at <75°C may cause sublethal injury rather than inactivation of the pathogens. Therefore, microwaves for pasteurization of milk involve a definite amount of risk unless excessive heating is allowed.

Effect of Microwave Processing on Nutrients and Shelf Life of Milk: The nutritional quality of microwave processed milk is better than that of conventionally treated milk due to rapid and uniform heating, and because of lack of hot surfaces in contact with the milk which would reduce thermal degradation of milk constituents. The microwave processed milk has shown lower â-lactoglobulin denaturation and lower furosine formation than that of milk processed with the conventional method. Microwave pasteurized milk (80.1°C, 15 s) has been found to have satisfactory quality, which remained better even after 10 days of storage, as compared to the milk heated in a plate heat exchanger.

Microwave processing of milk is yet to assume commercial significance due to non-availability of fool-proof microwave treatment and high equipment cost. However, developments in magnetron manufacture and equipment design are likely to make microwave processing of milk acceptable by dairy industry in the coming years. The instant heating capability of microwaves have resulted in processing of milk to very high temperatures such as 200°C in just 40 milliseconds, but commercialization of such processes seems to be a matter of future. Microwave heating has been suggested to be suitable for several dairy processing applications such as in-package paneer making, clarification of butter into ghee, thermization of yoghurt, cooking of cheese curd, and thawing of butter. But till date only the last application has found industry's acceptance.

6.10. Ultrasonication

The destructive effect of high-power ultrasound on microorganisms has been known for many years. It has potential for use in preserving foods but has not been used commercially for this purpose in the dairy industry.

Ultrasonication refers to the use of sound waves of frequencies higher than is audible by the human ear (>18 kHz). Ultrasound can travel through gas, liquid and solid materials and is therefore suitable for use in milk and milk products. It has application in the dairy industry in both its- high and low-power forms. The high-power form (10-1000 W cm^{-2}) at relatively low frequencies (20-100 kHz) causes changes in bacteria, the physical structure of food and food components, while the low-power form (1 W cm^{-2}) at high frequencies (0.1-20 MHz)is nondestructive and used for evaluation of the physical state of products and diagnostic purposes. This article is concerned only with the high-power form because of its ability to destroy bacteria and hence substitute, in part or in full, traditional heat treatments for preservation of milk and milk products.

Effect on Bacteria: The destructive effect of ultrasonic waves on microorganisms has been attributed to the combination of effects, namely cavitation and associated shear forces, localized heating and free radical formation. When ultrasonic vibrations are propagated in fluids, they cause the formation of microscopic bubbles, or cavities, and fluid appears to boil ('cold boiling'). The cavities rapidly collapse, emitting shock waves. This formation and implosion of bubbles, known as 'cavitation', can cause physical changes in the surrounding medium and disruption of organisms therein. The bubbles collapse with a range of intensities, and localized high local pressures (up to 100 MPa) and temperatures (up to 5000 K) which contribute to the destructive effect on cell walls momentarily produced.

The intensity of cavitation is affected by the frequency and amplitude of the ultrasound wave. At low frequencies (e.g. 20 kHz), large bubbles are produced and high energy forces result when they collapse. At higher frequencies, bubble formation becomes increasingly difficult and at frequencies greater than 2.5 MHz cavitation does not occur. The intensity of cavitation increases as the amplitude of the ultrasound waves increases.

The extent of ultrasonic cavitation decreases with the viscosity of the medium. However, the effectiveness of ultrasonication in viscous liquids can be increased by use of high-intensity, low frequency ultrasound, and by increasing the temperature of the medium. The effectiveness of ultrasound decreases as the level of solids (fat, protein, lactose, gums) in the food increases.

Application of ultrasound for example, to water can lead to the formation of the free radicals OH^*, H^{+*} and $H_2O_2^*$ species, which have bactericidal effects. The prime target of free radicals in cells is the DNA. Hydroxyl radicals are very reactive and can initiate the formation of peroxy radicals on amino acid residues, causing substantial losses of tryptophan, tyrosine and other amino acids. Subsequently, a chain reaction is initiated which, in the presence of oxygen, usually leads to protein fragmentation and, under anaerobic conditions, to the formation of higher molecular weight aggregates through crosslinking.

The bactericidal effects of ultrasonic treatment vary with the organisms, the time of treatment, the intensity of the ultrasound, protective effects of the medium and temperature. Cavitation fields contain a large number of eddies (small currents with a swirling motion) with a range of sizes, eddies smaller than a cell can exert shear stress on it. With the decrease in cell size, the number of eddies that can exert stresses which can cause cell disintegration also decreases. Conversely, the larger the bacterial cells, the more sensitive they are to ultrasound. Gram-negative bacteria are more sensitive than Gram-positive, and rod-shaped organisms are more sensitive than coccus-shaped organisms. The resistance of Gram-positive cells is attributed to their thicker cell wall which contains a tightly adherent layer of peptidoglycans.

Effect on Enzymes: The effect of ultrasonication on enzymes depends on the molecular structure of the enzymes and the nature of the medium, especially the presence of dissolved gases. Enzymes vary greatly in their response. For example, polyphenol oxidase and lysozyme are sensitive, while catalase and pepsin are not.

Inactivation of enzymes generally requires long treatment times and presence of oxygen. The effect of sonication has been attributed to splitting off the prosthetic groups (such as haem in haem proteins and the lipid portion in lipoproteins); fragmentation of the polypeptide chains; and oxidation or degradation of amino acid residues via a free radical mechanism. The loss of activity of pepsin and trypsin after sonication has been attributed to the oxidation of cyclic amino acids and sulphydryl groups: inactivation is significantly reduced when hydrogen is sustitutred for oxygen in the sonicating medium or when antioxidants are present.

Combination treatments with heat and pressure: Bacterial cells become more sensitive to heat treatment after ultrasonication. Sequential or simultaneously applied sonication and heat treatment (thermosonication) allow destruction of bacteria at much lower temperatures than would be required for heat treatment alone. Simultaneous application of pressure and ultrasound further enhances the susceptibility of bacteria to heat. Applying pressure with heat and ultrasound (manothermosonication) overcomes the loss of cavitation at high temperatures and enhances the bactericidal effect of the ultrasound.

The heat resistance of *Bacillus stearothermophilus* has been found to reduce ½ to 1/3 its original value after sonication. Thermoduric streptococci are also sensitive to this combined treatment. A mild increase in the temperature of the medium during ultrasonication increases its lethality for vegetative cells. The heat resistance of *Bacillus subtilis* to an MTS treatment has been observed to decrease to about 1/10 that of simply heating (100-110°C). The lethality of MTS treatment could be 6-30 times greater than that of the corresponding heat treatment at the same temperature depending on the microorganisms. The effect is greater for the yeasts than for spores. MTS can also be effective for inactivation of extracellular proteases and lipases with little or no damage to the nutritive and sensory quality of the milk resulting into the longer shelf life of UHT milk

6.11. Ionizing Radiation

The application of ionizing radiation (gamma-rays, X-rays, high-energy electrons) as an alternative to heat treatment of dairy products commenced in the 1940s. While it is possible to pasteurize and even sterilize milk, butter, cheese, yoghurt and other dairy products by ionizing energy, the process causes unacceptable flavour and colour changes and loss of certain vitamins. However, it has an application in several areas of dairy technology, such as sterilization of packaging materials and additives. It is recognized as an alternative method to fumigation of food/packaging materials to control the microbial contamination and can facilitate trade in fresh and dried foods. Compared with the energy required for canning, refrigeration, the energy used for irradiation preservation of food is very small. Irradiation is also a cost effective method of food processing for reducing the incidence of food-borne diseases. FAO/WHO has pronounced that food subjected to ionizing radiation treatment under properly controlled conditions is safe for human consumption.

Ionizing radiations such as gamma-rays or beta-particles are believed to cause microbial inactivation by both the 'direct' and 'indirect' mechanisms. According to the 'direct hit' or 'target' theory, a high energy particle / radiation traversing the food hits microbial cells, thereby affecting vital cellular components and producing lethality. The indirect or 'secondary effect' mechanism involves effects occurring via free radicals produced elsewhere in the medium or via chemical reactions originating outside the cells.

Low dose irradiation is effective in inactivating non-spore forming pathogenic bacteria and food-borne parasites. Most food-borne parasites may be inactivated or destroyed by a dose as low as 1 kGy. The total bacterial count of milk is reduced by around 99% (2 log reduction) by treatment with 2-5 kGy of ionizing radiation but doses of up to 10-20 kGy are necessary to achieve sterilization, that is, to achieve complete destruction of spore-forming bacteria.

Milk enzymes are more resistant to ionizing energy treatment than to heat treatments. Alkaline phosphatase loses less than 10% of its activity on irradiation with up to 10 kGy. Lipases and proteases which cause flavour defects and stability problems in dairy products during storage are also less susceptible to irradiation than to heat.

Application of Irradiation in Dairy Processing: Though the studies on irradiation preservation of milk stared long back, yet it has not found, to date, any commercial application because of off-flavour development accompanying the irradiation treatment. While certain components of the off-flavour originate in the serum fraction of milk, the most significant part of it seems to arise from milk fat. A dose as low as 1 kGy can give rise to this problem. Irradiation of milk at high doses causes browning, caramelization and off-flavours such as bitterness. The dose at which off- flavours become detectable is about one-hundredth of that required for sterilization, although the flavour threshold varies with the fat and moisture contents of the product. Irradiation of milk in a frozen state appears to provide the answer. Although the technique has not found any acceptance for processing milk, recently, successful sterilization of ice cream and frozen yoghurt by gamma irradiation at -78°C has been reported. Successful attempts have also been made to inactivate *Listeria* in soft cheeses by irradiation. A treatment dose of 2.6 kGy did not alter the organoleptic properties of camembert cheese and resulted in complete destruction of inoculated *L. monocytogenes*. Irradiation has been found to enhance the sensory quality of Domiati and Kareish cheeses.

Irradiation under inert atmosphere or vacuum, or in the presence of added antioxidants (ascorbyl palmitate or a combination of butylated hydroxyanisole and butylated hydroxytoluene) rduces the development of oxidative flavour defects. Although overall acceptability of the flavour of irradiated products is lower than that of the non-irradiated products, specific flavour notes are maintained in the strongly flavoured products after irradiation and these can even mask irradiation induced off-flavours.

Irradiation bleaches milk fat due to oxidation of the β-carotene. It also increases the sensitivity of the dairy products to non-enzymatic browning. However, this can be minimized by irradiating the food product in the frozen state. Ionizing radiation treatment causes considerably higher losses of certain vitamins in the dairy products than does heat treatment. The nutritive value of milk proteins is not significantly impaired by irradiation treatments of up to 10-15 kGy.

Combination treatments The combined effect of irradiation and other modes of preservation can be used to ensure microbial safety and also to prevent the development of undesirable sensory and chemical changes in dairy foods. Modified atmosphere packaging, vacuum packaging, barrier films, temperature manipulation before, during or after irradiation treatment and chemical preservatives can be used effectively in conjunction with irradiation treatment to extend shelf life.

References

Cheryan, M. 1998. Ultrafiltration and Microfiltration Handbook, Technical Publishing Co. USA.

Datta, N. and Deeth, H.C. 2003. High-pressure processing

Dharma Pal, 1993. Membrane technologies: Principles of ultrfiltration. *Encyclopaedia of Food Science, Food Technology and Food Nutrition*. Academic Press, London pp. 2975.

Jost, R. and Jelen, P 1997. Crossflow microfiltration- an extension of membrane processing of milk and whey. *IDF Bull.* 320:9.

Larsen, P.H. 1996. Microfiltration for pasteurized milk. *IDF Special Issue* 9602:232.

Roberts, J.J. 1994. Membrane Tech., Basic Principles, latest developments and applications. *Food Industries*, 47(4):24.

Samuelsson, G. , Dejmek, P., Tragarth, G. and Paulsson, M. 1997. rennet coagulation of heat-treated retentate from crossflow microfiltration of skimmilk. *Milchwissenschaft* 52:187.

□□□□

7

Packaging and Distribution of Milk

Packaging means a coordinated system of preparation of goods for distribution, storage, merchandizing and shipment at optimum cost compatible with the requirements of the product. It also includes the art, science and technique used, preparatory to and during transportations and selling of goods and technical methods and work processes related to the above preparations.

The broad range of dairy products necessitates that packaging equipment and materials encompass nearly all types from flexible to rigid and from high to low barrier. The general types of packaging and equipment are discussed below with a focus on fluid products but it must be recognized that other dairy products such as cheese have their own particular packaging requirements and technologies.

Role of packaging in distribution and sale: The essence of what makes milk and dairy products important source of human nutrition also causes rapid deterioration and high perishability. The major role of dairy packaging is to retard the deterioration by preventing microbial recontamination and excessive chemical deterioration. Fluid products are especially susceptible to microbial, enzymatic and chemical degradation. In addition to retarding quality loss, packaging must provide containment, facilitate use, identify products, communicate, and appeal to consumers, all with maximum production efficiency. The large volumes and low unit value means that these functions must be met with minimal economic cost and environmental impact. Because food packaging is generally highly regulated, legal requirements must also be understood and met.

Selection of packaging material: It is essential to know the nature and composition of the product, its desired shelf life under specified conditions of storage in terms of light, temperature, humidity, presence of oxygen and the types and causes of deterioration including mechanical stress, the product may undergo during handling and storage. The packaging material must not impart its own odour to the product. It should be inert to food and non-toxic. The consumer expects that the package should not only protect the product but also give information about the contents, storage conditions, methods of use, date of manufacture and expiry, price and nutritional considerations.

Product shelf life: Many dairy products including fluid milk can be classified on the basis of desired shelf life. Typically the package materials and processes are substantially different from each classification. For fluid milk the classifications are:

1. Conventionally pasteurized, refrigerated milk has a shelf life of approximately 10-20 days. The major issues include light protection, filling line speeds, size, prevention of recontamination and container and filling costs.
2. Pasteurized extended shelf life (ESL) milk (20-60 days) has the same considerations as above but the recontamination from both the container material and filling process become critical. Typically, containers and equipment may be pretreated with UV light, hydrogen peroxide baths, ionizing irradiation, or combinations prior to filling. Often the filling equipment is fully contained and treated with biocide agent prior to packaging.
3. UHT-aseptic ambient stored milks (shelf life up to 12 months) have an intended shelf life of months under ambient conditions and so in addition to recontamination, oxygen barrier considerations become critical. In most cases, containers for aseptically packaged milk are structured with a high-barrier material such as aluminium foil or high-barrier polymer.

Protection of product flavour: The nature of the product and its primary modes of deterioration must be considered. Packaging must protect the flavour of dairy products. This is most often a problem in fluid products. There are number of flavour package-related problems, the most common of which may be the development of off-flavours due to exposure to light. Light causes the formation of 'light-struck' off-flavours. Packaging can also allow the transfer of odours such as stored foods (onions) or distribution odours (diesel fumes). Packages made from substandard materials or overheated during formation can transfer odours to products. For example, ink can transfer solvent odours to products where the exterior of the material contacts the interior during container manufacture or storage. Polymer- based materials can transfer plastic-like odours if overheated.

In long shelf life aseptic products where oxidation is a problem very high- barrier materials may be required. All polymers permeate oxygen (and other vapours such as water) at a defined rate that varies over a three-magnitude range. The effect of oxygen ingress has been investigated for products such as aseptic milk and cheeses but the effect of barrier on refrigerated products is less defined. Inhibiting oxygen ingress in cheeses inhibits mould growth and oxidation in shelf-stable (i.e. long shelf life) milk. Shelf-stable milk is often packaged in materials containing a layer of aluminium foil to reduce ingress to a minimum.

Prevention of postprocessing contamination: Perhaps the most important consideration for selecting dairy packaging is its direct effect on product quality and safety. Many dairy products and especially fluid products such as milk are treated, usually by heat, to inactivate pathogenic and spoilage microorganisms. As mentioned above, packaging must not directly or indirectly allow postprocessing contamination with pathogenic or spoilage microorganisms. This means that microbiological considerations are important in the package manufacturing process and form of the package. For example, the spore load in polymer-coated paper board materials must be considered, especially if the cut edge of the material directly contacts milk. This could allow direct transfer of spores to the product. Bottles must be treated to prevent contamination after blow-moulding. This has become more critical in recent years as aseptic and ESL dairy products have become important. The equipment and materials must often have the capacity to be thoroughly sanitized or sterilized prior to filling.

Distribution: Packaging must reliably meet the rigours of distribution and have sufficient mechanical strength. This factor becomes more important as distribution time and distances become longer. Packaging systems are commonly subjected to laboratory analysis to determine their shock, vibration and crush resistance using standardized testing equipment.

Cost: Economic costs are made up of package unit costs, marketing costs (product distribution and storage costs) and packaging process costs (equipment and operation). Typically, higher barrier and higher container weight are most costly. Smaller containers are more costly than large on an equal unit of product basis because surface-to-volume ratio is higher in small than in large containers. Features such as reclosure, light barriers and unique shape further add to cost. Filling equipment represents large capital costs as well as a significant operating cost.

7.1. Packaging Materials for Fluid Milk

Milk has been packaged in several types of containers across the globe. The general requirements of a milk packaging container are as follows:

- It must be tamper-proof, so that it is protected against fraudulent practices between the time of packaging and consumption.
- It must be of such a size that the capacity always relates to the keeping quality of the product and that its contents correspond to the consumer's daily requirements.
- It must be clean and attractive.

Glass bottles for milk were introduced back at the beginning of the 20th century. Since 1960 other packages have entered the milk market, mainly paperboard packages but also plastic bottles and plastic pouches. It may either be used once (single-use) or may be returned to the processing plant for reuse.

Single-use packaging materials: These are also classified as flexible packaging. They, as the name suggests, are used to package milk once and are discarded after removing the product. The consumer is responsible for disposing off the packages. They have been in the news in recent times due to difficulty in their disposal and their role in environmental pollution.

Plastic pouches: Flexible plastic material can be made into pouch packs. As they are not self-supporting, they generally need some secondary packaging. The advantages offered by the plastic packages are: good barrier properties, visibility of the contents, light weight (thus reducing the cost of transportation), single–service, thus eliminating the need for return, washing and sanitation, easy to carry, economical and can be made more attractive.

The most commonly used plastic material for pouches is polyethylene (PE). There are several types of polyethylene available and are characterized by their density. These are low density (LDPE, 0.91-0.925 g/cm^3), medium density (MDPE, 0.926-0.941 g/cm^3) and high density (HDPE, 0.942-0.970 g/cm^3). The material has good moisture barrier properties, but poor oxygen barrier characteristics. HDPE is the least permeable to moisture. PE is suitable both for rigid and flexible packaging, though for some applications, it must be combined with an oxygen barrier. Sealed packages have the commonality of requiring an internal heat seal layer so that pouch can be heat sealed. The degree of barrier and thickness of each layer varies from approximately 25-75 μm. Most are transparent but in some cases opaque. They may be roughly divided on the basis of oxygen and/or water vapour transmission rates into high-, moderate- and low barrier materials.

Flexible pouches are also made from a derivative of polyvinyl chloride (PVC) in the plasticized form (PPVC). It contains plasticizers to render it flexible and stabilizers to prevent thermal and UV light degradation of the product. However, there has been some controversy regarding its toxicity owing to the high chloride content and additives present.

The use of plastic pouches eliminates noise pollution in the milk bottling plants and during delivery, and also reduces water pollution caused by milk residues and detergents used in the bottle washing. However, they have the disadvantage of poor recyclability and hence, their disposal is a problem.

Carton: The history of the beverage carton is closely associated to the development in milk distribution. The first carton was patented in 1915 in USA as a 'folded blank box'. Cartons generally have a squire or rectangular cross-section. Tetrahedral and other shapes are also seen, but very rarely. These are manufactured by well-developed systems. They are high-technology packaging formats and need well-trained operators to ensure efficient filling of the product. The serving size is also important while designing the package. A 200 or 250 ml single–service package may be marketed with a straw and if a multi-serve (say, 1 litre), some sort of reclosable feature should be provided. These kinds of packaging materials are normally used for long-life products that need not be refrigerated during storage.

The form-and-fill types of cartons are normally used for milk. They are normally received as rolls of heat-sealable packaging material. The material is laminated paper, consisting of duplex kraft paper coated with PE inside and wax outside. A sandwitched layer of thin aluminium foil between an outer craft paper and inner PE coating is also prevalent.

The advantages of carton packaging are as follows: They are lightweight and compact shape, thus increasing distribution efficiency, made from renewable raw material (wooden fibre), hygienic, one-way containers, so no need for cleaning before or after filling operation, hence decreasing water and detergent use, recyclable and easy to dispose off.

The distinct disadvantage also is the felling of trees for making the raw material. However, it is a renewable source and can be regenerated with the help of strict laws and effective management. In the forest of Scandinavia and North America, from where the raw material is procured, for every tree cut, three new trees have to be planted.

Paper and paper-board materials: The paper board has the advantage of being in most cases the least expensive structural material for packaging and a renewable source. A number of treatments are used to protect the paperboard in the high humidity environment. The most common is to coat with polyethylene on both sides. The material is commonly used in rigid and semirigid cartons for fluids and as wraps for solids. High-barrier layers such as foil or poly (vinylalcohol) (EVOH) are commonly added for products such as aseptic milk, which requires extended shelf life and protection from excessive oxygen ingress. These multilayer laminates are relatively complicated and may be composed of seven or more distinct layers. Recently, hybrid composite containers that may be part rigid polymer and part coated paperboard have appeared in the dairy case.

Several kinds of paper-based materials are used in the form of wrappers, cartons, boxes, bags and cups, while boards are used as carton and boxes. These materials are made of bleached or unbleached kraft paper, grease-proof paper, vegetable parchment paper, gassine paper, wax-coated paper, plastic-coated paper, straight or corrugated paper boards, solid fibre boards, liner boards and box boards. While boxes and cartons are used generally for packaging products other than fluid milk, they may sometimes be useful in constructing the outer casing material (secondary packaging) for long distance transportation of flexible pouches.

Multiple - use packaging materials: Of the possible pack-types, bottles are the most commonly used multiuse packages. They can be made of glass and plastic. Metal bottles have also recently emerged for specialist markets, but they are rare and expensive.

Glass: Glass is one of the earliest commercial dairy packaging materials and still used in some markets. Glass containers come in the form of bottles, jars, jugs and tumblers. They may be plain and transparent or coloured and opaque. While the plain glass bottle provides the advantage of direct viewing of the product contained in it, it has the disadvantage of exposing the milk to ultraviolet rays that deteriorate it. Glass has many virtues, but also has several disadvantages that limit its use as a packaging material for milk. The advantages are as follows: strong and inert material, good closure and decorative options, raw materials easily available, recycling possible, excellent gas and water barrier properties, quality image, product compatibility, good internal pressure resistance and reuse opportunity. The disadvantages of glass are that it requires large amount of energy to form, being heavy, brittle and leaving dangerous shards when broken.

Plastic: Plastic bottles for milk are generally made with ribs to add strength. This additional tenacity is needed for withstanding the vacuum on filling machines, for resisting the lateral forces that act within the pack and during transit. Plastic bottles for milk are common in the developed countries and are yet to catch up in India. Plastic has the distinct disadvantage of making recycling difficult.

The most common forms are made of high-density polyethylene (HDPE) blow-moulded jugs and single-serve containers. HDPE has the advantages of low cost, and is easily formed into containers of sufficient strength to make containers to hold several litres of product. HDPE is also used extensively for cups for yoghurt and similar products. HDPE is often filled with minerals such as calcium carbonate or titanium dioxide to make the material opaque and white. Blow-moulding has the advantage that proprietary shapes can be formed at relatively low cost.

Polyethyleneterphthalate (PET) which is the primary material for plastic soft-drink and water bottles, has recently become widely used for blow-moulded single-serve milk containers. PET is significantly more expensive than HDPE but has high clarity and consumer appeal. Polypropylene is similar in some ways to HDPE but withstands higher temperatures and is commonly used to form tubs and lids for products such as cottage cheese and yoghurt.

Polycarbonate is expensive relative to other materials but has been used for refillable jugs.

Polyacrylonitrile polymers have also been proposed for use with milk but costs and other factors have limited actual use. They have the following disadvantages:

- Poor oxygen barrier properties in polyethylene,
- Less clarity than PET, though not very apparent,
- PVC is brittle (especially at low temperature) and breaks on impact.

Materials used for bulk supply: Milk is packaged for bulk and institutional supplies in cans made of stainless steel or aluminium and of capacity of 20 or 40 litres. These are robust and offer excellent product protection. However, there is little opportunity to differentiate one product from the other and branding/labeling is the only alternative.

PET containers are also used in Western countries, but they require some form of separate strap or handle. Milk is also sold in cafes and caterers in the Western countries in large 22 or 40-litre packs in the form of bag-in box. The short life of fluid milk allows the bag to be produced from PE in two layers, each of 50 micrometer thickness.

7.2. Processes for Packaging Fluid Milk

Process for single-use packaging: The pouch filling machine is an integral part of modern fluid milk plants. Several types of plastic materials used in forming the pouches. The material generally comes in the form of rolls, which are loaded on to the machine. The layer of plastic is folded vertically and sealed. A horizontal sealer seals the bottom of the pouch. Simultaneously, milk from an overhead float tank is siphoned into the formed cylinder. It is then again horizontally sealed at the top and cut off to form a pouch filled with milk. These machines come in adjustable filling heads capable of filling several volumes of milk as the need be.

Processes for multiple-use packaging: The filling of milk in glass bottles was an important operation in the fluid milk plant till recent times when the sachet-packing systems gained popularity for several reasons. However, inspite of the weight of the bottle and the problems regarding the return and cleaning of bottles before refilling, it has several advantages such as ease of cleaning and ease of visual detection of spoilage and impurities.

The bottle- filling process is a cycle of events that follow one another. Clean bottles are filled in the bottle-filling machine and capped (generally with aluminium foil caps). The filled bottles are stacked in crates and sent to cold storage. The crates of empty bottles, after selling the product are returned to the plant. The crates are emptied and cleaned separately. The bottles go to the bottle washer, where the broken/chipped bottles are discarded and the cleaned, disinfected bottles are returned to the bottle-filling machine.

Processes for bulk supply: The milk for bulk supply is generally processed and filled in containers manually. These may be cans of PET containers. Bulk milk is also sometimes supplied in small tankers or vans fitted with SS tanks.

In the modern dairying countries where the bag-in-box-type of containers is used, the bags, which have a separate bung with a flexible tube attached, are supplied to the producers. The dairy owners use semi-automatic filling machines to fill directly into the box. When delivered to the caterers the filled box fits into a custom-built refrigeration unit with a pre-fitted, simple on–off tap. The tube on the bag is fed around the tap and cut off to open the bag and permit product to be dispensed.

Storage of processed milk: While designing a milk plant, adequate amenities must be provided for storing packaged milk in terms of area as well as facilities such as refrigeration. Space would also be required for storing packaging materials, whether they be empty bottles and crates or rolls of packaging films.

7.3. Storage of Bulk Milk

Insulated tanks: Bulk milk after processing, is stored in insulated storage tanks in the dairy plant till distribution. The milk remains in chilled condition. It is recommended that milk be transported to the place of delivery as soon as possible. However, due to limitations of infrastructure, milk is stored for periods ranging from 4-12 hrs after processing.

Cans: processed milk for bulk supply is also sometimes stored in cans. Since the beginning of the second half of last century aluminium milk cans have replaced mild steel cans that were used earlier. The most common are cans with lids which do not require rubber gaskets for sealing. An adequate sealing arrangement is achieved with sunken grip or mushroom lids. Lids attached to the cans by chains are no longer used owing to problems in mechanical washing. Lead or other seals can be applied through simple arrangements at the lid ring to avoid tampering and pilferage. Normally floor conveyors are used to transport cans from one place to another in the processing area of the dairy plant.

Full cans are stored in one layer, thus permitting about 320 to 360 litres of milk to be stored per square metre excluding movement and working space. Empty cans after washing are stacked in layers horizontally, up to a height of 1.5 metre. For storing and moving washed empty cans simple trolleys on which the cans can be stored in 4-5 layers are very useful.

Storage of milk packed in multiple-use packages

Storage in bottles: Bottles with wide necks (36-40 mm), suitable for sealing with aluminium foil caps are most commonly used for packaging of pasteurized milk in multi-use containers. The filled bottles are placed in plastic crates. These were earlier made of galvanized steel wires or strips, but plastic is in vogue these days. The crates have internal divisions so that the bottles are not in contact with one another to minimize risk of breakage. They are designed to interlock, so that a stable stack can be built. Crates with filled bottles are stacked 5 or 6 high for one-litre and half-litre bottles, respectively for manual handling. Two to three crates more can be put in one stack for empty bottles. Crates can generally hold twenty half-litre and twelve to fifteen one-litre bottles. The stacks can be moved manually or by hand trolleys. There is no international standards for the dimensions of pasteurized milk bottles and crates.

Bottles used for in-bottle milk sterilization have narrower necks (26 mm) than the pasteurized milk bottles so that a more effective seal can be made. Prefabricated crown seals are used to seal the bottles. The requirements with regard to sturdiness during mechanical and thermal shocks are higher than those of a pasteurized milk bottles. The bottles are packed in crates as is done for the pasteurized milk bottles. The bottles are packed in crates as is done for the pasteurized milk bottles. The stacking system and the resulting storage area required are also similar. As with pasteurized milk, dimensions differ from country to country but a neck diameter of 26 mm is universal.

Storage of milk in single-use packages: The common feature of single-use containers are that they are discarded after emptying. This fact has an important bearing on the milk plant construction, organization and on the economics of the whole business. There is no collection and washing of the milk packages. Only the crates that carry the filled milk packages are collected and washed. Single-service delivery wraps, trays and boxes may also replace these. Intermediate storage of packaging materials and filled packages has to be organized at the plant.

Storage in pouches: The pillow-shaped sachets of pasteurized milk are collected in tubs after they are cut and separated from the packaging machine. They are placed in rectangular plastic crates holding 20 packages each and the crates are then stacked. Thus with crates stacked 10-high containing ½ litre sachets the store capacity without space for entry, movement and working is about 500, 600 l/$m^{2.}$ Both 1-litre and ½ litre packages have the same width and thickness (0.09 m). Varying the distance between transverse seals facilitates changing the capacity. It is important that the film is free from pinholes so as to avoid leakage, particularly when subjected to pressure from the adjoining pouches in the crates.

Storage in cartons: In several countries, pasteurized milk is packaged in cartons on similar lines as UHT milk. These may shape as rectangular block or tetrahedron. Rectangular cartons are normally used for UHT milk, though this is not a strict regulation. The tetrahedral packages, after filling, are placed in hexagonal plastic crates holding 18 cartons each. The crates are then stacked normally 6-high. Thus with 6-high stack of crates containing ½ litre cartons, the storage capacity excluding the area required for entry and working is about 500 l/m^2.

Empty crates for tetrahedral cartons are normally stacked 15-high. The crates occupy less space when empty, as they are tapered. Rectangular crates occupy the same space empty or full. The quantity of raw stock to be stored depends on the location of the milk plant and the paper supplier and also the purchasing power of the producer. It is generally necessary to carry two to three months' stock.

7.4. Distribution of Processed Milk

There are many methods and regulations for the distribution or retailing of milk, depending on the country and type of milk that is being distributed. The dairy industry does not invest in liquid milk retailing in most countries, other than for promotion and demonstration centres and automatic vending machines. The grocers sell and some times distribute the milk delivered by the plant. They charge a little extra (the retail margin) over the milk plant price for their services. In countries where the milk plant delivers milk directly to consumers, the plant absorbs the retail margin. There is no common system for establishing retail margins. They vary considerably between countries and sometimes, even between localities within the same country due to variation in cost of labour, transport and capital.

Distribution of bulk milk

Distribution in cans: Bulk milk may be distributed to institutions such as catering establishments, university hostels and hospitals in cans. These cans are filled in the dairy plant directly from the tanks in which milk is stored, either by pumps or by gravity filling. They are then transported to the consumers in appropriate vehicles (tempos, trucks, *etc*). The consumer empty the cans into their own storage systems and return the cans immediately. Alternatively, the cans may be retained and the previous time's empty and cleaned cans are returned to the vehicle to transport to the dairy plant. This cycle is maintained. It is important that the cans are cleaned again in the dairy plant even if they have been cleaned at the consumer's location.

Distribution in automatic vending machines: The sale of milk in bulk through automatic vending machines has been introduced successfully in Mexico and India. The system does not involve retail packaging by the milk plant as the consumer provides his own container. Thus, the milk is handled in bulk up to the point of retail sale. This eliminates the cost of packaging and there is substantial saving in running cost. The milk plant sells milk directly to the consumer and so, there is no need for middlemen or a distribution network.

A tanker delivers the refrigerated pasteurized milk to the vending station housed in a simple building. This consists of a refrigerated room in which the milk storage tank of the requisite capacity is placed at a high level. A small service room for the clean-in place (CIP) equipment is essential. Office or storage facilities may also be required. The milk is pumped from the tanker to the storage tank. From there, it is discharged as required by the customer through the coin- or token operated dispensers as shown in Fig 7.4.1.

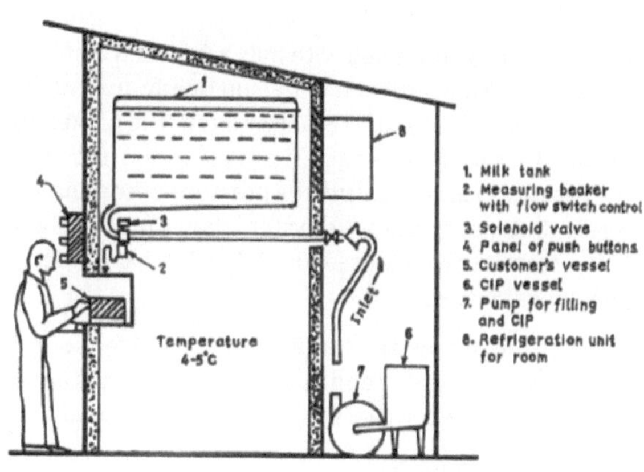

Fig. 7.4.1. Automatic milk vending equipment

Distribution of milk packed in multiple-use packages: The proper working of the distribution system involving reuse of containers, mostly glass bottles, depends entirely on how effectively the empty bottles are retrieved. There are normally three ways in which this is done:

In the first case, the milk may be delivered to the customer's doorstep and empty bottles recovered at the same time. This system has the advantage that it can work even in the customer's absence. The payment may be collected after a set period of time, say once per week.

Secondly, vehicles carrying the packaged milk may tour the customers' locality with many stops in each street. They normally announce their presence by blowing the horn or any other audible signal. The customers come to the vehicle bringing empty bottles. The customers need to pay a deposit on empty bottles, normally equal to the cost of the bottle. If they require more full bottles than the number of empties they return, extra deposits must be paid. If they require less a corresponding credit is allowed.

In the third method, milk may be sold only from shops to which the customer should go to purchase milk. A similar system as before, for paying a deposit on the bottles prevails here also.

Distribution of milk packed in single-use packages: Single-use packages offer the advantage of doing away with the cleaning-collecting-returning-cleaning routine that is needed for the multiple –use containers. Out of several distribution methods, the most commonly used is stacking of the filled packages in crates. Sometimes they are also wrapped in non-returnable materials. Crating has already been mentioned in the section dealing with pasteurized milk in tetrahedral cartons. For single-use transport packaging, shrink-film is most often used. This wrapping can be applied manually or mechanically. This system is used where short storage times and short distribution distances are involved. This has the disadvantage that the film does not give much mechanical support to the packages. Cartons wrapped in shrink-on film are often susceptible to damage, leakage and contamination, especially when handled manually. Special (perforated) shrink-films may be required in areas with high humidity to prevent condensation.

Rectangular cartons filled with milk are placed first on a flat tray blank in groups of twelve. The sides of the blank are then folded up tightly around the cartons. Thus, the pressure-absorbing ability of the filled cartons is fully utilized. The packed corrugated tray is then wrapped in shrink-on film, thus protecting against dust and moisture. It also presses the sides of the tray towards the cartons so as to improve the pressure-absorbing ability of the corrugated tray. This method is safe, but more expensive system than the shrink-wrap. The units can be handled manually. This system is normally used for UHT milk, which is to be stored for longer periods and distributed over longer distances.

Comparison of bulk and retail sale of milk: The merits and demerits of either of these systems depend on the locality and attitude of consumers and the type of milk being sold. Some of the differences between two systems are enumerated below:

1. Although pasteurized milk can be sold in bulk, sterilized and UHT milk cannot be sold without packaging.
2. Packaged milk is measured accurately.
3. Milk sold in bulk is amenable to adulteration at different levels such as during transportation as well as vending.

4. Keeping quality of pasteurized milk depends on maintaining a 'cold chain' throughout its distribution network. If milk that leaves the plant at temperatures much below 10°C in insulated vehicles and is kept by the retailer under refrigeration, the quality of milk is bound to be much better than the bulk-vended milk, particularly in cans.

The sale of milk in automatic vending machines ensures the continuity of the cold chain. However, there may be a need to redesign or reconstruct buildings to accommodate the equipment, which is often difficult in crowded cities. In Mexico and India, where this system is in operation, it is considered a success and has the full support of every group of customers. The equipment generally comes in capacities of 1000 and 2000 litres. The machine needs to be developed further, in order to make them more suitable to varying conditions and requirements.

Aseptic packaging

Aseptic packaging is a relatively new concept aimed at developing new product group, namely pre-sterilized and aseptically packaged foods. During aseptic packaging process, a pre-sterilized and sterile product is filled under sterile conditions into sterile packages in a sterile environment and then germ proof sealed.

Aseptic packaging is synonymous globally as brand for safe, hygienic, healthy, longer shelf life and nutritious food. Aseptic packages are the most environment friendly, energy efficient, recyclable, convenient to store, transport and handle. All the Good Manufacturing Practices (GMP) and HACCP procedures are strictly followed in aseptic processing and packaging.

The history of aseptic packaging goes back to the early 20th century. The first aseptic packaging of food specifically milk in metal cans was carried out in Denmark by Nielsen prior to 1913 and a patent for this process (termed aseptic conservation) was granted in 1921. In 1923, aseptically packaged milk from South Africa reached a trade fair in London, England in perfect condition. Aseptic processing first appeared in 1927 while the first patent was granted in 1936. It was in 1940s that the aseptic packaging industry moved into the worldwide market; aseptic technology provided safe, shelf-stable beverages to World War II troops across Europe. Commercial application of the technology was made extensively only after the introduction of aseptic packaging and flexible packages in the 1960s. Within a few years, the aseptic carton was to become a staple of food and beverage packaging around the globe. In the early 1960s, the Tetra Pak became the first company in the world to market aseptic packaging technology and more than 80% of aseptically packed products are from Tetra Pak systems.

Aseptic packaging system meets every requirement of food packaging, *viz.* product containment and protection, food safety, shelf life, a surface for the communication of information, sales appeal and a good value for the cost. Aseptic packaging offers advantages to the consumer (improved product quality, freshness) as well as to distributor (lower distribution and storage costs, more appropriate shelf life, relief of pressure on chilled cabinet, cost effective and free from additives). The aseptic packaging allows liquid foods and beverages to retain the colour, flavour, texture and nutrients that the nature intended, without the addition of preservatives. The growth of aseptically processed and packaged products is in part driven by the increasing cost of refrigeration and chilled storage space, as well as legislation that more tightly controls cold storage temperature fluctuation. Most products available today in retail and food service, aseptic packaging is applied for liquid based foods and beverages. For sometime, aseptic packaging has been associated with juice, milk, soy beverages and teas. Increasingly, other foods such as tomatoes, syrups and tofu are joining the ranks of aseptically packaged foods. The size of the global market for aseptic milk products has since grown rapidly and is now estimated to be in excess of 25 billion litres of product annually.

Requirements of Aseptic Packaging Systems: The major requirement of an aseptic packaging system is to prevent recontamination of the sterilized product. The principal consideration in this regard include the sterilization of the filling machine and packaging material by suitable physical and/or chemical means and maintaining aseptic barriers during filling and sealing. Besides the equipment and packaging, gas used to pressurizing the filling space is one of the sources of recontamination of the processed foods. Thus, mechanical failures such as inadequate heating of the gas, leaks in valves and pinholes in filters may cause recontamination and must therefore be checked.

Packaging Materials: The packaging materials for food products must provide containment, protection, preservation and consumer information. These basic requirements are true for all packaging methods, including aseptic process. Consumers and food-service providers are also looking for convenient, cost-effective, appealing and environmentally compatible packaging materials.

Paperboard cartons: Such packaging materials are commonly used in aseptic filling systems for milk, cream, fruit juices, soups, *etc*. The filling systems could be either of the following two types: those in which carton is formed within the filler from a continuous reel of material, and those in which cartons are supplied as pre-formed blanks, folded flat, which are assembled into cartons in the filler. The packaging material is mainly composed of printed-paper coated with aluminium foil and several plastic layers (polyethylene-paper board-polyethylene-aluminium foil-polyethylne) (Fig.7.4.2). The inner side of the finished package is coated with a special layer facilitating the sealing process. Each layer has specific function:

- The outer polyethylene layer protects the ink and enables the sealing process of the package flaps.
- The paperboard serves as a carrier of the décor and gives the package required mechanical strength.
- The laminated polyethylene binds the aluminium to the paper.
- The aluminium foil acts as a gas and light barrier.
- The inner polyethylene layer provides liquid barrier.

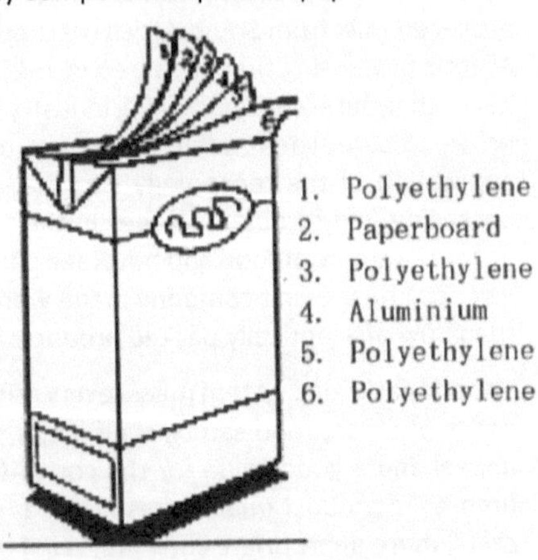

Fig. 7.4.2. Structure of a paperboard carton

The box shaped package is a laminate of up to four materials: high quality paperboard, polyethylene, adhesive polymer and aluminium foil. Each material plays a critical role in achieving the unique benefits of the aseptic package. Paper accounts for 70% of the package and provides stiffness, strength and the efficient brick shape. Twenty-four per cent of the package is polyethylene or adhesive polymer. The innermost polyethylene layer forms the seals that make the package liquid-tight, while an exterior layer keeps the package dry. The adhesive polymer acts as the glue layer between the aluminium foil and the inner polyethylene layer. Aluminium foil, at 6% of the package forms a barrier against light and oxygen.

These materials comprise the six layers of the package in the following order from the outside in: polyethylene, paper, polyethylene, aluminium foil, adhesive polymer and polyethylene, all of which are designed to work together to keep the products fresh. The inside layer of an aseptic package, which touches the product, is polyethylene not aluminium. The polyethylene used in the aseptic package- low density polyethylene (LDPE)- is a US Food and Drug Administration (FDA) – approved food-contact surface material. The aseptic packaging industry tests LDPE and has determined that LDPE does not leach into the product contained in aseptic cartons. Moreover, there is no leaching of aluminium or aluminium components through the plastic layer. It cannot degrade through exposure to heat or light. Residual monomer in any food packaging material must be minimized or eliminated, as any chemical transformations are unacceptable.

Aseptic packaging is a great example of up-front source reduction, reducing the amount of material produced at the source, so there is a less for the consumer to throw away or recycle. An aseptic package is typically 96% beverage to 4% packaging by weight. Compared with other types of packages, this product to package ratio illustrates that the aseptic carton is very efficient package that can help minimize solid waste. In fact, it also compares favourably to other single serve containers on a volume basis, accounting far less volume than many other single serve beverage packages: by weight, plastic bottles are 95% product to 5% packaging; steel cans are 87% product to 13% packaging; and glass bottles are 71% product to 29% packaging.

Many of the same characteristics that make aseptic packages an excellent example of source reduction also help conserve energy. Aseptic packages are among the most energy efficient beverage packages on the market today due to their lightweight, innovative brick shape, and unique filling process. These packages begin saving energy even before they are filled. Empty packages are stored flat or on rolls, rather preformed like glass, metal and most plastic containers. As a result, one standard semi-trailer truck can transport 1.5 million empty aseptic cartons versus only 1,50,000 glass bottles. In addition, because aseptic products do not need refrigeration, storage and distribution are cheaper and selling paths can be longer and more varied. Once filled, the aseptic carton's lightweight and compact shape conserves even more energy in transport. The block shape is space-efficient and, because the aseptic package is lightweight, more products can be shipped in fewer trucks. In addition, because aseptic packages preserve their contents without refrigeration, no refrigerated trucks, special warehouses, freezers or coolers are needed. This saves utility, shipping and warehousing cost. Aseptic packages use far less energy to deliver the same amount of beverage than other large containers. For example, multi-serve plastic and glass bottles can use three times more energy than aseptic cartons to deliver the same amount of beverage.

Glass: Glass bottles have been used for packaging of many liquid foods but it has not been a commercial success with aseptic filling plants. Glass as such offers protection against oxygen and light if it has been provided with anti-actinic compounds.

Cans: Aseptic canning is expensive, particularly for low cost product like milk. Cans are not preferred for packaging of UHT processed products as the processors and marketers of the product generally want to emphasize the newness of the process whereas cans are identified with conventionally retorted products. The cans may be of tinplate or drawn aluminium: the solder in tinplate cans may have to be of higher melting point than normal to withstand the can sterilization temperatures. Cans pass along a conveyor belt within a continuous tunnel. Tunnel temperature (200-220°C) for sterilization of cans is attained by steam (at atmospheric pressure), superheated with gas flames-sterilization time being 40s normally. Cans having passed through the sterilization tunnel continue through the filling chamber where they are filled with the product. The can lids are sterilized, again by superheated steam, in a separate unit. The lids are applied and seamed in a chamber kept sterile by superheated steam and a flue gas.

Sterilization of Packaging Material and Filler Environment: Three main sterilization processes for packaging material are in common use, either, individually or in combination: irradiation, heat and chemical treatments.

Irradiation

Ionizing radiation: Particle irradiation techniques using gamma rays from cobalt-60 or caesium-137 have been used to sterilize the interior of sealed but empty containers, especially those made of materials that can not withstand the temperature needed for thermal sterilization, or that, because of their shape, could not be sterilized by other means. A radiation dose of 25kGy (2.5 M rad) or more is generally accepted to be sufficient to ensure sterility. The packages are sealed into microbial-proof containers prior to the irradiation treatment. It is also possible to use low energy (100 keV), large area electron beam for the surface sterilization of packaging materials and containers.

Pulsed light: By storing electric energy in capacitor and releasing it in short pulses, high peak power levels can be generated. The use of intense and short-duration pulses of broad spectrum white light to sterilize aseptic packaging material underwent considerable research and development efforts in the 1990s. The duration of pulses ranges from 1μs to 0.1s, and the flashes are typically at the rate of 1-20 flashes per s. approximately 25% of the emitted light, which has an intensity of about 20,000 times that of sunlight at the earth's surface, is UV, 45% visible and 30% infrared. Generally, a few flashes applied in a fraction of a second provide high levels of microbial inactivation.

Heat: Heat sterilization process can involve either stream (moist heat) or dry heat. Steam is pure water with no air or other gases present. Dry heat is hot air in the absence of water molecules. The sterilization effect depends on time and temperature, and steam is much more efficient than dry heat. Steam sterilization at 121°C for 20 min is equivalent in effectiveness to dry heat sterilization at 170°C for 60 min.

Saturated steam: The most reliable sterilant is without doubt steam. However, in order to reach temperature sufficiently high to achieve sterilization in a few seconds, the steam (and thus the packaging material with which it comes into contact) must be under pressure, necessitating the use of a pressure chamber. Also any air that enters the pressure chamber with the packaging material must be removed otherwise it would interfere with the transfer of heat from the steam to the package surface. Finally, condensation of steam during heating of packaging material surface produces condensate, which may remain in the container and dilute the product.

Despite these problems, saturated steam under pressure is used to sterilize plastic containers. In order to limit the heating effect to internal surface of plastic cups, the exterior of the cups is simultaneously cooled.

Chemical treatments

Hydrogen peroxide: The lethal effect of hydrogen peroxide (H_2O_2) on microorganism (including resistant spores) has been known for many years. The first commercial aseptic filling system was devised in 1961, which used a combination of peroxide and heat to sterilize the surface of carton packaging material. To get rapid sterilization, high concentrations of H_2O_2 and high temperature are needed. Recognized minimum parameters are 30%, at 70°C and for 6 s.

The US Food and Drug Administration has ruled that the concentration of H_2O_2 that may be present in food products packed in material sterilized by H_2O_2 must be no greater than 500 ppb (500 parts in 10^9) at the time of filling and must fall to approximately 1 ppb within 24 h. Since peroxide cannot be measured accurately in food products because of the presence of reducing compounds which rapidly eliminate it. Checks of the initial level must be made on packs filled with water.

A number of systems have evolved to achieve faster peroxide sterilization process by combining heat and radiation. UV radiation has a wavelength of 100-400 nm and the lower part up to 280 nm is biologically active and named UV-C radiation. In terms of microbial destruction, it has peak at 240-280 nm. Mercury vapour lamps emit UV-C at 253.7 nm. UV irradiation and hydrogen peroxide act synergistically when used together, the UV irradiation promoting the breakdown of peroxide into hydroxyl radicals. The advantage of such combination of such that much lower concentrations of peroxide can be used (0.5-5% compared with 30-35% for peroxide and heat together) and the problems of atmospheric contamination by peroxide and residual peroxide in the filled product are reduced.

Peracetic acid: Peracetic acid (PAA) is a liquid sterilant that is particularly effective against spores. It is produced by the oxidation of acetic acid by hydrogen peroxide and is effective against resistant bacterial spores even at 20°C. It is used for sterilizing machine surfaces as well as packaging materials such as polyethylene terephthalate (PET) bottles prior to aseptic filling. The PET bottles are rinsed with sterile water rather than hot water.

Aseptic Packaging Systems: The aseptic packaging system must be capable of filling the sterile product in an aseptic manner and sealing the container hermetically so that the sterility is maintained throughout the handling and distribution processes. Commercial requirements of less than one faulty package out of 10,000 produced are common.

The type of packaging material used is influenced by the nature of the product, the cost of both the product and the package, and the preferences of the consumer. The most widespread consumer package for aseptic products is the paperboard carton. Five major categories of aseptic packaging equipment are available and their major features and characteristics are described below.

Carton systems

The carton material consists of layers of paperboard coated internally and externally with polyethylene, resulting in a carton that is impermeable to liquids and in which the internal and external surfaces may be heat-sealed. There is also a thin (6.3 μm) layer of aluminium foil, which acts as an oxygen, flavour and light barrier.

Form-fill-seal carton: The packaging material is supplied in rolls that have been printed and creased, the latter being necessary to ease the forming process. A plastic strip is sealed to one edge and the packaging material sterilized using one of two procedures: a wetting system or a deep bath system. In the wetting system, a thin H_2O_2 film (15-35% concentration) containing a wetting agent to improve the formation of a liquid film is applied on the inner packaging material surface. The material then passes through a pair of rollers to remove excess liquid and is formed and sealed into a cylinder. It then passes under a tubular electric heater, which heats the inside surface to about 120°C and evaporates the H_2O_2. In the deep bath system, the packaging material is fed through a deep bath containing H_2O_2 (35% concentration) at a minimum of 70°C, the residence time being 6 s. After squeezer rollers have removed much of the peroxide, air at 125°C is directed through nozzles on to both sides of the material to evaporate the peroxide.

The sterilized packaging material is fed into a machine where it is formed into a tube and closed at the longitudinal seal by a heat-sealing element. In the process, the strip that was added prior to sterilization is heat- sealed across the inner surface of the longitudinal seal to prevent contact between the outside and the inside of the carton. It also provides protection of the aluminium and paperboard layers from the product, which could corrode or swell the layers if such a strip were absent.

Product is then filled into the tube and a transverse seal made below the level of the product, thus ensuring that the package is completely filled. Alternatively, the packages may be produced with a head- space of up to 30% of the total filling volume by the injection of either sterile air or other sterile inert gases. The sterilization, filling and sealing processes are all performed inside a chamber that has undergone sterilization prior to production and is maintained at an overpressure of 0.5 atm with sterile air.

Prefabricated cartons: In systems of this type, prefabricated carton blanks are used, the cartons being die-cut, creased and the longitudinal seam completed at the factory of origin by skiving the inner layer of board and folding it back. The cartons are delivered to the processor in lay-flat form ready to be finally shaped in the filler and the top and bottom seams formed and bonded.

The aseptic area of the filling machine consists of several separate functional zones where operations are carried out in sequence. Sterility is maintained in each zone by a slight overpressure of sterile air. The inside surface of the carton is sterilized with a 35% solution of H_2O_2, delivered either as a fine spray or as peroxide vapour in hot air so that the vapour condenses as liquid peroxide on the carton surface. The peroxide is removed by a jet of hot air at 170-200° C.

After filling, the carton top is folded and closed, the seal being made either by heating or ultrasonic welding. The protruding flaps or 'ears' on each side are folded down and sealed to the package with hot air. The finished cartons are then discharged from the pocket chain on to a conveyor belt.

Plastics: For many years, blow-moulded plastic bottles made from high-density polyethylene or polypropylene have been used, sometimes with pigments added to give greater protection to the contents against light. It is also possible to mould bottles from multilayered materials, resulting in much improved barrier properties and thus longer shelf-lives for the products packaged in them. Very recently, aseptic PET systems capable of packaging dairy products have been commercialized.

Three different types of systems are in use:

Nonsterile bottles: After blowing (either immediately prior to the following steps or on a separate site) the plastic bottles are conveyed into a sterile chamber, which is kept at a slight overpressure with sterile air. The bottles are inverted and sprayed inside and outside with a solution of H_2O_2 or PAA. The H_2O_2 is evaporated by passing the bottles through hot air tunnel prior to filling. Bottles sterilized with PAA are rinsed with sterile water and then filled. A chemically sterilized, heat-sealable closure, such as a plastic film or cap, is then applied.

Sterile blown bottles: Bottles are extruded, blown with sterile air and sealed under conditions that ensure internal sterility. The sealed bottles are then introduced into a sterile chamber (maintained under a slight positive pressure) where the outside surfaces are sterilized with H_2O_2 sprays. The closed top of the bottle is cut away, the neck trimmed, the bottle filled and a foil cap or heat sealable closure that has been sterilized outside the chamber is applied.

Single station blowing, filling and sealing: In this mechanically complex system, the separate operations of parison (the extrusion-or injection-moulded tube from which the moulded containers are blown) extrusion, blow-moulding, bottle-filling and sealing all take place in sequence in a single mould. Sterility of the inside surface of the containers is ensured by the high temperature of the plastics material during extrusion of the parison, and the use of sterile air for blowing. The thermoplastics used for this type of container include high density polyethylene and polypropylene. After filling, the tube projecting from the bottle mould is vacuum-formed or sealed with jaws into a cap which closes the bottle. No special arrangements to ensure sterility are required since the filling and sealing are carried out within the closed mould.

Sachet and Pouch systems

Lay-flat tubing: This system uses a blown film polymer in the form of lay-flat tubing so that only a transverse seal is required to form the bag. The assumption is made that the inside of the tubing is sterile due to the temperature achieved during the extrusion process. Either a single film or a co-extrusion can be used. The tubing is fed from the reel into a sterile chamber in which an overpressure of air is maintained. The sachets are sealed at the bottom, cut and moved to a filling section. After filling they are sealed at the top and leave the chamber through a water seal.

Form-fill-seal pouches: In this system, a vertical form-fill-seal machine operates in a sterile chamber. The packaging material is passed through 35% H_2O_2 and then drained and dried with hot air. The film used is typically a laminate of linear low density polyethylene with a centre layer of ethylene vinyl alcohol copolymer and carbon black to give the pouch the required shelf-life. Typically, the pouch has fin seals on all four sides.

Cup systems

Preformed plastic cups: The cups are usually made from high-impact polystyrene (HIPS), polypropylene or co-extruded, multilayered material if improved barrier properties are required. The cups are fed onto a conveyor that is inside a sterile tunnel supplied with sterile air. The cups are sprayed inside with 35% H_2O_2 and after about 3s the solution is removed with compressed hot air at a maximum temperature of 400°C, depending on the material from which the cups are made. The inside surface of the cups reaches a temperature of about 70°C, which completes surface sterilization and reduces the peroxide residues to acceptable levels.

Cups can also be sterilized by carrying them through a 35% peroxide bath at 85-90° C before heating and passing through a water bath. The cups then enter a sterile chamber where sterilization is completed by spraying with sterile water and drying with hot air.

The sealing material (usually aluminium foil with a thin coating of a thermoplastic to provide sealability) is typically sterilized with a 35% peroxide solution, which is then removed either by radiant heat, hot sterile air or by passing the material over a heated roller. In some systems, UV radiation is used, either alone or in conjunction with peroxide.

Disposal of packaging waste: Packaging waste consists of paper and paper products, glass, metals and plastics. Strategies for handling these components include source reduction, recycling, recovery of energy and landfill. Currently about 10% is recycled, 10% incinerated and remaining 80% finds its way into landfills.

Source reduction: Reducing the input of raw materials and choosing materials that are not environmentally harmful helps to conserve natural resources. This method involves the reduction of both the amount and the toxicity of all materials going into the waste stream. Source reduction includes the use of lighter weight materials that does a comparable job such as cans with less wall thickness, or elimination of unnecessary packaging. For food or ingredient packagers, these can be cost effective measures, translating into lower product shipping costs. Source reduction efforts must be carefully examined since switching from one material to another may lead to only a shift in environmental problems.

Recycling: Recycling involves the collection of used and discarded materials, processing these materials and making them into new products. It reduces the amount of waste that is thrown into the community dustbins thereby making the environment cleaner and air fresher to breathe. Surveys carried out by the government and non-government agencies in the country have all recognized the importance of recycling wastes. The steps involved in the process prior to recycling include: a) collection of wastes from the doorsteps, commercial places, *etc*, b) collection of waste from community dumps, c) collection / picking of waste from final disposal sites.

This method helps in reducing waste going for landfills or incinerators and provides a source of raw materials. But the success of this method depends on the existence of a market for the recycled products. In some areas where recycling efforts are aggressive, there is a glut of scrap material.

When it comes to the recycling of the plastic wastes, there are many problems. A variety of different types of plastics are used. The plastics contain a wide range of additives as well as other materials. The sorting of plastics may be technically difficult, unhygienic and expensive. Recycling of plastic packaging, which makes up about 90% of municipal solid waste, is relatively new. Generally six types of resins are used: polyethylene terephthalate (PET) in soft drink bottles; high density polyethylene (HDPE) in boil-in bag pouches and milk jugs; polyvinyl chloride (PVC) in meat wrap; low density polyethylene (LDPE), polypropylene (PP) in syrup bottles and yoghurt tubs; and polystyrene (PS) in disposable dishes and cups. These plastics may be sorted by type before they can be recycled. To facilitate identification of type, the society of plastic industry has developed an easy to use numerical coding system for use by plastic container manufacturers. Market for recycled plastics include roofing material, package strapping, pipes, yard furniture, automotive parts and flower parts.

Recovery of energy: All packages incorporate energy, which can be extracted when the waste is incinerated. The potential yield depends on the type of packaging material. This method is extremely valuable since it can reduce the amount of waste land filled by 75% or more while generating electricity. Proper use of incineration does not cause air pollution. Burning of paper reduces its volume to about one-ninth, but heavy metals in the printing ink have raised concerns about emissions and ash produced during the process. Plastics burn cleanly when properly incinerated, releasing up to four times more energy than the typical components of solid waste. In spite of the advantages of incineration, the U.S. relies on this method for only about 10% of the solid waste stream. This is low in comparison with other countries such as Switzerland and Japan, which burn 70% of their solid waste for energy production. Paperboard packages are highly suitable for energy recovery. Wood and oil (the raw material for the plastic) are conventional source of energy, and it can be said that we simply borrow these raw materials for packages before using them as fuel. The incineration of two tons of packaging material yields as much energy as one ton of oil. Paperboard packages have very low weight, and their main component comes from a source that is renewable. Compared to most other packages, the amount of waste generated is small. A one-litre Tetra Brik pack weighs 27g and generates only that amount of waste.

Landfill: Although the least desirable method for waste disposal, landfill is the most commonly used. Landfills provide a means of merely getting solid waste out of site by entombing it in the ground devoid of water and oxygen required for decomposition. As a result, even organic waste that decomposes naturally takes years to do so. Plastics, take up only one-tenth the space of paper, hold some merit for land filling. But there is some concern about the possibility of heavy metals such as cadmium or lead being leached. Research is now focusing on development of two types of degradable plastics: photodegradable which degrade when exposed to sunlight, and biodegradable which contain corn starch or vegetable oils and breakdown into small pieces. While degradable plastics may prove to be effective above ground, enhanced degradability will have little effect, if any on landfills.

References

Burton, H. 1988. Ultra-high processing of milk and milk products. London. Elsevier Applied Scinces.

Hochkiss, J. H. and Meunier- Goddik, L. 2003. Packaging. Cited in *Encyclopedia of Dairy Sci.*, vol, IV: 2201.

IDF.1995. Technical guide for the packaging of milk products, 3rd Edn., International Dairy Federation Bull. No. 300, Brussels.

8

Special Milks

When natural constituents of whole milk are altered by addition, removal, exchange and / or treatment, the resultant milk is designated as special milk. Recent years have witnessed a large increase in market penetration of special milks into the total fluid milk market. In many countries, now a large portion of fluid milk is consumed in the form of special milks. Manufacturers of special milks offer numerous advantages that are broadly related to dietary, cost and scarcity aspects. Special milks provide an avenue to diversify the milk with variety of flavours and other characteristics.

Milk is considered as nature's almost perfect food. However, milk in its natural form is not considered suitable for many more healthy people who do not like the taste of milk as such. All these problems can be overcome by manufacturing special mllks such as dietetic milks, low fat milks, flavoured milks, etc.

Butterfat is the most expensive constituent of milk. Therefore, the cost of buffalo whole milk is very high and many people particularly the weaker section of our society cannot afford to buy it. Consequently, manufacture of low priced toned milk was introduced in many markets. This also enabled the dairy plants to meet the ever increasing demand of milk, particularly during lean season. Replacement of butterfat by vegetable fat could also help in reducing the cost of milk

Due to seasonal fluctuation in milk production, there is acute shortage of milk during the lean period in our country. In certain parts of the world fresh milk is not produced at all. Manufacture of reconstituted and recombined milk from anhydrous milk solids can overcome such whole milk shortage. These anhydrous milk solids could either be prepared from the domestic seasonal surplus or marketed from those countries that have surplus milk production. The machinery and manpower of a market milk plant can be fully utilized all the year round by such diversifications.

Classification: Depending on the ingredients used and process employed, special milks can be broadly classified as follows:

i. Plain special milks

ii. Flavoured milks

iii. Vegetable solid–based milks or simulated milks

iv. Miscellaneous milks, e.g. soft-curd milk, humanized milk, vitamin D-milk, etc.

8.I. Plain Special Milks

Plain special milks are also called as designated milks. These milks are prepared only from milk ingredients with or without addition of water, e.g. full cream milk, toned milk, double toned milk, standardized milk, reconstituted milk and recombined milk. These are prepared mainly to extend the fluid milk supply. In the present day situation, preparation of designated milks is inevitable for the market milk plant. These designated milks should confirm to the minimum legal standards prescribed for them.

Full cream milk: Full cream milk means milk, or a combination of cow or buffalo milk or a product which has been prepared by a combination of both, which has been standardized to a fat per cent of 6.0 and solids-not fat (SNF) per cent of 9.0 by adjustment or addition of milk solids. Full cream milk must be pasteurized. It should show a negative phosphatase test. Upon pasteurization, it should be packaged in clean and sanitary containers and should be properly sealed in order to prevent subsequent contamination.

Toned and double toned milk: The definition of toned and double toned milk is given in chapter-1. The toned and double toned milk are prepared as follows:

The toned and double toned milk can be prepared by standardization either by partially skimming the fat in the whole milk with a cream separator or by admixture with fresh or reconstituted skimmilk in a proper proportion. If surplus whole milk is available, calculated amount of fat is partially removed by adjusting cream separator to result in milk with requisite fat and SNF level in toned or double toned milk. The other method for preparation of toned and double toned milk is by mixing calculated amount of skimmilk and whole milk in a tank. The amount of skimmilk and whole milk is calculated by Pearson Square method. In case surplus whole milk is not available, then spray dried skimmilk powder is reconstituted with potable water and mixed with whole milk to give requisite amount of fat and SNF in resulting toned and double toned milk.

The calculated amount of potable water is received in pasteurizing tank equipped with an agitator. The water is heated while the agitator is kept in motion to 38-40°C. Then a calculated amount of skimmilk powder is slowly added at the point of agitation and the mixture is thoroughly agitated till it dissolves completely. A calculated amount of whole milk is now added and the mixture again agitated thoroughly till a homogenous mixture is obtained. The mixture is then filtered, homogenized, pasteurized at 63°C for 30 min, rapidly cooled to 5°C, packaged and kept at 5°C or below until distribution.

Recombined milk: Recombined milk refers to the product obtained when butter oil (also called dry anhydrous milk fat), low heat skimmilk powder and water are combined in the correct proportion to yield fluid milk. The milk fat may also be obtained from other sources, such as unsalted butter or plastic cream.

Recombination is an alternative method of supplying a product which closely resembles fresh dairy milk to markets where the genuine article is not available. The manufacture of recombined milk and milk products has been well established in many countries around the world and a variety of processes and items have been developed for this purpose.

Recombination process: Recombination normally consists of mixing skimmilk powder with water and emulsifying a suitable quantity of milk fat into the mixture. In a recombined milk plant it is possible to choose the proportions of fat and non-fat solids at will. However, the normal mix generally consists of: pure anhydrous milk fat, 3%; skimmilk powder (equivalent to 9.5 non-fat solids) and 87% water. This results in a well balanced drink with flavour and nutritional properties resembling those of fresh dairy milk.

Non-fat solids for recombined milk are usually supplied in the form of skimmilk powder. The powder can be stored for months, or even years, without being spoiled, and dissolves easily in water to form reconstituted skim milk. Low-heat powder is used for recombination purposes, the main reason being its ability to become completely dissolved without sedimentation. Apart from this it will normally have a less cooked flavour. Fat must be added in order to convert the reconstituted skimmilk into recombined whole milk. Butter oil, butter or cream are often used as fat source.

Whole milk powder, containing both proteins and fat, can also be mixed with water to make recombined milk. But it deteriorates quicker than skimmilk powder and does not dissolve as easily unless it has been 'instantized', i.e. specially heated during the drying process to improve its solubility. The flavour of recombined milk depends largely on the characteristics of the fat when used. It is particularly important that this should be free from all flavours and have a low peroxide value.

Water for recombined milk production must be of good drinking quality- free from harmful microorganisms and with a very low content of mechanical or chemical impurities. The use of hard alkaline water may affect the solution rate of milk powder and tends to give a chalky defect in the product, due to the reaction between calcium ions and the phosphate groups in the milk. When very hard water is used to reconstitute skimmilk powder, premature coagulation of proteins in the milk may occur if further heat treatment is applied. Too high content of copper and iron may cause off-flavours resulting from oxidation of the fat used.

Recombination temperature and hydration time: The wettability of the powder increases when the water temperature increases from 10 to 50°C. There is no increase between 50 and 100°C, possibly the opposite. It is important that the proteins obtain their normal state of hydration which is completed in less than 20 minutes at 50°C. As a rule fresh, high-quality powder requires the shortest hydration time. Insufficient hydration time may lead to a 'chalky' defect in the final product. It is possible to carry out reconstitution at 10°C and then store the milk at this temperature overnight in order to obtain maximum hydration. However, more powder particles remain undissolved at a mixing temperature of 10-20°C compared with 35-45°C, even if the mix is kept 24 hours. The air content in reconstituted milk increases at lower mixing temperatures.

Fat addition and emulsification: The fat should not be added to the reconstituted milk until the hydration period is complete. The addition of fat at the same time or before the addition of milk powder should be avoided as this can lead to processing problems and reduce product quality. Milk fat is added first together with emulsifiers, if used. The fat must be added at a temperature above its melting point. In order to safeguard this, the addition of AMF must be carried out above 40°C. When fat is added to the milk in a vat, it must be thoroughly agitated in order to ensure uniform composition when it is pumped to the homogenizer. The recombined milk should not be kept at high mixing temperature for more than 2 hours because of microbial growth.

Air content: Skimmilk powder normally contains about 40% air by volume. The mixing equipment affects the air content of the recombined milk. Tests indicate that the air content in reconstituted skimmilk, dissolved at 50°C and with 14 to 18% dry solids, is the same as in normal skimmilk. At a mixing temperature of 30°C, the air content is 50-60% higher even after holding time of 1 hour. Too much air in the recombined milk has the following disadvantages: a) foaming, b) burning-on in the pasteurizer, c) cavitation in the homogenizer, d) whey formation in cultured milk products, and e) increased risk of the oxidation of fat.

Powder handling: Proportioning of skimmilk powder is based on the simple rule that the weight of the powder is one-tenth of the weight of the produced milk. For small plants, manual emptying of the calculated number of sacks of a given weight into the mixing tank is the easiest and most practical solution, but production can be mechanized for higher capacities. Milk powder handling creates a lot of dust. Large scale sack emptying, therefore, requires special equipment, including a dust control unit.

Reconstituted milk: Reconstituted milks can be prepared either from skimmilk powder (SMP) or from whole milk powder (WMP) by addition of water. But in industry it is generally prepared from low heat SMP. The fat : SNF ratio is adjusted equal to that of fresh skimmilk or fresh whole milk (approximately in proportion of 1 part of powder to 7-8 part of water).

For preparation of reconstituted milk calculated amount of potable water is received in pasteurization tank equipped with agitator. The water is heated to 40-45°C and calculated amount of spray dried whole milk powder is slowly added at the point of agitation. The mixture is thoroughly mixed, filtered and left for sufficient time (preferably 1 hr) for proper hydration of powder particles. The mixture is then pasteurized at 63°C/30 min and promptly cooled to 5°C or below until distribution.

8.2. Flavoured Milks

Preparation of flavoured milk is becoming an integral part of market milk plant because this milk has good consumer acceptance as refreshing and nourishing milk beverage. According to PFA rules, flavoured milk may be defined as cow or buffalo milk or any one of the designated milks to which flavour either natural or synthetic has been added. Sugar and colour may or may not be added depending on the requirements. If the flavoured milk is prepared from such milk which does not conform to any minimum legal standard in respect of fat and SNF, it is called as flavoured drink or flavoured dairy drinks. They can be commercialized in the form of pasteurized, UHT or sterilized products.

Types of flavoured milks

- Chocolate milk / drink
- Fruit flavoured milk / drink
- Sterilized flavoured milk / drink

Chocolate milk: Chocolate milk consists of milk or skimmilk, sugar and cocoa or chocolate, in addition it usually contains a suspending agent, vanilla and salt, and occasionally malt and spices. The main problem involved in this product is the selection of cocoa and other ingredients to obtain a desirable flavour, creaming, and cocoa sedimentation. Chocolate milk and chocolate drink are usually prepared with cocoa, which contains 6.5 to 22 per cent of fat. As the flavour is not materially influenced by the milk-fat content, a fat content of 2% is preferred.

Preparation: The milk on receipt is standardized to 2% fat level for preparation of the drink. Standardized milk is then preheated to 35-40°C and filtered; alternatively, after standardization it is preheated to 60°C, homogenized at 2500 psi and then clarified. To the warm milk, cocoa powder (1-1.5%), sugar (5-7) and stabilizer (sodium alginate- 0.2%) are slowly added and stirred to dissolve them properly. The mixture is then pasteurized at 71°C/30 min, cooled rapidly to 5°C, packed and kept under refrigeration (5°C) until used.

Defects: one of the problems in making chocolate milk is the creaming of the product; the cream layer will contain enough cocoa particles to give it a darker colour than the main body of the product. With some aging this darker cream layer will become mottled and uneven in colour, a condition that may be mistaken for souring. Even if this does not occur, the darker cream layer is not attractive as cream, and it makes the product appear lighter in colour, because of the colour contrast involved, and because of the actual removal of the coloured particles from the main body of the product. This creaming is, therefore, not considered desirable, and at present most of the chocolate milk that is sold is non-creaming.

The creaming of the product can be prevented by pasteurizing the milk at a high temperature, e.g. 70 -75°C for 15-30 min. Another method is to homogenize the milk. The addition of suspending agents to prevent cocoa sedimentation also prevents creaming.

Cocoa sedimentation is another problem of chocolate milk. Cocoa contains 3.0-3.7% crude fibre, which does not dissolve. Unless effective preventive methods are applied the suspended cocoa particles will settle out as a sediment layer of appreciable thickness. This detracts from the appearance of the product and causes inconvenience in serving.

Homogenization has been tried as a means of reducing the particles to a size sufficiently small to prevent settling. Homogenization of the syrup has been found ineffective; apparently the fibrous particles are too tough to be subdivided by this process. Homogenization of the finished product actually increases sedimentation. Where the milk is to be homogenized to prevent creaming, it should be done before the syrup or dry ingredients are added. The other method to control sedimentation is to add 0.2% sodium alginate.

Fruit flavoured milk: The method of preparation of fruit flavoured milk is similar to that used for chocolate milk/drink. Instead of coca powder, permitted fruit flavours/essence, together with permitted colours (matching) and sugar are used. The common flavours used are strawberry, orange, lemon, pineapple, banana, vanilla, etc.

Consumption of fruits along with milk has long been considered beneficial for health. In India, mango and banana are commonly used in preparation of milk shakes, particularly in summer months. Fruit flavoured milks are prepared by adding either the fruit pulp or fruit juice along with sugar to the milk. When fruit pulp is used as such a suitable pretreatment to avoid discoloration of pulp is essential.

Use of fruit juice is now preferred over natural fruits in the manufacture of fruit beverages. More and more dairies in Europe and America offer a wide range of fruit juice-based milk beverages these days. The general procedure of manufacturing these beverages involves: blending milk solids (either liquid whole/ skimmilk, whey, butter milk or their counterpart concentrated or anhydrous form) with fruit juice, sugar solution, stabilizer (generally pectin, carrageenan, CMC, gelatin, etc) and an edible acid (citric, lactic, malic or tartaric acid). The choice of various ingredients and their quantity depends on their preference of consumers. The final product may be either pasteurized or sterilized, but UHT processing is favoured for long shelf life of the product.

It is now possible to produce lactose reduced or sugar-free milk beverages suitable for persons suffering from diabetes or lactose intolerance. For preparing these milks either fructose or aspartame is used to replace lactose or milk is subjected to ultrafiltration treatment. Use of hydrolyzed lactose in preparation of flavoured milk beverages is now gaining tremendous consumer acceptance.

In order to obtain good results, the following precautions should be taken:

- No acid (citric or tartaric) should be added to the fruit syrup, as this may cause curdling of milk.
- Excessive fruit syrup should be avoided. The best sugar content of the syrup is 45-55 per cent.
- Add 1 part of fruit syrup to 5 parts of milk.
- Care should be taken to see that there is a pleasant blend of sweet, fruity, and milky flavours (together with an appealing colour).

Sterilized flavoured milk: The raw milk, upon receiving, should be strictly examined by the prescribed physicochemical and bacteriological tests and only high quality milk should be used for manufacture of sterilized flavoured milk. The incoming milk should be promptly cooled to 5°C for bulk storage in order to check any bacterial growth. The milk should be preheated to 35-40°C for filtration, so as to remove visible dirt, etc. Flavour / essence, permitted colour (matching), and sugar (syrup) are added to clarified milk and mixed well. The fruit flavoured milk is now filled in clean and sanitized bottles and then capped properly. The filled bottles are then sterilized at 108-111°C for 25-30 min. The sterilized milk bottles should be gradually cooled to room temperature. Finally, the sterilized milk is stored in a cool place.

8.3. Vegetable Solids-based Milks

Vegetable solid–based milks or simulated milks can broadly be divided into two groups: a) those that use one or more components of milk as ingredients, and b) those without milk components. The flavour, consistency, nutritional value and appearance of both must be similar to natural milk. The main advantage of preparing these milks are their low cost, special dietetic role and as milk replacer during scarcity. Some common examples of such milks are described as follows:

Filled milk: The main objective of preparing filled milk is to replace expensive butterfat with less expensive vegetable fats. Filled milk is prepared either by combining fresh skimmilk or reconstituted skimmilk with vegetable oils. The choice of oil will depend on economics, flavour preference and dietary considerations. A vegetable oil even after homogenization will not remain properly dispersed in skimmilk without special aids, it is, therefore, necessary to add emulsifiers and stabilizers to filled milk. In certain countries these emulsifiers and stabilizers are marketed as 'imitation milk base mixes'.

Imitation milk: This type of milk is prepared largely from non-dairy ingredients. However, they may contain certain derivatives of milk, e.g. sodium caseinate. Sucrose is used as a source of sweeteners but whey products are also sometimes used mainly as a source of lactose, to provide solids and to supplement sweetness. Apart from sodium caseinate, the other sources of protein is soy protein isolate (SPI) which is highly refined, bland, water dispersible and water soluble protein. Sometimes, it may also be supplemented with groundnut protein. Emulsifiers and stabilizers are added to improve the fat emulsion and consistency. The method of manufacturing imitation milk is essentially the same used for recombined and filled milks.

Soy milk: Regrettably the quantum jump in human population over the years has led to milk scarcity especially in certain regions of the country aggravating the intensity of demand specifically in and around cosmopolitan centres. In order to redeem the situation, it calls for augmentation of fluid milk through substitutions obtainable from non-conventional sources, viz. soy milk, groundnut milk, etc. which could possibly be incorporated with fluid milk in desired ratios and used for supplementing market milk supply besides being converted to basal products.

It is well known that protein yield per hectare by growing soybean is the highest among all sources of vegetable protein or animal protein. The protein content of soybean is about 40% which is higher than the value obtained from the other natural sources of protein. Nutritionally, soy protein is the most balanced plant protein for human consumption. The amount of protein in 1 kg soy bean seed is equivalent to 12 litre milk and soy bean comes 10 times cheaper than milk. Each 100 g soy bean contains 710 IU of vitamin A, 0.75 mg of thiamine, 240 mg calcium, 700 mg of phosphorus, 11.5 mg of iron and yields 432 calories.

Besides being rich in protein, vitamins and minerals soy milk is very economical, free of lactose, highly digestible and nutritious alternative dairy diet. It is cholesterol-free product, has very low fat content and is rich in polyunsaturated fatty acids (PUFA), especially linoleic acid and lecithin.

Generally soy milk contains about 7-8% total solids. Adding 3-4% sugar and around 0.05% salt brings it to a sugar, salt and total solid level to approximately close to toned cow milk, i.e. about 12-13% total solids.

Nelson, et al. (1976) developed 'Illinois Process' which is most commonly used for the preparation of soy milk. This process involves hydration of whole soy bean by soaking in 0.5% sodium bicarbonate solution (1:3 bean: solution) for 8-12 hr till the weight of beans gets doubled. The soak solution is then drained and the soaked beans are blanched by dropping directly into the boiling water having 0.5% sodium bicarbonate for 30 min to inactivate the lipoxigenase enzyme. This is followed by draining, tap water rinsing for cooling, disintegration with water and finally heating the slurry to 90°C. After filtering, the whole mass is homogenized (3500 psi), pasteurized (71°C / 15 sec) and chilled to 4°C, packaged and stored under refrigeration till distributed.

8.4. Miscellaneous Milks

Soft-curd milk: Soft-curd milk is milk that forms a soft curd when coagulated with rennet or pepsin under standardized procedures. Mother's milk forms a soft curd when coagulated in the stomach and is apparently more quickly digested by infants than cow's milk, which forms a harder curd. Methods for modifying cow's milk for infant feeding include procedures that reduce the curd tension; diluting with water, acidification with lactic or other acid, and boiling will all reduce the curd tension of milk.

The curd tension of milks from individual cows varies from 0 to about 200 grams. The vast majority of samples will fall within the range of 20 to 90 grams, and herds milk commonly range from 50 to 70 grams (Hill, 1923). Hill regards milk with a curd tension of 30 grams or under as soft-curd milk, and this standard has been adopted by several boards of health. On an average the curd tension of buffalo milk is significantly higher at 40 g than that of Indian cow milk which is 24 g (Kuchroo and Ganguli, 2006). The curd tension of milk is affected by such factors as the species of the milch animal, individuality of the animal, breed, stage of lactation and udder infections. Species of the animal has great effect on the curd tension of milk. The breed plays an important role in the curd tension of milk. For example, the milk of Jersey cows showed higher curd tension than that of Holstein. The curd tension of milk is higher during the early and late stages of lactation than during the middle stages.

The curd tension is mainly controlled by the casein, calcium phosphate and fat content of milk. The hard curd milk containing more casein should furnish more coagulating centres after peptic action and hence give a more rapid coagulation. In such event the micelles of casein would probably form a closely woven network from which the water would be squeezed out, resulting in a rather dense mass. The soft curd on the other hand having less casein would furnish fewer coagulating centres; the micelles would extend farther before interlocking so that a relatively loose structure would result.

The colloidal calcium phosphates severed from the protecting action of the casein by the pepsin in themselves may furnish coagulating centres, hence the greater the concentration of calcium phosphates, the more rapid the coagulation, the more compact the micellar structure, and the harder curded the milk.

The fat may contribute to the determination of the curd character by interrupting the growth of the micellar threads of protein and so modify the structure. It will be apparent from this viewpoint that the manner in which the fat is dispersed would be as important as its concentration. Another possibility is that the amount of protein adsorbed by the fat varies considerably from individual milk to milk and that this influences the micellar structure which results from peptic coagulation.

Methods of preparing soft–curd milk: A number of methods are available for the preparation of soft-curd milk. With the exception of the natural soft-curd milk, they require special processing procedures, viz the addition of enzymes or salts to milk, or the removal of calcium and phosphorus by base exchange. Since their legality is not established, it is not advisable to undertake soft-curd production.

Normal individual cow's milk varies in curd tension; because this is apparently a fairly constant characteristic, it is possible to test cows and assemble a herd that will produce milk with a curd tension of 30 grams or lower. Certain cows in all breeds of dairy cattle produce naturally soft-curd milk. Holsteins, however, more commonly produce soft-curd milk followed by Jerseys (Doan, 1938). Natural soft-curd milk is invariably low in total solids, solids-not-fat, and fat.

The curd tension of milk can also be lowered by application of heat processing above the pasteurization temperature. Boiling lowered the curd tension by 79.5 and 78% for buffalo and cow milk, respectively. By simmering the milk for 3 min, very little further lowering in the curd tension of cow milk was observed as compared to that of boiled milk. In case of buffalo milk this difference was noticeable. Pasteurization caused a reduction of 10% in both cow and buffalo milk (Rao, et al., 1964). Modified milk for infant feeding is usually heated to the boiling point. This procedure reduces the bacterial content and produces soft-curd milk. Evaporated milk, because of its heat-treatment and because it is homogenized, frequently exhibits no curd tension. This fact accounts for much of the increased use of evaporated milk for infants. Homogenization also markedly reduces the curd tension of milk. Pressure of 2,500 to 3,000 are used for marked reductions.

Milk as functional food: Functional foods may be defined as the foods containing significant levels of biologically active components which impart health benefits beyond basic nutrition. They are also referred to wellness foods, health foods or neutraceuticals. It is now scientifically accepted that foods play role in the prevention of diseases such as coronary heart disease, atherosclerosis, stroke, diabetes, cancer and liver ailments.

Milk has been described as nature's nearly perfect food as it provides vital nutrients including proteins, essential fatty acids minerals and lactose in balanced proportions. Milk and milk products are recognized as important constituents of a well-balanced and nutritionally adequate diet. Milk and milk products complement and supplement nutrients available from grains, legumes, vegetables, fruits, meat, seafood and poultry.

The dairy industry has provided the consumer with choice of products lower in fat and sodium. In addition, dairy foods with supplemented calcium, potassium, micronutrients, protein, prebiotics, probiotics, phytosterols, omega fatty acids and fibre have been made available for the informed consumers.

Fortified milk: Milk and milk products provide an excellent medium for fortification with various nutrients. Traditionally, milk has been fortified with vitamins A and D. Now, popular ingredients of functional significance are being incorporated to enhance market value of dairy foods and dairy-based foods. Some of these ingredients designed to enhance consumer appeal are: Calcium, claimed to prevent osteoporosis and cancer and to control hypertension. Antioxidants (vitamins C and E) are claimed to prevent cancer, cardiovascular disease and cataracts. In addition, plant sterols for cholesterol reduction, dietary fibre (psyllium, guar gum, gum acacia, oat fibre, and soy components) as well as multivitamin-mineral mixes are being incorporated in fat-free milk. In addition to infant food formulae, there is a proliferation of energy and weight reduction shake drinks for consumer segments ranging from adult to geriatric populations. Other products in the market contain hydrolyzed milk proteins and their peptides targeted to athletes for improving their performance. Some products are touted for control of weight and blood pressure, and some for the digestive and immune health (Chandan, 2009).

Vitamin D Milk: vitamin D, called the 'anti-rachitic vitamin' is one of the most important food accessories, especially in the diet of infants and young children, for it regulates the absorption and metabolism of the bone-forming elements, calcium and phosphorus. Most of the vitamin D in regular diet comes from fish, meat, egg, milk, and milk products. In general, milk is not a rich source of this vitamin unless special procedures are followed in its production or processing.

For many years, it was known that sunshine and cod-liver oil tended to prevent or cure rickets, a common disease among children. It was reported that sterols developed anti-rachitic potency on exposure to ultraviolet rays. The skin contains the sterol, cholesterol, and this develops anti-rachitic properties when exposed to ultraviolet rays either from sun light or from an artificial source. Through further research it was learnt that a number of sterols act as 'provitamins,' yielding vitamin D upon activation by any of several methods. The two of major commercial importance are ergosterol (provitamin D 2) which is derived chiefly from yeast and 7-dehydrocholesterol (provitamin D3) which is widely distributed in animal tissues.

Photosynthesis of precholecalciferol occurs in the skin during exposure to sunlight. The high-energy UV B photons with energies between 290 and 320 nm penetrate into the skin, where they are absorbed by epidermal and dermal stores of 7-dehydrocholesterol (vitamin D3). When the sky is clouded, exposure to this radiation is only 30% and via glass it decreases to about zero. Only 2 hours after precholecalciferol is formed in the skin it is converted to cholecalciferol. Once formed, cholecalciferol exits the skin into the dermal capillary bed where it is bound to the vitamin D-binding protein.

Cod-liver oil had long been used as a additional vitamin D for children. However, because rickets still remained prevalent, many nutritionists suggested that some food regularly consumed by the public be used, to convey increased amounts of this vitamin. Milk, the best single food source of calcium and phosphorus, is almost universally recognized as the best logical food for this purpose, since it can supply vitamin D automatically, when and where it is most needed.

Sources: The main food sources of vitamin D are fish, fish products, eggs (many of which contain 5-15 μg /100 g; 1 μg = 40 IU) and food to which vitamins have been added. Milk is not a good source of vitamin D. The whole milk contains only 0.7- 1.0 μg / litre. Even a high-fat dairy product like butter does not contain more than 0.75 μg / 100g. Also human milk does not contain much vitamin D but, from this little amount, at least 70% of total activity is available as calcidol. Total activity in human milk is about 0.4-0.6 μg / litre, which does not fulfill the daily requirement of infants. An extra supply is required either via exposure to sun light or by vitamin D supplementation.

Enrichment of milk: Several methods of enrichment of milk were investigated, viz. metabolized, irradiated and fortified milk. However, only last method of fortification was found to be feasible and economical.

Production of metabolized vitamin D milk involved feeding of irradiated yeast to cows. Yeast is rich in ergosterol and develops a high potency of vitamin D_2 upon irradiation with ultraviolet light under suitable conditions. The irradiated dry yeast was mixed with the grain ration, so that it was automatically fed in amounts proportional to the milk production. This method was not found suitable because of its high cost. This high cost was unavoidable because of the poor efficiency of the cow in transferring vitamin D from feed to milk. Only about 2% of the ingested vitamin D appeared in the milk.

Production of irradiated vitamin D milk involves exposing a thin rapidly flowing film of milk to an intensive source of ultraviolet radiation. As a result of this treatment, the milk develops an increased vitamin D potency. However, there is danger of development of off-flavour in milk.

Production of fortified vitamin D milk was found to be low in cost, flexible, and simple. This method involves adding a definite amount of standardized vitamin D concentrate to the proper amount of milk and mixing thoroughly to secure uniform distribution.

At first, the vitamin D concentrates were emulsified in vegetable oil, but later, cream or butterfat, with or without added milk solids, was used as a carrier. In recent years, the trend has been toward the use of irradiated ergosterol (vitamin D_2) instead of cod-liver oil concentrate, because of the much lower cost and greater availability. The concentrates are packed in different sized, hermetically sealed containers and sterilized. They are then ready for use. The size of the container and potency of the concentrate are adjusted so that the entire contents of the container, when added to the standardized-sized batch of milk (usually at the start of pasteurization), will give a finished potency of 400 U.S.P. units per litre, plus an additional amount as a factor of safety.

Humanized milk: The ideal food for the human infant is human breast milk, which has the important nutritional advantage that it is secreted ready warmed, sterile and perfectly balanced in proteins, fats, carbohydrates, vitamins and minerals. Human milk is not only a complex fluid adopted to the needs of the young once but in addition and in contrast with the processed cow milk preparations, it is also a live secretion with active enzymes, hormones and functional corpuscles. Of this fluid the healthy infant consumes 2.5 fl. Oz. per pound of body weight per day and as human milk has a calorific value of 20 cal / fl. Oz., this represents daily intake of 50 cal for each lb. of body weight.

There are occasions when a substitute for breast milk must be found. In recent years, technological developments, notably in dairy forming, food processing, pediatric nutrition, environmental hygiene and socio-economic and educational levels have made wide spread artificial feeding of human babies practical, particularly in industrialized countries with a parallel decline in breast feeding.

For artificial feeding of infants various formulae have been developed. In all these formulae, attempts are made to adjust the composition of baby food as close to human milk as possible. If the milk of any mammal is modified in such a way that it resembles in its behaviour in the digestive tract of infants to the human milk, the resulting product is called humanized milk. Generally cow milk is used as an alternative to human milk in one form or the other. Although cow milk also has a calorific value of 20 cal per fl. Oz., it is not suitable as a direct substitute for breast milk, because its composition differs significantly in several ways.

Apart from the fact that the nature and constitution of the proteins differ in the different species, there is a higher proportion of protein and a lower proportion of sugar in cow milk as compared with human milk. Furthermore, human milk contains nearly three times as much albumin and a rather less than a third of the less digestible casein that is present in cow milk. On an average the cow milk contains more protein (3.3 g / 100 ml) than human milk (1.2 g / 100 ml). Human milk constitutes 40% casein, mainly β- and κ-casein and 60% whey proteins mainly α-lactalbumin. In addition, human milk contains lactoferrin, serum albumin and lysozyme. Human milk contains 7 g lactose / 100 ml which represents 40% of energy and cow milk contains 4.8 g / 100 ml which supplies about 30% of total energy value of milk. Cow milk is richer in vitamins of the B-group, but has less of vitamin A, C and E. Neither human nor cow milk is good source of fat soluble vitamin D. Moreover, cow milk is deficient in iron and in vitamin D, so far as the nutrition of human infant is concerned, and as cow milk is always boiled or otherwise subjected to heat before use as in infant food, a considerable proportion of the vitamin C content may be destroyed. It is, therefore, apparent that cow milk must be modified and supplemented in order to make it suitable for feeding to infants. So far as supplementation is concerned, vitamin C is usually supplied to artificially fed infants in the form of fruit juices such as orange, tomato or lemon and vitamin D is given as a fish liver oil or a synthetic vitamin concentrate. After the first few weeks when the reserves of iron present in the body at birth have been used up, this element is usually prescribed separately as one of its salts. The modification of cow milk to make its composition in respect of proteins and carbohydrates approximate more nearly to that of human milk must be discussed separately, depending upon the particular form in which the milk is obtained. The ultimate aim of all methods of modifying cow milk is to produce a well balanced fluid containing about 20 cal per fl. Oz in order to supply the necessary quota of body building materials and to secure at the same time a minimum fluid intake of 2.5 fl. Oz. / day for each lb of body weight.

Milk and its preparations for infant feeding: Whenever whole milk, either as fresh liquid milk, as full cream powder or as a full cream evaporated milk is used as a basis for infant feeding, it can be made to approximate in composition, at least sufficiently for all practical purposes to that of human milk. This can be done by simple dilution with water in order to reduce the proportion of protein, and then adding sufficient carbohydrate to bring the sugar content nearer to that of human milk. For this purpose cane or beat sugar is most commonly used.

A fresh liquid cow milk which has been boiled to rid it off pathogenic organisms and allowed to cool forms a satisfactory basis for infant feeding. A commonly employed formula is as follows:

1.	Fresh boiled cow milk	-1.75 fl. Oz.	= 35 cal
2.	Boiled water	-	0.75 fl. Oz.
3.	Sugar (level teaspoonful)	- 1.0 drachm	= 15 cal
	Total	**2.5 fl. Oz.**	= **50 cal**

In India more than 55% of total milk production comes from buffaloes. Buffalo milk differs from cow milk not only in composition but also in its major protein, i.e. casein of buffalo milk differs significantly from that of cow milk. Buffalo milk contains higher protein content than cow milk (3.6 vs. 3.4%). Casein content is higher in buffalo milk, micelles bigger in size and contained more calcium and phosphorus as compared to cow casein. Unlike in cow casein, â-casein was the predominant component, while k-casein was lower in buffalo casein. Kuchroo and Ganguly (2006) attempted to evolve a method for the manufacture of infant food from modified buffalo milk simulating human milk. Buffalo milk being richer in calcium, protein, fat and higher in curd tension than human milk myriad technological approaches have been made to modify it. Modifications in the manufacture of this new product to simulate human milk were: (a) calcium in skimmilk was reduced by 50% by electrodialysis which decreased curd tension and improved heat stability; (b) milk proteins particularly á$_{s-}$ casein was degraded by regulated proteolysis of milk with trypsin; (c) vegetable oil and milk fat in distinct proportions were incorporated resulting in improved PUFA profiles; and (d) fortification with lactose and vitamin mixture. The spray-dried powder obtained from the modified buffalo milk contained 3.1 g protein, 3.5 g fat, and 628 mg of linoleic acid per 100 calories with Ca/P ratio of 2.2. These data satisfy the standards for the infant food formula according to FAO/WHO (1955, 1966).

References

Chandan, R.C. 2009. Functional foods – An Overview. XXXVII Dairy Industry Conference held at Goa, Feb 7-9, Souvenir:33.

Doan, F.J. 1938. Soft-curd milk. A critical review of the literature, *J. Dairy Sci.*, 21: 739.

Hill, R.L. 1923. A test for determining the character of the curd of cow's milk. *J. Dairy Sci.*, Vol 6: 509.

Kuchroo, C. N. and Ganguly, N.C. 2006. Technological approaches for infant food manufacture from modified buffalo milk. *J Food Sci.*, 45(5):1333.

Nelson, A. I., Steinberg, M.P. and Wei, L.S. 1976. Illinois process for preparation of soy milk. *J. Food Sci.*, 41:57.

Rao, R.V., Chopra, V.C., Stephen, J. and Bhalerao, V. R. 1964. Studies on curd tension of milk. *J. Food Sci. and Tech.*, 1:19.